PATHOLOGIES OF POWER

CALIFORNIA SERIES IN PUBLIC ANTHROPOLOGY

The California Series in Public Anthropology emphasizes the anthropologist's role as an engaged intellectual. It continues anthropology's commitment to being an ethnographic witness, to describing, in human terms, how life is lived beyond the borders of many readers' experiences. But it also adds a commitment, through ethnography, to reframing the terms of public debate—transforming received, accepted understandings of social issues with new insights, new framings.

SERIES EDITOR: Robert Borofsky (Hawaii Pacific University)

CONTRIBUTING EDITORS: Philippe Bourgois (UC San Francisco), Paul Farmer (Partners in Health), Rayna Rapp (New York University), and Nancy Scheper-Hughes (UC Berkeley)

UNIVERSITY OF CALIFORNIA PRESS EDITOR: Naomi Schneider

PATHOLOGIES OF POWER

HEALTH, HUMAN RIGHTS, AND THE NEW WAR ON THE POOR

with a new preface by the author

PAUL FARMER

WITH A FOREWORD BY AMARTYA SEN

UNIVERSITY OF CALIFORNIA PRESS
Berkeley · Los Angeles · London

University of California Press
Berkeley and Los Angeles, California

University of California Press, Ltd.
London, England

Material included in Chapters 1 to 7 and 9 has been adapted from earlier
work by the author, which appeared in the following publications: "On
Suffering and Structural Violence: A View from Below," *Daedalus* 125,
no. 1 (1996): 261–83; "On Guantánamo," in *The Uses of Haiti*, by P. E.
Farmer (Monroe, Maine: Common Courage Press, 1994); "A Visit to
Chiapas," *America* 178, no. 10 (1998): 14–18; "TB Superbugs: The
Coming Plague on All Our Houses," *Natural History* 108, no. 3 (1999):
46–53; "Medicine and Social Justice," *America* 173, no. 2 (1995):
13–17; "Listening for Prophetic Voices in Medicine," *America* 177, no. 1
(1997): 83–85; "Cruel and Unusual: Drug-Resistant Tuberculosis as
Punishment," in *Sentenced to Die? The Problem of TB in Prisons in East
and Central Europe and Central Asia,* edited by V. Stern and R. Jones
(London: International Centre for Prison Studies, King's College, 1999);
"Pathologies of Power: Rethinking Health and Human Rights," *American
Journal of Public Health* 89, no. 10 (1999): 1486–96.

For use of the quotations in the epigraphs in this book, grateful acknowl-
edgment is made to the authors and publishers, as listed on pages 379–81
and deemed part of this copyright page.

Library of Congress Cataloging-in-Publication Data

Farmer, Paul
    Pathologies of power : health, human rights, and
the new war on the poor: with a new preface
by the author / Paul Farmer ; with a foreword by
Amartya Sen.
        p.   cm. — (California series in public
anthropology ; 4)
    Includes bibliographical references and index.
    ISBN 0–520–24326-9 (Pbk. : alk. paper)
    1. Social stratification.   2. Equality.   3. Poor—
Medical care.   4. Discrimination in medical care.
5. Right to health care.   6. Human rights.
I. Title.   II. Series.
HM821.F37   2005
305—dc22   2004010906

Manufactured in the United States of America

14   13   12   11   10   09   08   07   06   05
10   9   8   7   6   5   4   3

Our system is one of detachment: to keep silenced people from asking questions, to keep the judged from judging, to keep solitary people from joining together, and the soul from putting together its pieces.

Eduardo Galeano, "Divorces"

FOR OPHELIA, LOUNE, JIM, AND TOM,
MY PARTNERS IN HEALTH

Sometimes the lack of substantive freedoms relates directly to economic poverty, which robs people of the freedom to satisfy hunger, or to achieve sufficient nutrition, or to obtain remedies for treatable illnesses, or the opportunity to be adequately clothed or sheltered, or to enjoy clean water or sanitary facilities.

In other cases, the unfreedom links closely to the lack of public facilities and social care, such as the absence of epidemiological programs, or of organized arrangements for health care or educational facilities, or of effective institutions for the maintenance of local peace and order.

In still other cases, the violation of freedom results directly from a denial of political and civil liberties by authoritarian regimes and from imposed restrictions on the freedom to participate in the social, political and economic life of the community.

Amartya Sen, Development as Freedom

Rats and roaches live by competition under the law of supply and demand; it is the privilege of human beings to live under the laws of justice and mercy.

Wendell Berry

CONTENTS

FOREWORD

AMARTYA SEN

"Every man who lives is born to die," wrote John Dryden, some three hundred years ago. That recognition is tragic enough, but the reality is sadder still. We try to pack in a few worthwhile things between birth and death, and quite often succeed. It is, however, hard to achieve anything significant if, as in sub-Saharan Africa, the median age at death is less than five years.[1] That, I should explain, was the number in Africa in the early 1990s, *before* the AIDS epidemic hit hard, making the chances worse and worse. It is difficult to get reliable statistics, but the evidence is that the odds are continuing to fall from the already dismal numbers. Having made it beyond those early years, it may be difficult for us to imagine how restricted a life so many of our fellow human beings lead, what little living they manage to do. There is, of course, the wonder of birth (impossible to recollect), some mother's milk (sometimes not), the affection of relatives (often thoroughly disrupted), perhaps some schooling (mostly not), a bit of play (amid pestilence and panic), and then things end (with or without a rumble). The world goes on as if nothing much has happened.

The situation does, of course, vary from region to region, and from one group to another. But unnecessary suffering, debilitation, and death from preventable or controllable illness characterize every country and every society, to varying extents. As we would expect, the poor countries in Africa or Asia or Latin America provide crudely obvious illustrations of severe deprivation, but the phenomenon is present even in the richest countries. Indeed, the deprived groups in the "First World" live, in many ways, in the "Third." For example, African Americans in some of the most prosperous U.S. cities (such as New York, Washington, or San Francisco) have a lower life expectancy at birth than do most people in immensely poorer China or even India. Indeed, location alone may not enhance one's overall longevity.

EXPLANATION AND REMEDY

How can we come to terms with the extensive presence of such adversity—the most basic privation from which human beings can suffer? Do we see it simply as a human predicament—an inescapable result of the frailty of our existence? That would be correct had these sufferings been really inescapable, but they are far from that. Preventable diseases can indeed be prevented, curable ailments can certainly be cured, and controllable maladies call out for control. Rather than lamenting the adversity of nature, we have to look for a better comprehension of the social causes of horror and also of our tolerance of societal abominations. However, despite many illuminating studies of particular aspects of these general problems, investigators tend to shy away from posing the questions in their full generality. To confront the big picture seems like an overpowering challenge.

Paul Farmer, however, is not easily overpowered. He is a great doctor with massive experience of working against the hardest of diseases in the most adverse of circumstances, and, at the same time, he is a proficient and insightful anthropologist with far-reaching discernment and understanding. Farmer's knowledge of maladies such as AIDS and drug-resistant tuberculosis, which he fights on behalf of his indigent patients, is hard to match. This he combines with his remarkable expertise on culture and society, acquired not just by learning from a distance but also from actually living and working in different parts of the deprived world. In addition, Paul Farmer is a public health interventionist with a dogged determination to work toward changing iniquitous institutions and mismatched arrangements. As the co-director of Harvard's Program in Infectious Disease and Social Change (working with Dr. Jim Yong Kim, another remarkable public health expert), Farmer has led several major initiatives in changing the direction of health care and intervention (for example, in tackling drug-resistant TB).

But what is particularly relevant in appreciating the contribution of this powerful book is that Paul Farmer is a visionary analyst who can look beyond the details of fragmentary explanations to seek an integrated understanding of a complex reality. In his earlier publications, including *AIDS and Accusation* (1992), *The Uses of Haiti* (1994), and *Infections and Inequalities: The Modern Plagues* (1999), he has already done much to illuminate important features of global deprivations. Now, in this remarkable book, which is hard to put down, comes the big picture, firmly linked with informationally rich illustrations of individual examples.

Farmer points to what he calls "structural violence," which influences "the nature and distribution of extreme suffering." The book is, as he explains, "a physician-anthropologist's effort to reveal the ways in which the most basic right—the right to survive—is trampled in an age of great affluence." He argues: "Human rights violations are not accidents; they are not random in distribution or effect. Rights violations are, rather, symptoms of deeper pathologies of power and are linked intimately to the social conditions that so often determine who will suffer abuse and who will be shielded from harm." Those "social conditions" and their discriminatory effects are the subject matter of this general investigation and the specific case studies that establish the overall picture of powerlessness and deprivation.

CONCEPTS AND METHODS

Some will undoubtedly ask whether this is not too general, too grand, and perhaps even too ambitious an inquiry. Also, are the questions absolutely clear? How exactly is "power" defined? Does Farmer delineate the "social conditions" precisely? Does he provide an exact definition of "structural violence"? In fact, that is not the way Paul Farmer proceeds, and it is important to understand the methodology that distinguishes this wonderful study.

A phenomenon can be either characterized by a terse definition or described with examples. It is the latter procedure that Farmer follows. That procedure is, of course, quite standard when we learn certain basic words (such as "red" or "smooth"), as Ludwig Wittgenstein (arguably the greatest philosopher of our times) has famously discussed:

> An important part of the training will consist in the teacher's pointing to the objects, directing... attention to them, and at the same time uttering a word; for instance the word "slab" as he points to that shape.... This ostensive teaching of words can be said to establish an association between the word and the thing.[2]

Though not so primitive as "red" or "smooth" or a "slab," terms like "power" or "violence" can also, often enough, be helpfully communicated through examples.

This is not to deny that we can try to explain these complex terms in other ways as well, in particular by proposing a precise definition through the use of other words. That indeed is the usual procedure, widely used, in the social sciences. And yet, as we know from experience, this is sometimes highly misleading, since the capacious content of a social concept or its diverse manifestations may often be lost or diminished through the maneuver of trying to define it in sharply delineated terms. The expressions "power," "structure," and "violence" are not eccentric inventions of Paul Farmer; they have figured extensively in the literature on social inequality.[3] But attempts at defining them exactly by other words have typically been inadequate and unclear (and sometimes they have also generated the kind of "sociological jargon" that can sound arrestingly weird). For this reason, among others, the alternative procedure, by exemplification, has many advantages in epistemology and practical reason in parts of the social sciences. The epigrammatic definition, which many social scientists seek, often cannot escape being misleadingly exact; it can be precise but precisely inaccurate. A rich phenomenon with inherent ambiguities calls for a characterization that preserves those shady edges, rather than being drowned in the pretense that there is a formulaic and sharp delineation waiting to be unearthed that will exactly separate out all the sheep from all the goats.

Farmer does not fall for the temptation of a make-believe exactness. While keeping his eyes firmly on the general picture as he sees it, he goes from one case study to another to explain what "structural violence" is like (or how disparity of "power" may operate). We see the evident similarities as well as the rich variations of form and expression. By learning from Farmer's book as a whole, we get an overall understanding that draws together the diverse details spread across these harrowing accounts.

ACÉPHIE'S POWERLESSNESS

For example, in discussing deprivations in Haiti, Farmer observes that "political and economic forces have structured risk for AIDS, tuberculosis, and, indeed, most other infectious and parasitic diseases" and adds that "social forces at work there have also structured risk for most forms of extreme suffering, from hunger to torture and rape." He discusses in each case exactly how this structuring of risk, in distinct forms, blights the lives of many, without touching the affluence of others. He moves from Haiti to Mexico, then to Russia, then to Peru, then to the United States, and right across the world, looking for—and insightfully identifying—institutional structures that push some into the abyss, while others do just fine. The carefully chosen details in each case help us to understand Farmer's notion of "structural violence" through a process that is not altogether dissimilar to the teaching of the idea of a "slab."

Indeed, power inequalities can work in many distinct ways. Take the case of Acéphie, the comely woman born in the small village of Kay through which runs Rivière Artibonite, Haiti's largest river. She is lucky to be born into a prosperous peasant family, but her luck does not last for long. When the valley is flooded to make room for a reservoir, the villagers are forced up into the stony hills on the sides of the new lake. Their voice does not receive a hearing. The displaced people—the "water refugees"—seek whatever jobs they can get (no longer able to grow the rice, bananas, millet, corn, or sugarcane they grew so abundantly earlier), and Acéphie's family ceases to make ends meet. Nevertheless, Acéphie—like other young women in families of water refugees—carries the family's agricultural produce (miserable as it is) to the local market. The soldiers, stationed on the way, watch the procession of girls who walk to the market and often flirt with them. The girls feel lucky to get such attention, since soldiers are powerful and respected men.

When Captain Jacques Honorat woos the tall and fine-featured Acéphie, with her enormous dark eyes, reciprocation eventually follows (even though Acéphie knows that Honorat is married and has several other partners). The sexual relation does not last long, but it is enough to disrupt Acéphie's life, while Captain Honorat dies of unexplained fevers. After trying to qualify herself as a domestic servant in the neighboring town of Mirebalais, the twenty-two-year-old Acéphie moves to Port-au-Prince and finds a servant's job, at a tiny wage. She also begins seeing Blanco Nerette, who comes from a similar background (his parents were also water refugees) and now chauffeurs a small bus, and they plan to marry. However, when Acéphie becomes pregnant, Blanco does not welcome the news at all. Their relationship founders. Also, thanks to her pregnancy, Acéphie loses her job. The battle for economic survival turns intense and is now joined by disease. Acéphie dies of AIDS—loved still by her own family but uncared for and unhelped by society. She leaves behind a daughter, also infected with the virus. That is the beginning of another story, but not a long one.

The inequalities of power that Acéphie faced in her brief life involved *bureaucracy* (beginning with displacements to make room for the new reservoir without adequate rearrangement), *class* (reflected in Acéphie's relations with her employer and with Captain Honorat), *gender* (related to her standing vis-à-vis the males she encountered—from the soldiers to Blanco), and of course the *stratified society* (with the absence of public facilities for medical attention and care for the poor). Acéphie did not encounter any physical violence, but Farmer is persuasive in seeing her as a victim of structural violence.

POVERTY, INEQUALITY, AND POWER

The asymmetry of power can indeed generate a kind of quiet brutality. We know, of course, that power corrupts and absolute power corrupts absolutely. But inequalities of power in general prevent the sharing of different opportunities. They can devastate the lives of those who are far removed from the levers of control. Even their own lives are dominated by decisions taken by others. In one chapter after another, Paul Farmer illustrates the diversity and reach—and also the calamitous consequences—of structural violence. The basic theme and the theses become firmly established through these disparate but ultimately blended accounts. The whole draws on the parts, but firmly transcends them, in the integrated understanding that Farmer advances.

That understanding also suggests lines of thinking about ways of remedying the deprivations and the disparities. For example, if inequality of power, in different forms, is central to deprivation and destitution, then little sense can be made of the frequently aired and increasingly popular slogan, "I am against poverty, but I am really not bothered by inequality." That attempt at a putative dichotomy can be disputed from different perspectives, for example, through an appreciation of the powerful effects of social and economic inequality on the unfreedoms that the subjugated experience.[4] The proposal to distance inequality from poverty is severely challenged by Farmer's many-sided documentation of the impact of inequality of power on the lives that the subjugated can live. This diagnosis does not, of course, yield any instant solution of the problems; but it does indicate the difficult—and often ignored—social and economic issues that must be firmly faced to eliminate preventable morbidity and escapable mortality.

We live in an age of science, technology, and economic affluence when, as Farmer points out, we can, for the first time in history, deal effectively with the diseases that ravage humanity. And yet the reach of science and of globalization has stopped short of bringing reasonable opportunity for survival within the grasp of the deprived masses in our affluent world. This is where the pathologies of power take their toll. As Farmer argues, "Anyone who wishes to be considered humane has ample cause to consider what it means to be sick and poor in the era of globalization and scientific advancement."

Depressing as Farmer's case studies are, their overall message is constructive and optimistic. The solutions are by no means easy, but they are not beyond the reach of our informed and resolute effort. This volume is a major contribution to the understanding that is needed for a determined encounter. We must avoid being like the man, to quote Dryden again, who "trudged along unknowing what he sought, / And whistled as he went for want of thought." Paul Farmer teaches us how to stop whistling and start thinking. We have reason to be grateful.

PREFACE TO THE PAPERBACK EDITION

Most human rights organizations are modeled after Northern watchdog organizations, located in an urban area, run by a core management without a membership base (unlike Amnesty International), and dependent solely on overseas funding. The most successful of these organizations only manage to achieve the equivalent status of a public policy think-tank, a research institute, or a specialized publishing house. With media-driven visibility and a lifestyle to match, the leaders of these initiatives enjoy privilege and comfort, and progressively grow distant from a life of struggle.

In the absence of a membership base, there is no constituency-driven obligation or framework for popularizing the language or objectives of the group beyond the community of inward-looking professionals or careerists who run it. Instead of being the currency of a social justice or conscience-driven movement, "human rights" has increasingly become the specialized language of a select professional cadre with its own rites of passage and methods of certification. Far from being a badge of honor, human rights activism is, in some of the places I have observed it, increasingly a certificate of privilege.

"Why More Africans Don't Use Human Rights Language"
Chidi Anselm Odinkalu

-1-

In central Haiti's largest town, a dusty and beaten-down place, there stands, at the entrance to the city, a military checkpoint. For most of the twentieth century, chains barred the way and the station was manned by heavily armed soldiers. During the 1980s, I was stopped there on many occasions, as the town was home to central Haiti's chief referral hospital, to which we would sometimes transport patients or bring medical supplies. Usually we were just waved through the checkpoint without a search. But during the military coup that lasted from 1991 to 1994, we were often harassed and threatened, one time in the presence of some American nuns who were searched, more carefully than is respectful, for papers, tapes, and what the soldiers termed "contraband documents." The military men had guessed, correctly, that the good sisters were part of a human rights delegation and had interviewed the victims of harassment far worse than that meted out at any roadside search.

But a short while later the Haitian army, established through an act of the U.S. Congress during the American occupation of Haiti (1915–1934), was disbanded. Nobel Laureate Oscar Arias, former president of Costa Rica, describes how this occurred in an opinion piece published in the *Washington Post*. It's worth citing at length:

> The 1991 coup against Haiti's first democratically elected president was definitive proof of the army's predatory role. Even though the 1994 agreement returning Jean-Bertrand Aristide to office called for a reduction of the army from 7,500 to 1,500 troops, a force that size was still a clear threat to democratic governance. In 1995 I visited Haiti to discuss with President Aristide the benefits of doing away with the army entirely [as had been done in Costa Rica]. He readily agreed that the army was a problem, but he doubted he would have the political mandate to tackle it.

Arias continues his recounting of events:

> Since Aristide said that he could not abolish the army without the support of the Haitian people, the Arias Foundation for Peace and Human Progress commissioned an independent polling firm to gauge popular support for the idea. The results were stunning: 62 percent of Haitians were strongly in favor of abolition and only 12 percent were against. These figures were key in convincing Aristide that demilitarization was an idea whose time had come. He cut the army's funding and set in motion a legislative process to have the abolition of the army enshrined in Haiti's constitution.[1]

Since the modern Haitian army had never known, in the long years of its existence, a non-domestic enemy, it's easy to see why there was so much popular support for its abolition. Early results of the abolition were evident in 1996, when Jean-Bertrand Aristide became the first president in Haiti's almost two-hundred-year history to peacefully hand over power to another elected civilian, René Préval. President Arias attended Préval's inauguration ceremony and recalled that "Aristide happily noted that the only members of the army still on the government payroll were twenty marching band musicians."

Cut to the same city in early March 2004. The military checkpoint is back, but now the soldiers' uniforms are different. Although an international peacekeeping force now resides in Haiti, these aren't foreign troops. They're Haitians, several of them former army officers. They are sporting what one assumes is army surplus, because "US

ARMY" is emblazoned on much of their gear. The lapels bear distinctly un-Haitian names—"Fletcher," for example, is not a moniker I've encountered in two decades of seeing patients in rural Haiti.

How did this unpopular army suddenly return to its former haunts and checkpoints? It wouldn't have happened without the mechanics of a coup. Amy Wilentz, writing in *The Nation,* put it succinctly:

> One thing about coups: They don't just happen. In a country like Haiti, where the military has been disbanded for nearly a decade, soldiers don't simply emerge from the underbrush; they have to be reorganized, retrained and resupplied. And of course, for something to be organized, someone has to organize it.[2]

As Wilentz suggests, many questions remain unanswered. We know that U.S. funds overtly financed Aristide's opposition. But did they also fund, even indirectly, the rebellion that so prominently featured high-powered U.S. weapons only a year after 20,000 such weapons were promised to the Dominican Republic,[3] next door? Senator Christopher Dodd is urging an investigation into the U.S. training of six hundred "rebels" in the Dominican Republic, and also wants to investigate "how the International Republican Institute spent $1.2 million of taxpayer money" in Haiti. Answering these and related questions would take an intrepid investigative reporter with great latitude rather than a physician working, with some trepidation these days, in central Haiti. It would take a reporter willing to take on hard questions about U.S. policies in Latin America.

These recent events were the brutal upshots of policies made far from central Haiti and far, in fact, from Port-au-Prince. In the postscript to Chapter 2 of *Pathologies of Power,* I described the longstanding embargo on humanitarian and development aid to the hemisphere's poorest country. Aristide was reelected at almost precisely the same time that the current president of the United States was elected, although there's evidence that only one of the two won his country's popular vote (to get no more technical than that about the U.S. results). Be that as it may, one of these two men was called to lead the Western world's poorest country, while the other leads the most powerful nation in human history. Anyone interested in pathologies of power would be able to predict the impact of an aid embargo on Haiti's fragile, cash-strapped government. In any case, the aid through official channels had never been very substantial. Counted per capita, before the embargo the United States was giving

Haiti one-tenth what it was distributing in Kosovo. But claims heard
since the overthrow from the mouths of former ambassadors and
the Bush administration—that hundreds of millions of dollars
flowed to Haiti—are correct, though misleading. Aid did flow, just
not to the elected government. Most of it went to non-governmental
organizations, and some of it went to the anti-Aristide opposition.
U.S. organizations like the International Republican Institute and
the National Endowment for Democracy funneled hundreds of
thousands, perhaps millions, of dollars to the opposition.[4]

The cuts in bilateral aid and the diversion of monies to the opposition meant that little effort could be made, in a country as poor as
Haiti, to rebuild schools, health care infrastructures, roads, ports,
telecommunications, or airports. But this entire affair was not considered newsworthy until after Aristide's overthrow at the end of
February 2004, a coup effected by armed rebels now sporting U.S.
army surplus uniforms and carrying weapons, it would seem to this
untutored eye, of U.S. manufacture. It was not until March 7 that
one could read, in the U.S. daily press, about the ties between the
coup and the practices of the "international community," as it's
called. In its one and only investigative piece about the three-year
aid embargo, the *Boston Globe* finally stumbled upon the facts:

> For three years, the US government, the European Union, and interna-
> tional banks have blocked $500 million in aid to Haiti's government,
> ravaging the economy of a nation already twice as poor as any in the
> Western Hemisphere.
>
> The cutoff, intended to pressure the government to adopt political
> reforms, left Haiti struggling to meet even basic needs and weakened the
> authority of President Jean-Bertrand Aristide, who went into exile one
> week ago.
>
> Today, Haiti's government, which serves 8 million people, has an
> annual budget of about $300 million—less than that of Cambridge
> [Massachusetts], a city of just over 100,000. And as Haitians attempt
> to form a new government, many say its success will largely depend on
> how much and how soon aid will flow to the country.
>
> Many of Aristide's supporters, in Haiti and abroad, angrily contend
> that the international community, particularly the United States, aban-
> doned the fledgling democracy when it most needed aid. Many believe
> that Aristide himself was the target of the de facto economic sanctions,
> just as Haiti was beginning to put its finances back in order.[5]

In Chapter 2, I sought to present a shred of good news from the
front lines of the struggle against impunity by recounting the suc-

cessful prosecution of the perpetrators of the Raboteau massacre. But that optimism proved premature. Even a brief study of the curriculum vitae of the "rebels" now manning military checkpoints shows many of them to have been the authors of this and other massacres; they and their accomplices are now at large.[6]

The post-coup government was assembled, it would seem, with help from the U.S. government, which has issued contradictory statements about the rebels, now praising them, now disavowing them. Other press reports, and the turn of events, lead us to believe that the former military is back to stay. In his first public statement, the man sworn in as Haiti's new prime minister, Gerard Latortue, announced that Aristide's order to replace the military with a civilian police force violated Haiti's constitution; he promised to name a commission to examine the issues surrounding its restoration. The de facto prime minister also named a former general to his new government. A ceremony in Gonaïves had this prime minister sharing the stage with rebels and gang leaders: the headline in the *Jamaica Observer* (21 March 2004) read: "Latortue praises gang leaders, gunmen." And in the *New York Times*—not in an editorial but in a news article—we find that "Mr. Latortue and his cabinet, which are installed this week, are trying to send a clear message of stability after several months of bloody revolt and three years of a corrupt Aristide administration that have left the public sector in tatters and exhausted the people's trust." The same story informs us that Mr. Latortue and his entourage flew in a U.S. Army Black Hawk helicopter and a Chinook transport helicopter, escorted by U.S. troops, to meet the "rebel" army leaders Guy Philippe and Jean Tatoune, a convicted mass murderer.[7]

Today, the Central Plateau is completely in the hands of former military men. There are no police and no foreign troops, only the armed men in army surplus. It's hard not to argue that the conventional human rights groups missed the boat on the entire story. Illegally blocking humanitarian assistance to one of the world's poorest countries surely ranks among the most vicious abuses of power in the modern toolkit. Yet the aid embargo didn't even register on the radar of most human rights groups. Many of these groups are now back in Haiti on "fact-finding missions," long after what observers of structural violence would recognize as the decisive facts. One such mission concluded that "international human rights organizations, especially Human Rights Watch and Journalists Without Bor-

ders, and to a lesser extent Amnesty International, have taken the
NCHR [National Coalition for Haitian Rights] reports uncritically
and failed to develop other impartial human rights contacts in
Haiti." That is, the international community—the funders, it must
be noted—were relying overmuch on local and overseas partisan
groups with overt political agendas but little in the way of expertise
in or commitment to documenting rights abuses.[8]

These lessons from Haiti's painful experience have wide resonance elsewhere. Writing from Africa, Chidi Anselm Odinkalu offers a damning assessment of conventional human rights work there:
"The current human rights movement in Africa—with the possible
exception of the women's rights movement and faith-based social
justice initiatives—appears almost by design to exclude the participation of the people whose welfare it purports to advance." The
people excluded are of course the poor majority, who are not held to
be part of "civil society" in much of Latin America and Africa.
Odinkalu hazards a guess as to why so many human rights groups
mirror the inequalities of our world:

> Local human rights groups exist to please the international agencies that
> fund or support them. Local problems are only defined as potential pots
> of project cash, not as human experiences to be resolved in just terms,
> thereby delegitimizing human rights language and robbing its ideas of
> popular appeal.[9]

-2-

This book is about the struggle for social and economic rights, the
neglected stepchildren of the human rights movement. Because social and economic rights include the right to health care, housing,
clean water, and education, they are sometimes called "the rights of
the poor." As noted in these pages, debates about the relative merits
of one set of rights over another seem arcane outside of the rather
insular world of the mainstream "human rights community." But
say you choose to focus, as a physician might, on AIDS and tuberculosis. These are the two leading infectious causes of adult death in
the world today. The argument that the afflicted deserve access to
care for these ailments is an argument for social and economic
rights. Here too one looks for good news along with the bad. In the
final chapter of *Pathologies of Power*, I mentioned that Physicians
for Human Rights, focusing on Africa, had launched a campaign to

make access to HIV care a human right. Theirs was, to my knowledge, the first human rights group based in the United States to start a campaign to press for the right to treatment, even though the broader movement's sacred text, the Universal Declaration of Human Rights, was pretty straightforward on these points. More than once in these pages, I cite Article 25 of the Universal Declaration, which states that "Everyone has the right to a standard of living adequate for the health and well-being of himself and of his family, including food, clothing, housing and medical care and necessary social services, and the right to security in the event of unemployment, sickness, disability, widowhood, old age or other lack of livelihood in circumstances beyond his control." Article 27, similarly, argues that everyone has the right "to share in scientific advancement and its benefits."

Rights declarations are, of course, exhortatory and largely unenforceable. And the bad news is that very few enjoy these rights. AIDS and other problems of poverty in Africa remain the obvious cases in point, so why are human rights groups not focusing on these most pressing issues? Odinkalu's penetrating analysis echoes that advanced in *Pathologies of Power*:

> In Africa, the realization of human rights is a very serious business indeed. In many cases it is a life and death matter. From the child soldier, the rural dweller deprived of basic health care, the mother unaware that the next pregnancy is not an inexorable fate, the city dweller living in fear of the burglar, the worker owed several months arrears of wages, and the activist organizing against bad government, to the group of rural women seeking access to land so that they may send their children to school with its proceeds, people are acutely aware of the injustices inflicted upon them. Knowledge of the contents of the Universal Declaration will hardly advance their condition. What they need is a movement that channels these frustrations into articulate demands that evoke responses from the political process. This the human rights movement is unwilling or unable to provide. In consequence, the real life struggles for social justice are waged despite human rights groups—not by or because of them—by people who feel that their realities and aspirations are not adequately captured by human rights organizations or their language.[10]

This is a terrible irony of good intentions.

Certainly, the amount of resources available to do AIDS work has likely trebled in the year since this book was published. But these resources will this year be delivered to a grand total of 150,000 out of an estimated 6 million patients who need therapy. (In Africa alone,

28 million people are living with HIV, but not all of them need such therapy—yet.) In addition to declining life expectancy, Botswana, South Africa, and other, poorer countries in southern Africa may also experience shrinking populations because of AIDS deaths.[11] "AIDS alone is devastating the heart of these countries, affecting people in the prime years of not only their economic production, but the prime years of reproduction," said the president of the Population Research Institute, a Virginia-based group that opposes population controls as a way to curb growth. "Population control efforts make no sense in the face of the AIDS epidemic."[12]

AIDS has killed more than 20 million people since the epidemic began two decades ago. More than twice that many now live with HIV. Unless treatment is made available, most of these people are expected to die within the coming decade. It is thus good news that the prices of antiretroviral drugs continue to drop dramatically.[13] But even if treatment becomes much more widely available, the absence of a rights-based approach will mean that these life-saving therapies will be made available only to those who can pay for them.

What of the number two infectious killer? Tuberculosis is predicted to maintain that position in the coming years, even though a rights-based approach to tuberculosis has been adopted more widely, if timidly, of late. Tuberculosis treatment is regarded as a "public good." But in settings of scarce resources—which is to say, in all those places where tuberculosis is prevalent—the world of public health continues to be split by debates. For example, there are those who argue vehemently that only infectious tuberculosis of the lungs—"smear-positive disease" in the jargon—should be a priority, since that's the form thought to lead to epidemic transmission. It's "cost-effective" to think of this airborne disease as a public-health problem requiring public resources, goes the argument; other forms of tuberculosis are not infectious and not the ranking priority. How unfortunate for the cost-effectiveness ideologues that this rule of thumb has not proven true. In one recent study from Canada, fewer than 31 percent of all tuberculosis cases were "smear-positive," and epidemic transmission was associated with patients who did not have laboratory evidence of infectious tuberculosis when this "cost-effective" diagnostic tool was used.[14] Wouldn't a rights-based approach—taking as its basis that all persons with tuberculosis deserve access to care—have served us better?

Also on the rise is multidrug-resistant tuberculosis (MDRTB), much discussed in this book. Again, public health nihilists have long argued that MDRTB is too expensive and too difficult to treat. *Pathologies of Power* predicted that we'd wake up to this threat, and we did: about one month ago. After years of discouraging any focus on treating MDRTB, the World Health Organization recently concluded that "multi-drug resistant tuberculosis poses a major threat to the European Union." The report, released in March 2004, predicted 300,000 new cases of MDRTB cases each year, and noted that the epidemic would be fanned by HIV. According to the report, some 70 percent of MDRTB cases are likely to be caused by the "superbugs" described in Chapters 4 and 7.[15]

-3-

The world is full of bad news, and you don't have to be working in rural Haiti to hear it. In Chiapas, Guatemala, and Rwanda, the struggle against impunity continues, with reports from each place reminding us that the glass is best viewed as half empty.[16] Even the luckier part of the world provides scarce solace. Instead we read about terrorism, ethnic violence, and the slow burn of racism reflected in, say, handgun violence in the United States. A single day's headlines include the following, if you're in rural Haiti on March 19, 2004 and looking at news sites on the Internet:

- Taiwan's President Re-Elected a Day After Being Shot
- Army Drops All Charges Against Muslim Chaplain
- Canadian Feed Mills Blamed for Mad Cow Infection
- Whites-Only Scholarship Stirs Rhode Island School
- Town Remembers One of the First to Die in Iraq

If you have a broadband connection, a service called CNN Newspass will inform you that a "Grade School Murder Was Foiled" in Forsyth, Montana.

It is the central thesis of *Pathologies of Power* that a rising tide of inequality breeds violence. Perhaps the only silver lining out there is that violence, terrorism, and war—both episodic and structural violence—may yet provoke an international debate and even some soul-searching about the cost of our peculiarly modern inequalities. Two wire stories from today offer discrepant readings on violence and terror:

Blood and flesh splattered on the walls. Nearby windows shattered. Only a charred metal seat and two twisted wheels were left of Yassin's wheelchair, and a blood-soaked brown shoe lay in the street. Lying in tatters nearby was the brown blanket in which Yassin—a quadriplegic—was nearly always wrapped.[17]

.   .   .   .   .

The meeting Monday comes as Spain's incoming Socialist government begins to pressure European allies and the United States for a new approach to fighting terrorism—based less on military force and police measures and more on rooting out social and economic inequities blamed for turning Muslim countries into breeding grounds for young men prone to terrorism.[18]

From rural Haiti, both violence and disease have always appeared as pathologies of power. Structural violence was at the heart of Haiti's creation, and this former slave colony is as good a reminder as any of the intimate ties between those who are victims of violence and those who are shielded from it. More guns and more repression may well be the time-honored prescription for policing poverty, but violence and chaos will not go away if the hunger, illness, and racism that are the lot of so many are not addressed in a meaningful and durable fashion.

Central Haiti
March 22, 2004

NOTES

1. Oscar Arias, "Only the marching band," *The Washington Post,* March 12, 2004.

2. Amy Wilentz, "Haiti's occupation," *The Nation,* April 19, 2004.

3. "[A] senior US military official said a small number of US special forces conducted antiterrorism exercises, called Operation Jaded Task, with the Dominican military in February 2003. . . . The US official said 20,000 M-16s were provided to the Dominican forces to help the country guard its border with Haiti and that all the weapons could not be accounted for." Bryan Bender, "Aristide backers blame US for ouster," *The Boston Globe,* March 1, 2004.

4. For more on Washington's ongoing war on Haiti, see the Council on Hemispheric Affairs's report *Unfair and indecent diplomacy: Washington's vendetta against Haiti's president Aristide,* January 15, 2004. Available at: http://www.coha.org/NEW_PRESS_RELEASES/New_Press_Releases_2004/04.03_Haiti_Aristide.htm.

5. Farah Stockman and Susan Milligan, "Before fall of Aristide, Haiti

hit by aid cutoff," *The Boston Globe,* March 7, 2004.

6. Paul Farmer, "Who removed Aristide?" *London Review of Books,* April 15, 2004: 26(8).

7. Kirk Semple, "Haiti's new cabinet and rebels hit the road," *The New York Times,* March 21, 2004.

8. The report continues: "Although they were the only human rights group in the country adequately funded and having trained monitors throughout Haiti, the NCHR became completely partisan: anti-Lavalas, anti-Aristide. This is simply not proper for a group calling itself a "Haitian Rights" organization. During the final month before the coup, they abandoned any pretext of impartiality, joining calls for the ouster of Aristide, without reference to the means. After February 29, they continue to cite abuses by "chimère," whom they call simply "Aristide gangs," without documenting the connections. Though they told our group they had "heard about" violence against unarmed Lavalas [members], including the possible complicity of U.S. Marines in the Bel Air incident, the NCHR said they "lacked access" to the pro-Lavalas shantytowns. Of course they lacked access: they lacked any shred of credibility as a human rights monitor." Tom Reeves, "Return to Haiti," *ZNet,* April 15, 2004.

See also the report from the National Lawyers' Guild, which reached the same conclusions: Thomas Griffin, *Summary Report of Haiti Human Rights Delegation—March 29 to April 5, 2004,* National Lawyer's Guild, April 11, 2004.

9. Chidi Anselm Odinkalu, "Why more Africans don't use human rights language," *Human Rights Dialogue: Human Rights for All? The Problem of the Human Rights Box,* Carnegie Council on Ethics and International Affairs, Winter 2000: 2(1). Available at: http://www.cceia.org/viewMedia.php/prmTemplateID/8/prmID/602.

10. Ibid.

11. United States Census Bureau, *Global Population Profile 2002,* March 22, 2004. Available at: http://www.census.gov//ipc/www/wp02.html.

12. Genaro C. Armas, "Fertility rates, AIDS slow world population growth," AP, March 22, 2004.

13. In early April 2004, the Global Fund, the World Bank, UNICEF, and the Clinton Foundation announced agreements that will make it possible for developing countries to purchase high-quality AIDS medicines and diagnostics for less than $140 per patient per year.

14. E. Hernández-Garduño, V. Cook, D. Kunimoto, R. K. Elwood, W. A. Black, J. M. FitzGerald, "Transmission of tuberculosis from smear negative patients: a molecular epidemiology study," *Thorax* 2004; 59:286–290.

15. World Health Organization, *Third global report on anti-tuberculosis drug resistance in the world* (Geneva: World Health Organization, 2004). Available at: http://www.who.int/gtb/publications/drugresistance/2004/.

16. For more recent updates from each of these places, see the following works: Victoria Sanford, *Violencia y Genocidio en Guatemala* (Guatemala: F&G Editores, 2003); Victoria Sanford, *Buried Secrets: Truth and Human Rights in Guatemala* (New York: Palgrave Macmillan, 2003); Africa Rights,

Rwanda: Broken Bodies, Torn Spirits: Living with Genocide, Rape and HIV/AIDS, Kilgali, April 15, 2004; Jan Rus, Rosa Aida Hernandez Castillo, Shannon L. Mattiace, eds., *Mayan Lives, Mayan Utopias: The Indigenous Peoples of Chiapas and the Zapatista Rebellion* (Lanham, MD: Rowan & Littlefield, 2003).

17. Lara Sukhtian, "Hamas founder's killing sparks calls for revenge: Israel assassinates Palestinian as he leaves mosque; Arabs outraged," AP, March 22, 2004.

18. Mar Roman, "Spain arrests four more suspects in Madrid bombings," AP, March 22, 2004.

ACKNOWLEDGMENTS

Because these chapters are grounded in the experience of specific communities, I have many debts to people on three continents and on a couple of very special islands. In Haiti, I am, as ever, grateful to Didi Bertrand, Fritz and Yolande Lafontant, Flora Chipps, and Loune Viaud as well as to the people of Cange and to the large number of victims of human rights abuses who came to me seeking my help as a physician. Several of my patients requested specifically that their stories be told; I hope they will forgive the lag time. Of course, it takes a village to care for patients, and so I would like to thank some of my colleagues—friends, really—in Haiti: Fernet Léandre, Jean-Hughes Jérôme, Cynthia Orélus, Jessye Bertrand, Marie-Sidonise Claude, Wesler Lambert, Maxi Raymonville, Maxcène Oréus, Jean Germeille Ferrer, and other clinicians at the Clinique Bon Sauveur. In Port-au-Prince, I am indebted to William Smarth, Antoine Adrien, Michèle Pierre-Louis, Mildred Trouillot Aristide, and to all those working for social and economic rights in Haiti. Thanks also to Hervé Razafimbahiny and Brian Concannon (who, in addition to working on major projects, are never too busy to help get innocent people out of jail), as well as Michelle Karshan and the rest of the small human rights community in Haiti. They know that the path is paved with thorns.

In Cuba, I thank my great friend Jorge Pérez Ávila, who will forgive me, I hope, for taking his patients out drinking (they were only *mojitos*). I am also grateful to Gustavo Kourí, Jorge González Pérez, Guadalupe Guzmán, and the community of those living in Santiago de las Vegas. In addition, I add special thanks to Jesús Valle, Eduardo Campo, Fernando Mederos, and others good enough to spend so much time recounting their own experiences.

In Guatemala, I am especially obliged to Blanca Jiménez, Jesús Gaspar Jerónimo, Juan Alberto Jiménez, and Santiago Pablo Diego. In spite of their terrible losses during a war financed in part by my country of origin, they have offered me nothing but hospitality and kindness. In Mexico, deep appreciation goes to Julio Quiñones Hernández; Leonel González Ortiz; Dagmar Castillo; Jorge Gabriel García Salyano, and all of the staff of EAPSEC; Demóstenes Martín Pérez Urbina; Father Eliberto; and Pablo and Patricia Farías. Gratitude and admiration to the valiant people of many different communities in the autonomous zones, who, given current conditions, wisely prefer to go unnamed. The Fray Bartolomé de Las Casas Human Rights Center is an invaluable source of important documentation, and I am grateful for its hospitality.

In Russia, I thank Oksana Pomonarenko, Alexander Goldfarb, Ekaterina Goncharova, Alexander Pasechnikov, and many others at both Partners In Health–Russia and the Public Health Research Institute (PHRI). Thanks also to Sergei Borisov, Mikhael Perelman, and other colleagues involved in the care of patients with tuberculosis. Valery Sergeyev, regional director of the Moscow office of Penal Reform International, has been a patient source of unbiased information. Within the Ministry of Justice, I am grateful to Alexandr Kononets, Yuri I. Kalinin, Vladimir Yu. Yalunin, and Minister Yuri Chayka. It has been striking to me that I had readier access to prisons in Russia than I did in my own country. All my trips to the Russian Federation were related, in one way or another, to the Open Society Institute; and I thank my many interlocutors in New York and in Moscow, including George Soros, Mia Nitchun, Srdjan Matič, Nina Schwalbe, Nancy Mahon, Miriam Porter, and Ekaterina Yurievna. Most of all, I thank Aryeh Neier, a visionary in several realms, not the least of them human rights.

In Peru, I thank Jaime Bayona and the entire "DOTS-Plus" team, especially the *promotores* and nurses; Rocío Sapag; the parish of Cristo Luz del Mundo; Brother Lenny Rego of Centro Óscar Romero; Benedicta Serrano; Gustavo Gutiérrez and the staff of the Instituto Bartolomé de Las Casas; Maria van der Linde and the staff of DEPAS; Emma Rubín de Celis; and Francisco Chamberlain. The impact of Peru and Peruvians is not evident in this book, which contains few case materials from Peru. This is misleading, however, since much of what I have written in these pages has been shaped by my association with Socios En Salud and other groups there.

In Boston, my primary appointment is in Harvard Medical School's Department of Social Medicine, with which I have been affiliated for my entire adult life. It's been an exceptionally fruitful association, at least from my point of view. Arthur Kleinman encouraged this work on human rights when many department chairs would have ruled it out of order; the same could be said for Dean Joe Martin, who has exhorted faculty members to become more interested in such matters. That the Department of Social Medicine affords me such a hospitable home is no doubt a result of its leadership: prior to Arthur came Leon Eisenberg, and before him Julius Richmond; they continue to exude goodness within the walls of the department—and their influence extends, happily, far beyond those walls. Byron and Mary Jo Good and Allan Brandt are continuing the tradition, which I regard as very much in keeping with the spirit of Rudolph Virchow. Within the Department of Social Medicine, I am particularly grateful to the staff of the Program in Infectious Disease and Social Change, especially our students, several of whom shared some of the experiences described here. I hope I may be forgiven for singling out David Walton, Kedar Mate, Raul Ruiz, Marshall Fordyce, Evan Lyon, Giuseppe Raviola, Sierra Washington, and Mehret Mandefrou.

At the Brigham and Women's Hospital, my other Boston home, I thank Marshall Wolf and Victor Dzau as well as Jamie Maguire, Elliott Kieff, Paul Sax, Johanna Daily, Sigal Yawetz, and other members of the Department of Medicine and its Infectious Disease Division.

Partners In Health (including its Institute for Health and Social Justice) is more a concept than a place and is not based in any one city. But I again turn to Boston in thanking my partners there: Aaron Shakow, for all-round scholarly assistance with this and other projects; Annie Hyson, for help with Chiapas documentation; Jennifer Singler, for her interest in liberation theology (and for serving as my left arm, connected to her heart, after Joia Mukherjee broke the former); Chris Douglas, for materials used in the chapter on ethics; Lydia Mann-Bondat, for her interest in health and human rights; and, finally, Laura Tarter and Nicole Gastineau, for their able assistance on research and documentation and also for their cheerful assistance in completing the innumerable tasks that arise in bringing a book to press. Joyce Millen, Siripanth Nippita, and Carole Mitnick have kept the Institute going in one form or another for several years, in the process keeping us accountable and up to date. I'm especially grateful to Carole for her close reading of the material on tuberculosis in prisons, and also for her company during inspections of prisons. I look forward to working ever more closely with Joia Mukherjee, Mary Kay Smith-Fawzi, Serena Koenig, Cynthia Rose, Melissa Gillooly, Ed Nardell, and Arachu Castro (whose help was invaluable in editing Chapters 2 and 3) as we seek to extend the notion of social and economic rights to more of the destitute sick.

Co-inhabiting several worlds—the Brigham, Partners In Health, Harvard Medical School—are a few friends worth their weight in precious gemstones. Heidi Behforouz, Sonya Shin, Jennifer Furin, Keith Joseph, and Carole Smarth are the best that one could ask for in clinical colleagues. By treating patients with dignity, compassion, and great competence, they promote human rights on a daily basis. Howard Hiatt, the godfather of Partners In Health and a discerning consumer of human rights discourse, has often been the sounding board against which I have developed some of these ideas. Most of all, I thank Mercedes Becerra, without whom, as they say, this book would not exist.

Less easy to classify are free-floating friends and colleagues who have helped me in one way or another, usually to see something that I would have otherwise missed. This group includes Jean Gabriel *fils;* Tracy Kidder; Kris Heggenhougen; Joy Marshall; Ken Fox; Nancy Dorsinville; Mark Pavlick; Nalini Visvanathan; Erica James; Noam and Carol Chomsky; Jeff Sachs; Gene Bukhman; Jody Heymann; Vivien Stern; Hernán Reyes; Nancy Scheper-Hughes; Mirjam J.E. van Ewijk and Paul Grifhorst; Paul Rabinow; Philippe Bourgois; David Simmons; Charlie Everett; Gilles Peress; Nick Vogenthaler; Bill Schultz; Len Rubenstein; Ama Karikari; Lino Pertile and Anna Bensted; Emilio Travieso; Amartya Sen; Bryan Stevenson; Bob Bilheimer; Leslie Fleming; Lorena Barberia; Johannes Sommerfeld; Didier Fassin; Alaka Wali; Henry Steiner and other members of the University Committee on Human Rights; Richard Smith; Don Berwick; Annie Dillard; Jack Coulihan; Moupali Das; Carolyn Keiper; Karen Bos; Janice Leung; Deogratias Niyizonkiza; an anonymous reviewer for the University of California Press, from whom I learned a great deal; and, most of all, Barbara Rylko-Bauer, who was good enough to turn her editor's eye—and her poet's heart—to this book. It's no exaggeration to add that Barbara has shaped both content and form of *Pathologies of Power.* Indeed, I'm convinced I would not have finished the book without Barbara's encouragement, counsel, and assistance.

My deepest debt in the project of putting into words a number of distressing experiences is without question Haun Saussy, my most critical reader. For bibliographic materials and all-round inspiration, I thank Virginia Farmer (my first instructor in human rights, who in living by the Golden Rule passed it on to her brood). Catherine Bertrand Farmer has also provided invaluable help with editing, documentation, and translating documents from five languages. Without her knowledge of Tzotzil and Tzeltal, some of my materials from Mexico would have been useless. Gratitude also to her team of even younger assistants, Gabriel and Pablo Bayona Sapag (whose familiarity with Quechua helped more than they know), and Thomas Jei Kim (whose critical rereading of the notion of "Asian values" has been indispensable).

It is impossible to write a book about health and human rights without invoking the memory of Jonathan Mann, whose spirited responses to—and critiques of—the ideas presented here are sorely missed. Pierre Bourdieu shaped my understanding of social theory, and I am saddened that he will not see this book in print.

Such a long list of thank-yous might suggest that this should be a text without errors, and, indeed, I do hope that it is free of factual inaccuracies. Yet I am not a specialist in the conventional sense. I write about Haiti with a certain assurance, since I have lived and worked here for all of my adult life and know its rural reaches as an anthropologist and as a doctor who cares for the destitute sick. But the same cannot be said for my work in Peru or my visits to Cuba, Russia, or Mexico. I have looked at these places through the eyes of a physician-anthropologist who knows Haiti best. I believe this perspective is useful, because it brings into relief the importance, in each setting, of social and economic rights. This is no doubt because Haiti's infamous poverty stands as both rebuke and interrogation—and, if we are lucky, as revelation—in virtually any setting.

Finally, I have a long and fruitful history of work with the University of California Press. Stan Holwitz introduced me to the world of writing books and seeing them published; Rob Borofsky and his series, Public Anthropology, encouraged me to finish this one; Naomi Schneider is as gracious and supportive an editor as one could hope to meet; Mary Renaud works magic with her editorial scalpel.

This book is dedicated to my chief co-conspirators, Ophelia, Loune, Jim, and Tom. Without them, perhaps I would be reduced to being either a frustrated physician, lacking the tools necessary for social justice work, or a bitter seminar-room warrior, lacking the experience of service to the poor. My gratitude to them, and to all of the Partners In Health family, knows no bounds. But I cannot close these acknowledgments without recalling the example offered by Jean-Marie Vincent, Chouchou Louis, Amos Jeannot, and Armando Mazariegos. One could say that their deaths—by murder, all of them—have been instructive and somehow redemptive, since their sacrifice has inspired others to ask hard questions about human rights. But I have found these deaths to be haunting, irrevocable, and for me and many others they have inspired largely pain; this book does little to ease that pain. In the end, then, I cannot really view their loss as redeemed.

INTRODUCTION

Fleas dream of buying themselves a dog, and nobodies dream
of escaping poverty: that one magical day good luck will
suddenly rain down on them—will rain down in buckets. But
good luck doesn't rain down yesterday, today, tomorrow, or
ever. Good luck doesn't even fall in a fine drizzle, no matter
how hard the nobodies summon it, even if their left hand is
tickling, or if they begin the new day with their right foot, or
start the new year with a change of brooms.

   The nobodies: nobody's children, owners of nothing. The
nobodies: the no ones, the nobodied, running like rabbits,
dying through life, screwed every which way.

   Who are not, but could be.

   Who don't speak languages, but dialects.

   Who don't have religions, but superstitions.

   Who don't create art, but handicrafts.

   Who don't have culture, but folklore.

   Who are not human beings, but human resources.

   Who do not have faces, but arms.

   Who do not have names, but numbers.

   Who do not appear in the history of the world, but in the
police blotter of the local paper.

   The nobodies, who are not worth the bullet that kills them.

                    Eduardo Galeano, "The Nobodies"

The people in a number of the stories are of the kind that
many writers have recently got in the habit of referring to as
"the little people." I regard this phrase as patronizing and
repulsive. There are no little people in this book. They are as
big as you are, whoever you are.

                    Joseph Mitchell, *McSorley's Wonderful Saloon*

In the summer of 1999, in the company of friends and co-workers, I
crossed the border between Mexico and Guatemala. The frontier was
heavily militarized on the Mexican side. We were searched there, as we
had been searched elsewhere in Chiapas: with up to seventy thousand

troops stationed in the region, the Mexican government can readily do a good deal of rummaging.[1]

We walked across the frontier uneventfully and there, close to the appointed hour, met our friend. Call her Julia. A broad smile broke over her face, a beautiful and reflective one; long black hair fell over her back, and she wore the traditional attire (a braided multicolored sash and frock) of her people, the Mam. The smile belied the great suffering Julia had seen. Her husband, a health worker, had been "disappeared" by Guatemalan security forces on the Mexican side of the border and had never been heard from again. Her nineteen-year-old brother, a rebel soldier, had been killed in combat, his body displayed as a grisly trophy for the Guatemalan army. She herself had lived a long decade of mourning and exile in Mexico. But now her smile spoke of new and restorative projects.

All of us—friends from the States, from Mexico, and from Guatemala—were bound together, most of us for over a decade, by our work in health care. Julia was also an international visitor, in a sense: like so many from the region, she had lived for years in refugee camps in Mexico, where she and others had worked to improve the health first of fellow refugees and, later, of the poor of Chiapas.[2] Now that she had returned to her home in highland Guatemala, we were to meet her surviving family and to discuss a community health project with Julia and her *compañeros* from the refugee camps.

Soon after we reached the outskirts of the town of Huehuetenango, we parked our pickup truck near a small cement house, pale blue. We found Julia's family engrossed in a movie, perhaps of Mexican or European provenance, about Guatemalan refugees. We signaled our interest in watching along. I didn't catch the name of the film, but it was clear that it treated the worst years of the killing—the years during which Julia lost her husband. In the course of almost four decades of armed violence, some two hundred thousand died in Guatemala, the majority of them civilians killed by the army.[3] The bit of the movie we caught brought foreign involvement into relief. Judging from the accent, one of the actors was meant to represent a *gringo*.

After half an hour or so, Julia's father stopped the movie—it was a videotape—and put on an impromptu concert for us. He and two of his sons stood together and played the marimba (a percussion instrument that looks like a giant xylophone). They later showed us pictures of Julia's martyred brother and proudly underlined his name on the "honor roll of heroic guerrillas." It was chill and damp in the house, which was warmed only by bare lightbulbs, but we all felt a great warmth, as if being welcomed back after a long and unforeseen separation.

The next morning, we were to meet Julia and the leadership of the renascent health project. But first we were invited to attend part of a workshop. It was being held in a parish school at the end of a muddy road that led up one of the small mountains looming over Huehuetenango. The topic of the workshop: gender relations. The pupils were natives, the instructors two young women from the capital city. The instructors were slender and wore jeans; they looked a lot like those of us who'd come from Boston. And since they spoke the language of U.S. universities, or its echoes in foundations and international bureaucracies, they sounded a lot like us, too.

More specifically, the women from Guatemala City were conducting a "gender-sensitivity workshop." They had asked each of those present—about twenty locals, mostly young women, although Julia's father was there, too—to draw a scene from childhood. The adult pupils sat crammed into children's desks, supplied with crayons. One of the facilitators would hold aloft a drawing and ask the artist, and occasionally the audience, questions about it. The theme of the questions was gender relations.

It was difficult to know how all this was being received—the participants were impassive and spoke only when the women from Guatemala City addressed them. Some, it was clear, did not speak Spanish well; at least one young woman needed a translator. Furthermore, the prominence of dramatic biographical events—deaths, most notably, but also violence that had little to do with gender relations within the indigenous communities—kept pushing the discussion off the course charted by the facilitators. One young woman explained that the death of her mother in childbirth meant that at the age of ten she had by necessity assumed a great deal of responsibility for the care of her younger siblings:

> *Facilitator* (expectantly): "So your father treated you differently because you were a girl?"
>
> *Respondent* (matter-of-factly): "No, not really. He loved us all the same."

A stilted silence followed. I felt uncomfortable, and so, I could tell, did my co-workers. (Ophelia's cheeks were flaming.) It was not the silence that rankled. It seemed to us that the exercise was demeaning—the participants, having survived genocide and displacement, were now being treated like children. They were being asked to respond to an agenda imported from capital cities, from do-gooder organizations like ours, from U.S. universities with the "right" answers to their every question. No harm done, perhaps, and the topic was important—but how helpful was this exercise, with its aim of changing the mentality of the locals, who were, after all, the victims of the previous decades of violence? A change in mentality was needed, certainly, but it was needed in the hearts and minds of those with power—and they were not here but in Guatemala City and Washington, D.C.

Julia signaled that it was time to leave the workshop and meet with the health committee. I was relieved. As we walked across a courtyard into a low, dark cooking area with a dirt floor, I whispered to Ophelia that I hoped we were not going to receive a proposal for "workshops designed to change the mentality of the victims." We had not come all the way to Guatemala to seek to reform the minds or the culture of the victims.

I should not have worried. The scarred but passionate veterans of the health committee were not about to field inane proposals. The next hour was bracing. The air, thick with smoke from the fires bubbling under two nearby cauldrons, was electric; and the discussion had a rare clarity, as Julia and the small group of survivors laid out their plans. They wanted to continue the work they'd begun before the war: promoting community health through training, education, and service. And the project they wanted our help with was a *mental* health project for which they had despaired of securing funding.

They wanted to exhume the dead. They wanted to locate and disinter those buried in mass graves by the army. Why? Because the victims had been "buried with their eyes wide open." And neither they nor their kin would know peace until they were buried properly. "So that their eyes may close," explained Miguel, who, along with Julia, spoke as their leader.

My own eyes were stinging, but not from the smoke. Again, a silence fell over us, this time a silence of complicity and solidarity. Ophelia spoke first, saying that we who would never know their suffering would try to do our part, and also that we would bear witness in the hope that such crimes could not be committed so readily in the future.[4]

In the sunny courtyard, the noise of Spanish mixed with local tongues drifted into hearing: the gender workshop was over. Our private meeting gave way to a meal of tortillas, tough beef, and beans. As I got up to fill my bowl, a poster caught my eye. It bore the imprimatur of the Catholic Church. Its message, though consonant with Catholic social teachings, would have struck Bostonian parishioners as out of place: "Down with neoliberalism," it said in rainbow colors, "Up with humanity!" Next to it hung a small portrait of the recently martyred Bishop Juan José Gerardi. Two days before he was bludgeoned to death in 1998—by officers in the army, according to our hosts—the bishop had released a massive report indicting the army as responsible for 85 percent of the deaths and disappearances during the conflict. Releasing the report was risky, he noted in the last speech he was ever to make, but it was the only way to begin any meaningful process of healing:

> In our country, the truth has been twisted and silenced. God is inflexibly opposed to evil in any form. The root of the downfall and the misfortune of humanity comes from the deliberate opposition to truth, which is the fundamental reality of God and of human beings. This reality has been intentionally distorted in our country throughout thirty-six years of war against the people.[5]

The images and events we experienced during these twenty-four hours—rummaging Mexican soldiers, a martyred teenager and a martyred bishop, the workshop of well-meaning elites from the capital, a mental health project involving exhumation, a cry against neoliberalism—encapsulate as well as anything can the heart of what I hope to write about in these pages. But how are these images and themes related to health and human rights? Take the term "neoliberalism," which, like the related word "liberal," admits to many meanings, some of them contradictory. Neoliberalism generally refers to the ideology that advocates the dominance of a competition-driven market model. Within this doctrine, individuals in a society are viewed, if viewed at all, as autonomous, rational producers and consumers whose decisions are motivated primarily by economic or material concerns. But this ideology has little to say about the social and economic inequalities that distort real economies.

In Latin America, neoliberal policies and ideologies have generally called for the subjugation of political and social life to a set of processes termed "market forces."[6] As a physician who has worked for much of my adult life among the poor of Haiti and the United States, I know that the laws of supply and demand will rarely serve the interests of my patients.[7] And so they and others in their position—globally, this would be hundreds of millions—have fought to construe as a basic human right access to health care, education, and other social services. Indeed, many would argue that most of Latin America's conflicts have been fought over neoliberalism; in the region today, far too many human rights abuses are committed in the name of protecting and promoting some variant of "market" ideology.[8]

This interpretation is at odds, I know, with U.S. notions of liberalism. Aren't "liberals" the great defenders of human rights? friends there ask, exasperated. They are defenders of my rights and yours, I respond, but people like us are in a distinct minority, as Immanuel Wallerstein reminds us:

> Liberals have always claimed that the liberal state—reformist, legalist, and somewhat libertarian—was the only state that could guarantee freedom. And for the relatively small group whose freedom it safeguarded this was perhaps true. But unfortunately that group always remained a minority perpetually en route to becoming everyone.[9]

The liberal political agenda has rarely included the powerless, the destitute, the truly disadvantaged. It has never concerned itself with those popularly classified as the "undeserving" poor: drug addicts, sex workers, illegal "aliens," welfare recipients, or the homeless, to name a few. It is even less concerned with populations beyond national borders. And yet the poor in the countries with which I am most familiar are struggling, and often failing, to survive:

> To put it in systematic terms poverty in the First World is understood in terms of a relative distance from certain standards of human well-being that have been realized in the past but that are now seen less and less frequently. The frame of reference continues to be positive—a degree of well-being attained once upon a time and still attainable. In Latin America, however, the most obvious and spontaneous frame of reference for the concept of poverty is not something positive, but something negative in the extreme: death. In our countries, concrete poverty is misery verging on death. The poor are those whose greatest task is to try to survive.[10]

This book is a physician-anthropologist's effort to reveal the ways in which the most basic right—the right to survive—is trampled in an age of great affluence, and it argues that the matter should be considered the most pressing one of our times. The drama, the tragedy, of the destitute sick concerns not only physicians and scholars who work among the poor but all who profess even a passing interest in human rights. It's not much of a stretch to argue that anyone who wishes to be considered humane has ample cause to consider what it means to be sick and poor in the era of globalization and scientific advancement.

Pathologies of Power uses case studies to examine the struggle for social and economic rights as they are related to health. Since a physician must have access to medicines and supplies in order to work on behalf of the victims of human rights violations thus defined, you would think that physicians would be deeply involved in pressing for social and economic rights. And since anthropologists often work in settings of violence and privation, you would think that anthropologists might have contributed heavily to our understanding of the dynamics of human rights violations. To date, however, human rights scholarship has been largely the province of lawyers and juridical experts; reports and documentation have been more likely to come from church groups and nongovernmental organizations than from academics. With a few notable exceptions (many of them cited in these pages), physicians and anthropologists have had far too little to say about human rights. But as a physician to the poor, I have seen what has happened, and what continues to happen, to those whose rights and freedoms—particularly freedom from want—are not safeguarded. As an anthropologist, I can discern the outlines of many of the ideologies used to conceal or even justify assaults on human dignity.

This training also helps to reveal that such assaults are not haphazard. The stage is set for more of the same, even though we are reassured by the powerful that the age of barbarism is behind us. It is disingenuous, surely, to affect surprise each time we learn of the complex and international processes that lead to another Haiti, another Chiapas, another Rwanda.[11] One is reminded of the old joke: What is the definition of a liberal? Someone who believes all the bad things that happen in the world stem from accidents.[12] Human rights violations are not accidents; they are not random in distribution or effect. Rights violations are, rather, symptoms of deeper pathologies of power and are linked intimately to the social conditions that so often determine who will suffer abuse and who will be shielded from harm. If assaults on dignity are anything but random in distribution or course, whose interests are served by the suggestion that they are haphazard?

·   ·   ·   ·   ·

We live in a time in which violence is right before our
very eyes. The word is applied to extremely varied contexts, but each is marked by open violence—by violent
acts, fury, hatred, massacres, cruelty, collective atrocities—but also by the cloaked violences of economic
domination, of capital-labor relations, of the great
North-South divide, to say nothing of all of the "every-

day" violences perpetrated against the weak: women,
children, all those excluded by the social system.

Françoise Héritier, De la violence

The term "human rights abuse" has been used to describe many offenses. There are, of course, the conventionally defined violations outlined in the various treaties and charters to which the guilty parties—nation-states, by and large—are so often signatories. But I will also discuss other forms of violence I have observed.

For well over a decade, I have grappled, as have many others, with conditions that could only be described as violent—at least to those who must endure them. Since the misery in question need not involve bullets, knives, or implements of torture, this misery has often eluded those seeking to identify violence and its victims. Decades ago, and at about the same time, liberation theologians and scholars such as Johan Galtung began writing of "structural violence."[13] In this book, as elsewhere, I use this term as a broad rubric that includes a host of offensives against human dignity: extreme and relative poverty, social inequalities ranging from racism to gender inequality, and the more spectacular forms of violence that are uncontestedly human rights abuses, some of them punishment for efforts to escape structural violence, as the Jesuit Jon Sobrino notes:

> Statistics no longer frighten us. But pictures of the starving children of Biafra, of Haiti, or of India, with thousands sleeping in the streets, ought to. And this entirely apart from the horrors that befall the poor when they struggle to deliver themselves from their poverty: the tortures, the beheadings, the mothers who somehow manage to reach a refuge, but carrying a dead child—a child who could not be nursed in flight and could not be buried after it had died. The catalogue of terrors is endless.[14]

Amartya Sen has referred to such destructive forces as "unfreedoms." Sen helps us to move beyond "liberal" notions of nominal political freedoms—most victims of structural violence have such freedoms on paper—without falling into the trap of economic reductionism: "Development requires the removal of major sources of unfreedom: poverty as well as tyranny, poor economic opportunities as well as systematic social deprivation, neglect of public facilities as well as intolerance or overactivity of repressive states. Despite unprecedented increases in overall opulence, the contemporary world denies elementary freedoms to vast numbers—perhaps even the majority—of people."[15]

Referring to violations of social and economic rights as well as civil and political ones (for it is my claim that the former abuses permit the latter), I ask questions about death by starvation or AIDS in central Haiti; about death from tuberculosis within Russian prisons; about the causes and consequences of coups d'état and low-intensity warfare in Chiapas, Haiti, and Guatemala; and about the practice of medicine in settings of great structural violence. In each of these situations, acts of violence are perpetrated, usually by the strong against the weak, in complex social fields. In each of these situations, a set of historically given and, often enough, economically driven conditions—again, here termed "structural violence"—guarantee that violent acts will ensue. In each of these situations, actions could have been—still can be—taken to protect the vulnerable. But the actions in question include more than legal protection of civil and political rights. For surely we have learned that the right to vote, for example, has not protected the poor from dying premature deaths, caused as often as not by readily treatable pathogens. The "nobodies" discussed by Eduardo Galeano are the victims of structural violence, and a physician working in post-Duvalier Haiti—or post-apartheid South Africa—would necessarily want to know why structural violence takes more and younger lives than ever before.

In short, civil rights cannot really be defended if social and economic rights are not. But in fact there is heated opposition to any enlargement of the rights concept. Some of it comes from the expected quarters. Jeane Kirkpatrick, one of the architects of Ronald Reagan's Central American policies, which helped finance the Guatemalan army's genocidal spree, termed the Universal Declaration of Human Rights "a letter to Santa Claus,"[16] in large part because the Declaration pressed for social and economic rights.[17] But even those who protect, rather than abuse, human rights seem to feel discomfort about social and economic rights. Pressing for social and economic rights, even those outlined in the Universal Declaration, is seen as "asking for too much." Thus even staunch supporters of civil and political rights may regard economic and social rights as better suited to a letter to Santa Claus, since they argue that more can be accomplished by defining our mission in a "pragmatically" narrow manner.[18]

Pragmatism assuredly has its role even in utopian struggles: to attempt too much is often to achieve too little. But the hesitation of many in the human rights community to cross the line from a rights activism of pure principles to one involving transfers of money, food, and medicine betrays a failure, I think, to address the urgent needs of the people we are trying to defend. The proponents of harsh market ideologies have never been afraid to put money—and sometimes bullets—behind *their* minimal and ever-shrinking conception of rights and freedoms. But one alarming feature of structural violence is that bullets are increasingly unnecessary when defenders of social and economic rights are silenced by technocrats who regard themselves as "neutral." In an acid commentary entitled "Professional Life/3," Galeano lays bare the lineaments of this new and effective form of terrorism:

> The big bankers of the world, who practice the terrorism of money, are more powerful than kings and field marshals, even more than the Pope of Rome himself. They never dirty their hands. They kill no one: they limit themselves to applauding the show.
>
> Their officials, international technocrats, rule our countries: they are neither presidents nor ministers, they have not been elected, but they decide the level of salaries and public expenditure, investments and divestments, prices, taxes, interest rates, subsidies, when the sun rises and how frequently it rains.
>
> However, they don't concern themselves with the prisons or torture chambers or concentration camps or extermination centers, although these house the inevitable consequences of their acts.
>
> The technocrats claim the privilege of irresponsibility: "*We're neutral,*" they say.[19]

Galeano links the "terrorism of money" to technocrats who describe themselves as neutral. I suspect this commentary has a certain resonance for anyone who moves easily between a rich university and a poor village, between a world-class teaching hospital and a dirt-floored dispensary, between the gleaming towers of international agency headquarters and the sprawling slums of a Latin American city. Human rights cannot be easily defended in a time of widespread, indeed growing, terrorism of the sort Galeano describes. Although it may seem impolitic to underline the inadequacy of existing measures, it is necessary, at some point, to acknowledge what the poor have been saying all along: that their rights cannot be protected while the "present economic and social structures foist" injustice and exploitation "upon the vast majority of our people under the guise of law."[20] These laws, even those designed to protect human rights, don't feel neutral at all.

While appreciating the need for high-minded charters, conventions, and legislation, it is also important to ask why it is so difficult to demonstrate the efficacy of these measures. This critique is offered in a constructive manner. If laws and charters are inadequate—and they clearly fail to perform under any but the most favorable conditions—what additional measures might be taken? From the point of view of a physician, it seems obvious that tackling poverty and inequality is central to any good-faith effort to protect the rights of the poor. The terrorism of money thus far evades and is abetted by existing legislation. It may well prove to be the biggest threat to recent gains in both health and human rights.

. . . . .

The headlong stream is termed violent
But the river bed hemming it in is
Termed violent by no one.

The storm that bends the birch trees
Is held to be violent
But how about the storm
That bends the backs of the roadworkers?

Bertolt Brecht, "On Violence"

This is also a book about the dynamics of rights violations. The struggle to develop a human rights paradigm is one thing; a searching analysis of the mechanisms and conditions that generate these violations is quite another. Without understanding power and connections, how do we understand why rights are abused, and when and where such events are likely to occur? Often enough, identifying victims and aggressors is the easy part—and leads to no real understanding. It's not that things are "not so black and white," as academics and pundits are wont to say, usually dismissively. They are plenty black and white. But they are also gray, and every shade of gray, so that strange and often veiled alliances form a bridge between aggressors and victims.

Take, for example, the case of Rwanda. In a study titled *Aiding Violence,* Peter Uvin argues that development and humanitarian aid to Rwanda in the years *prior* to the genocide helped to set the stage for what was to occur: "the process of development and the international aid given to promote it interacted with the forces of exclusion, inequality, pauperization, racism, and oppression that laid the groundwork for the 1994 genocide."[21] Of course, the development enterprise, like the human rights community, has defined its mission narrowly. The technocratic approach to development aid has mandated that some issues are brought to the fore while others are ignored. As Uvin, commenting on his own and others' blindness, notes:

Like almost all other players in the development community, I did not have any idea of the destruction that was to come. The pauperization was omnipresent, the racist discourse loud; fear was visible in people's eyes, and a militarization was evident, but that was none of my business, for I was there for another Rwanda, the development model.[22]

How, one wonders incredulously, could anyone working on behalf of the Rwandan poor have failed to anticipate the oncoming cataclysm? But such blinkered analyses are common in most settings in which massive human rights violations are about to occur. As Uvin suggests, these visual-field defects stem in part from the disciplinary division of labor so important in our times. The social fields in which human rights are violated are complex beyond the understanding of any one view or discipline. These contexts are also laden with symbolic complexities, and actions taken within them are often undergirded by baroque ideological justifications—in short, this is the stuff of conventional anthropological interest. But if I have persuaded you that human rights discourse might be examined profitably by an anthropologist, it is important to add that anthropologists have also neglected to examine structural violence and the abuses it inevitably breeds. In a now classic essay, Orin Starn deplores the failure of his fellow Andeanists to consider the terrible suffering all around them, even though a guerrilla war was soon to wrack Peru for a decade:

> Ethnographers usually did little more than mention the terrible infant mortality, minuscule incomes, low life expectancy, inadequate diets, and abysmal health care that remained so routine. To be sure, peasant life was full of joys, expertise, and pleasures. But the figures that led other observers to label Ayacucho a region of "Fourth World" poverty would come as a surprise to someone who knew the area only through the ethnography of Isbell, Skar, or Zuidema. They gave us detailed pictures of ceremonial exchanges, Saint's Day rituals, weddings, baptisms, and work parties. Another kind of scene, just as common in the Andes, almost never appeared: a girl with an abscess and no doctor, the woman bleeding to death in childbirth, a couple in their dark adobe house crying over an infant's sudden death.[23]

As one might expect, Starn's essay provoked fairly heated riposte. Umbrage was taken. In meetings and subsequent articles, anthropologists protested that they had written of such conditions.[24] But almost a decade later, Linda Green, in her compelling study of Mayan widows in the western highlands of Guatemala, still complains of "anthropology's diverted gaze"—diverted, of course, from structural violence:

Systematic inquiry into human rights violations remained elusive. Despite an alarming rise in the most blatant forms of transgressions, repression, and state terrorism, the topic has not captured the anthropological imagination until recently. Overwhelming empirical evidence demonstrates that state-sponsored violence has been standard operating procedure in numerous contemporary societies where anthropologists have conducted fieldwork for the past three decades.[25]

Green's study, unlike many of its predecessors, explores the "macrologics of power" without sacrificing ethnographic depth.[26] To study Mayan widows without exploring the mechanisms that transformed them from wives to widows would be to miss the opportunity to reveal the inner workings of structural violence (and to bury the dead with their eyes wide open). This machinery is transnational as much as it is local. It has a history. And yet I have sat through conferences in which the fate of Mayan orphans is discussed at great length with no mention of what happened to their parents. Indeed, a focus on atomistic cultural specificities is usually the order of the day. This is what anthropologists are expected to do. So it is with "anthropological" commentary on human rights. I use quotation marks because, as often as not, such commentary is made by non-anthropologists who draw on the concept of cultural relativism, a concept that many consider—incorrectly, in my view—anthropology's chief contribution to human rights debates.[27]

Allow me to give another example of how the concept of culture may be abused, and how power and transnational connections may be overlooked in contemporary examinations of human rights abuses. It arises from Haiti, the case I know best. By adopting the conventional Haitian manner of asking a riddle or pointed question—the riddler asks *Krik?*, the audience unleashes the riddle by exclaiming *Krak!*—let us examine some facts from the 1991 coup d'état that resulted in the most massive human rights violations in recent Haitian memory.

Krik? Who said this? "The foreign powers who dominate Haiti have for more than a century refused to acknowledge the integrity of Haitian culture and our right as the world's first independent black nation to steer our own ship of state."

Krak! "General" Raoul Cédras, in a 1991 radio address delivered in French shortly after he overthrew Haiti's first democratically elected president.[28]

What, one might ask, does such a high-minded statement (coming from such a source) reveal about power and transnational connections? First, it offers us a chance to recall that the modern Haitian army led by Cédras had been created by an act of the U.S. Congress during our nineteen-year military occupation of that country earlier in the twentieth century. Second, it reminds us that Cédras was himself the beneficiary of training, including workshops on human rights, at military institutions within the United States.

Third, we can note that his comments, delivered in a language that 90 percent of the Haitian population cannot speak, were crafted with an international audience in mind. This audience is ostensibly concerned with human rights and also with such matters as "cultural integrity" and "racial pride." To the extent that anyone was swayed by such comments—and the record shows that some were—the thousands of Haitians who had been killed outright in the weeks prior to Cédras's address could be impugned as traitors and stooges. As long as Cédras dominated the airwaves, they were silenced beyond the grave. To use the Guatemalan metaphor yet again: they had been buried with their eyes wide open.

To heap irony upon irony, and again playing to an international audience, the authors of the coup d'état chose as their first prime minister a certain Jean-Jacques Honorat—"a leading human rights figure," said the *Boston Globe*.[29] Known in Haiti as a stooge of power, Honorat did not disappoint. He claimed that the Haitian army had done the nation a great service in doing away with the dangerous riffraff who were calling for a more just distribution of Haiti's resources and in dispatching their loony leader, Father Jean-Bertrand Aristide. Honorat—who was indeed a member of the "human rights community," which says a great deal about said community—painted Aristide as the primary violator of human rights in Haiti, an allegation that, though baseless, found ready echoes in the corridors of power and in the U.S. press.[30]

The initial response of the human rights community to the Cédras-led coup was faltering, at best. With powerful friends and lobbyists abroad, the Haitian army could succeed in convincing some that the overthrown president had been Haiti's chief human rights violator. And sectors of the foreign press—notably, U.S. television and print media—echoed, without much further inquiry, the claims of the army. Thus many within the human rights community subsequently sought an impossible balance-point between two adversaries: the demonstrably violent Haitian army and the allegedly violent and unstable deposed president-in-exile. Such studied "neutrality" led some to believe that truth and justice lay somewhere between the victims and the aggressors, rather than on the side of the real victims. The problem was that no data ever existed to suggest that the deposed president had violated human rights, whereas a growing pile of evidence, and of bodies, demonstrated clearly that the military had.

We can make similar observations in considering the case of Chiapas, where the rebellion has pitted the rural poor against the Mexican government. Was this "ethnic revitalization"—most of the Zapatista rebels were indigenous people—or a broader movement for social and economic rights? Many statements from the rebels would seem to indicate the latter. On January 18, 1994, Zapatista leaders responded to the Mexican government's offer of conditional pardon with the following retort: "Who must ask for pardon and who can grant it?"

> Why do we have to be pardoned? What are we going to be pardoned for? Of not dying of hunger? Of not being silent in our misery? Of not humbly accepting our historic role of being the despised and the outcast?... Of having demonstrated to the rest of the country and the entire world that human dignity still lives, even among some of the world's poorest peoples?[31]

Many argue that it is no coincidence that Mexico's first uprising in decades began on the day that NAFTA—the North American Free Trade Agreement—was signed. It was also no surprise that poor health figured strongly among the complaints of the peasants in rebellion. In a declaration at the outset of the revolt, the Zapatistas noted that, "in Chiapas, 14,500 people die a year, the highest death rate in the country. What causes most of these deaths? Curable diseases: respiratory infections, gastroenteritis, parasites, malaria, scabies, breakbone fever, tuberculosis, conjunctivitis, typhus, cholera, and measles."[32] The declaration further noted that all of this misery was expanding right under the noses of tourists and others who visited the region: "While there are seven hotel rooms for every 1,000 tourists, there are 0.3 hospital beds for every 1,000 Chiapans."[33]

But scholarly observers tended to frame the rebellion as an ethnic uprising. Indeed, "anthro lite" seemed to abound among those who cheered for ethnic pride while ignoring, or being confounded by, the rebels' calls for social and economic rights *for the poor,* regardless of ethnicity. One can find lots of treatises about "ancient Maya secrets" and other arcane lore, but few about maternal mortality, high rates of tuberculosis, or the government's ongoing failure to deliver on promised land reform. No more than the aid workers in Rwanda and the Andeanists in South America, the anthropologists in Chiapas were not there to study structural violence. After one of the conflict's bloodiest civilian massacres, in December 1997, the lead editorial of the *Gaceta del Tecolote Maya,* a monthly publication for Mexican anthropologists, asked simply "*¿Antropología para qué?*"[34] Anthropology to what end?

What about the observations of powerful governments? In this arena, we have long known that it is best to examine not what they say—in declarations, for example—but what they do. This book focuses primarily on Latin America, for it is here that we can most easily discern the effects of our own country's stance on human rights. Such an exercise is less common than one might imagine, in large part because close scrutiny of human rights abuses in Latin America brings to light embarrassing connections: "For the U.S.A., the Western hemisphere is the obvious testing ground, particularly the Central America–Caribbean region, where Washington has faced few external challenges for almost a century. It is of some interest that the exercise is rarely undertaken, and when it is, it is castigated as extremist or worse."[35] Why should one be castigated as an extremist for pointing out the obvious connections between U.S. foreign policy—which, unlike the weather, is subject to human control—and human rights abuses? Perhaps because we do not want to know that U.S. aid "has tended to flow disproportionately," as Lars Schoultz notes, "to Latin American governments which torture their citizens."[36]

This rings especially true in Haiti, to which aid flowed freely during almost all years of the Duvalier dictatorships and during much of the violent military rule that followed the collapse of the dictatorship in 1986. Now, however, during the rule of a democratically elected government, the United States has orchestrated an international aid embargo against the Haitian government, freezing an estimated $500 million in promised and greatly need assistance.

The "neoliberal era"—if that is the term we want—has been a time of looking away, a time of averting our gaze from the causes and effects of structural violence. Whatever term we use to describe our times, we cannot avoid looking at power and connections if we hope to understand, and thus prevent, human rights abuses. And when we look at and listen to those whose rights are being trampled, we see how political rights are intertwined with social and economic rights, or, rather, how the absence of social and economic power empties political rights of their substance. In each of the places discussed at any length in this book—whether Chiapas or a U.S. military base in Cuba or a prison in western Siberia—the same sort of erasure is readily documented. Some of this erasure is a result, certainly, of the distortions introduced by a disciplinary focus. No one discipline could ever hope to capture the complexity, social and biological, of the assaults on health and human rights that I hope to document. But much of the erasure has a far more pernicious origin: hiding this suffering, or denying its real origins, serves the interests of the powerful. The degree to which literate experts, from anthropologists to international health specialists, choose to collude with such chicanery should be the focus of brisk and public debate. The persistence of such suffering, rooted in structural violence, concerns all of us, as the poet Wisława Szymborska has observed. "There is nothing more animal-like," she writes, "than a clear conscience."[37]

.   .   .   .   .

We have maintained a silence closely resembling
stupidity.
Revolutionary Proclamation of the
Junta Tuitiva, La Paz, July 16, 1809

In some countries, dissidents are driven into exile; in others, they are driven to television talk shows. In the poor communities discussed here, those who challenge established privilege may be driven to the edge of a pit they themselves have been forced to dig and there dispatched with a bullet at close range. The central thesis of this book is that human rights abuses are best understood (that is, most accurately and comprehensively grasped) from the point of view of the poor. This too is a relatively novel exercise in the human rights community. In no arena is it more needed than in that of health and human rights.

The field of health and human rights has grown quickly, but its boundaries have yet to be traced. More than fifty years after the Universal Declaration of Human Rights, consensus regarding the most promising directions for the future is lacking; moreover, outcome-oriented assessments lead us to question approaches that rely solely on recourse to formal civil and political rights. Similarly unpromising are approaches that rely solely on appeals to governments. Careful study reveals that state power has been responsible for most human rights violations and that violations are usually embedded in contexts rife with structural violence—again, social and economic inequities that determine who will be at risk for assaults and who will be shielded from them.

But the dynamic is changing in much of the world: as international financial institutions and transnational corporations now dwarf the dimensions of most states, the former institutions—and the small number of powerful states that control them—come to hold unfettered sway over the lives of millions. International human rights organizations, accustomed to looking for villains in the upper reaches of bureaucracies of banana republics, also need to turn their gaze back toward the great centers of world power in which they reside.[38] Only through careful analysis of growing *transnational* inequalities will we understand the complex social processes that structure not only growing disparities of risk but also what stands between us and a future in which social and economic rights are guaranteed by states or other polities. This is especially poignant when one considers the concept of the right of the world's poor to modern medical care, because in the "neocolonial" era, the rich countries are even less likely to accept responsibility for better stewardship, as James Galbraith notes:

> It is not increasing trade *as such* that we should fear. Nor is technology the culprit. To focus on "globalization" as such misstates the issue. The problem is a process of integration carried out since at least 1980 under circumstances of unsustainable finance, in which wealth has flowed upwards from the poor countries to the rich, and mainly to the upper financial strata of the richest countries.
>
> In the course of these events, progress toward tolerable levels of inequality and sustainable development virtually stopped. Neocolonial patterns of center-periphery dependence, and of debt peonage, were reestablished, but without the slightest assumption of responsibility by the rich countries for the fate of the poor.[39]

This book attempts to advance an agenda for research and action grounded in the struggle for social and economic rights, an agenda suited to public health and medicine and whose central contributions to future progress in human rights are linked to the equitable distribution of the fruits of scientific advancement. Such an approach is in keeping with the Universal Declaration but runs counter to several of the reigning ideologies of public health, including those favoring efficiency over equity.[40]

Indeed, many of the concepts currently in vogue in public health—from "cost-effectiveness" to "sustainability" and "replicability"—are likely to be perverted unless social justice remains central to public health and medicine. A human rights approach to health economics and health policy helps to bring into relief the ill effects of the efficacy-equity trade-off: that is, only if unnecessary sickness and premature death don't matter can inegalitarian systems ever be considered efficacious.

Pathologies of Power suggests that a broad biosocial approach, when anchored in careful examination of specific cases, permits a critical re-assessment of conventional views on human rights. To make this case, I link detailed case histories of individuals to broader analyses of health and human rights. The book charts the experience of several "communities on the edge"—HIV-positive Haitians detained on a U.S. military base, villagers in Haiti and Chiapas during military crackdowns, Russian prisoners with untreated or ineffectively treated tuberculosis—in order to explore the strengths and limitations of conventional approaches to human rights.

As noted, human rights discussions have to date been excessively legal and theoretical in focus. They seek to define rights, mandate punishment by appropriate authorities for the violators, enforce international treaties, and so on. A focus on health alters human rights discussions in important and underexplored ways: the right to health is perhaps the least contested social right, and a large community of health providers—from physicians to community health workers—affords a still-untapped vein of enthusiasm and commitment. Furthermore, this focus serves to remind us that those who are sick and poor bear the brunt of human rights violations. In making this argument, I draw freely on the critiques that a doctor to the poor is well placed to make.

Pathologies of Power is divided into two parts. The first four chapters rely heavily on my own experience in Latin America and Russia. That is, I have been an eyewitness to the events and processes described. Because all eyewitness accounts are both partial and "dated," I have dated Chapters 2, 3, and 4 and also the postscripts that follow them. The second half of the book also draws on this experience, but it aims to lay out the framework of a critique of "liberal" views on human rights, since such views rarely serve the interests of the poor.

Chapter 1 presents the basic themes of the book, as delineated in this introduction, by arguing that the social determinants of health outcomes are also, often enough, the social determinants of the distribution of assaults on human dignity. "On Suffering and Structural Violence" asks how large-scale social forces become embodied as sickness, suffering, and degradation in rural Haiti, where the same forces that structure risk for human rights abuses are also those shaping epidemics of tuberculosis and

AIDS. Conventional readings of human rights violations fail to draw on current understandings of the social determinants of a wide variety of ills, lending a random appearance to what is, in fact, a highly predictable set of outcomes.[41] Cultural relativism can further muddy these waters when it is linked to moral relativism and shoddy social analysis—as often occurs with the "identity politics" regnant in the United States. Because human rights violations are usually symptoms and signs of deeper pathologies of power, anthropology, sociology, history, political economy, and other "resocializing" disciplines have important roles to play if we are to understand how best to protect human rights. *Pathologies of Power* draws on social theory—and even liberation theology—to reintroduce the concept of structural violence and to link it to the acute violence of war crimes and systemic assaults against human rights.

I argue that equity is the central challenge for the future of medicine and public health. It is easy to document a growing "outcome gap" between rich and poor and show that it is caused in part by differential access to increasingly effective technologies. Drawing on the work of many, I underline the pathogenic role of inequity. That is, it is a striking fact that wealthy societies riven by social inequality have poorer health indices than societies in which comparable levels of wealth are more evenly distributed. At the same time, it is important to sound a warning about the habit of conflating the notion of society with that of nation-state. We already live in a global society. Thus, calls of a right to equity must necessarily contend with steep grades of inequality across as well as within international borders. The same holds for analyses of human rights abuses. Nationally framed analyses of human rights—such as those appearing in, for example, reports from human rights watchdog organizations—may obscure their fundamentally transnational nature.

Part I of the book then explores these themes through specific cases. Chapter 2, "Pestilence and Restraint," details the experience of HIV-positive Haitian refugees fleeing a brutal military coup. Detained by the U.S. government on its base in Guantánamo, Cuba, the voices of these refugees went largely unheard. Meanwhile, elsewhere on the same island, the attention of the international media was drawn to another small group of people living with HIV: Cubans who found themselves in AIDS sanatoriums. Contrasting the experience of the two groups, and the attention each received, brings into sharp focus the forces shaping both the underlying policies and international responses to them.

Chapter 3, "Lessons from Chiapas," reports on the situation in Mexico's poorest state some four years after the Zapatista rebellion. Originally written in the days before the Acteal massacre of December 1997, this account explores what is at stake in the varied interpretations of the *campesinos'* ongoing struggle for dignity. The experience of one community in quest of health suggests that the Zapatistas and their noncombatant supporters may have something to teach the human rights community.

Chapter 4, "A Plague on All Our Houses?" exposes prison epidemics of tuberculosis in Russia, showing that structural violence is again central to determining who is most likely to be imprisoned, who is most likely to become infected and sick once detained, and who is most likely to receive delayed or inappropriate treatment. This largely overlooked epidemic of multidrug-resistant tuberculosis will soon be too large to be hidden. The only way to halt what amounts to tuberculosis-as-punishment is to provide prompt and effective treatment to all prisoners. Even amnesty will be inadequate, if prisoners are released to a dismantled public health system that cannot cure them.

Part II of the book returns to general questions but remains closely tied to specific instances and places. "Health, Healing, and Social Justice" (Chapter 5) explores the differences among three approaches to development work. In comparing charity, development, and social justice approaches, it is important to note that only the latter encourages privileged actors such as physicians and academics to adopt a moral stance that would seek to expose and prevent pathologies of power. Chapter 6, "Listening for Prophetic Voices," reports with alarm the combined effects of the expanding influence of a market ethos and a growing social inequality on the practice of medicine. With an "outcome gap" that widens whenever an effective intervention is not made available to those who need it most, it is clear that greater and faster medical progress can lead paradoxically to worse outcomes. Conventional medical ethics, mired as they are in the "quandary ethics of the individual," do not often speak to these issues, because of the fact that the bulk of their attention is focused on individual cases where massive resources are invested in delivering services unlikely to ever benefit most patients.

Chapter 7, "Cruel and Unusual," offers a more in-depth consideration of the prison-tuberculosis association. In addition to examining the obvious correlation between overcrowding and transmission of an airborne pathogen, this chapter asks how the constraint of agency through imprisonment is related not only to increased risk for sickness and death—which are not supposed to be part of the punishment package—but also to risk of the sort of erasure documented throughout this volume. In New York a decade ago and in Russia at this writing, social inequalities (including racism) and economic policies came together to produce epidemics of drug-resistant tuberculosis. Thus does drug-resistant tuberculosis come to constitute a human rights violation, a fact ignored by many in the human rights community.

These themes are explored more fully in Chapter 8, "New Malaise." Although the quandaries of the sick in industrialized countries are important and should never be dismissed, the failure of ethics to grapple with the tragedy of the modern era's *destitute* sick is nothing short of obscene. Obscene but not surprising. The same blind spots mentioned earlier are those that afflict today's medical ethicists. Surely it is an ethical problem, for example, that in the coming year an estimated six million people will die of tuberculosis, malaria, and AIDS—three treatable diseases that reap their grim harvest almost exclusively among populations without access to modern medical care. These deaths are reflections of structural violence and should be a central concern for the human rights community.

The final chapter, "Rethinking Health and Human Rights," reflects on the implications of the book's central arguments for an emerging field of inquiry and action. The divorce of research and analysis from pragmatic efforts to remediate inequalities of access is a tactical and moral error—it may be an error that constitutes, in and of itself, a human rights abuse. A brief Afterword includes a personal postscript, a reflection on what it was like to bear witness to a decade of violence in Haiti and to hear outsiders—including some in the human rights community—offer erroneous interpretations of what was happening there.

In 1994, following the publication of a book in which I explored the roots of political violence in Haiti, the military government declared me persona non grata. This prevented me from fulfilling my obligation to patients in great need of medical services. It was an unpleasant exercise for other reasons: the book alienated some people whose opinions I value. All in all, it was an experience far less gratifying than direct service to the destitute sick; and I concluded that I would not write another book about human rights and structural violence. But the rest of the decade convinced me that such exercises, though unpopular, are important. When it is a matter of telling the truth and serving the victims, let unwelcome truths be told. Those of us privileged to witness and survive such events and conditions are under an imperative to unveil—and keep unveiling—these pathologies of power.

PART I
BEARING WITNESS

When it is genuine, when it is born of the need to speak, no one can stop the human voice. When denied a mouth, it speaks with the hands or the eyes, or the pores, or anything at all. Because every single one of us has something to say to the others, something that deserves to be celebrated or forgiven by others.

Eduardo Galeano, "Celebration of the Human Voice/2"

IN PRAISE OF SELF-DEPRECATION

The buzzard has nothing to fault himself with.
Scruples are alien to the black panther.
Piranhas do not doubt the rightness of their actions.
The rattlesnake approves of himself without reservations.

The self-critical jackal does not exist.
The locust, alligator, trichina, horsefly
live as they live and are glad of it.

The killer-whale's heart weighs one hundred kilos
but in other respects it is light.

There is nothing more animal-like
than a clear conscience
on the third planet of the Sun.

Wisława Szymborska

Dr. Plarr was a good listener. He had been trained to
listen. Most of his middle-class patients were accustomed to spend at least ten minutes explaining a simple
attack of flu. It was only in the *barrio* of the poor that
he ever encountered suffering in silence, suffering
which had no vocabulary to explain a degree of pain,
its position or its nature. In those huts of mud or tin
where the patient often lay without covering on the dirt
floor he had to make his own interpretation from the
shiver of the skin or a nervous shift of the eyes.

Graham Greene, The Honorary Consul

YOU DON'T HAVE TO BE a doctor to know that the degree of injury, of
suffering, is unrelated to the volume of complaint. I have seen the sullen,
quiet faces in waiting rooms in Peru, say, or in prison sickbays in Russia. I have seen these faces in the emergency rooms of the United States.
I have seen the impassive faces of the silent women trudging across the
public spaces of the towns of Chiapas. But their silence is of course imposed from above. Perhaps if Greene's Dr. Plarr had been an even better
listener, he might have heard the true cacophony of the barrio. For underneath this silence lies the pent-up anger born of innumerable small
indignities, and of great and irremediable ones. Underneath this silence
lie the endless jeremiads of the suffering sick. Structural violence generates bitter recrimination, whether it is heard or not. And given that residents of the barrio and the cities and neighborhoods like it are those
who endure most of the world's misery, they are precisely those most
likely to have a "vocabulary to explain a degree of pain, its position or
its nature."

One could almost say that there are two ways of knowing, and thus
two ways of bearing witness. The first—to report the stoic suffering of
the poor—is in every sense as genuine as another, more freighted form
of knowing. That is, it is true that members of any subjugated group do
not expect to be received warmly even when they are sick or tired or

wounded. They wouldn't expect Dr. Plarr to invite a long disquisition about their pain. They wouldn't expect the sort of courtesy extended so effortlessly to the privileged. The silence of the poor is conditioned. To describe it as stoic, as Greene's character does, is not to be wrong, but rather runs the risk of missing the great eloquence beneath the silence.

Sometimes it is the job of a physician to scratch at this surface silence, to trigger that painful eloquence. It is the self-appointed job, often, of the anthropologist to do so. But sometimes it is more respectful not to scratch at the surface silence; it is respectful to note it, as does Dr. Plarr, and to do one's job quietly. This is a second silence, then, and I have at times maintained it. Even in this book about human rights abuses, relevant events and details have been omitted. It had been my plan to write about them, and I began to do so in earlier drafts; I had all the necessary formal clearance. But in the end I did not always wish to break this second silence. These details, had they been included, would not have changed the basic theses and conclusions of this book.

I am therefore somewhat uneasy about calling the first half of this volume "Bearing Witness." Some of my anxiety has legitimate sources: the boundary between bearing witness and disrespectful (or self-interested) rooting is not always evident, even to those seeking to be discerning. And, to be honest, writing of the plight of the oppressed is not a particularly effective way of assisting them. As Philippe Bourgois notes, paraphrasing a warning issued by Laura Nader years ago: "Don't study the poor and powerless, because everything you say about them will be used against them."[1] I hope to have avoided lurid recountings that serve little other purpose than to show, as anthropologists love to do, that I was there.[2]

I've also hinted at another source of concern: any account is necessarily a partial one, and I have been a partial witness in every sense. It took me a relatively short time in Haiti to discover that I could never serve as a dispassionate reporter or chronicler of misery. I am openly on the side of the destitute sick and have never sought to represent myself as some sort of neutral party. (Indeed, I have argued that such "neutrality" most often serves, wittingly or unwittingly, as smokescreen or apology for the structural violence described here.) Also, I have sometimes found, especially in recent years, that the second silence is not worth breaking. Pragmatic solidarity may strike some as a far more prosaic task than reporting. But the protests of the poor—inaudible, remember, to many—serve as a stern reminder of the priorities of the oppressed.

I am less proud, however, of another source of trepidation: using terms such as "bearing witness" is considered passé in much postmodernist thinking.[3] And I suppose that if one can use a term as easily to describe a testimonial given during a church service or an Alcoholics Anonymous meeting as to describe surviving and later denouncing a massacre, then there is reason enough to worry about its utility. Nonetheless I use "bearing witness" to describe the first half of this book because it consists of chapters that draw heavily on personal experience. These are things I have seen with my own eyes. They are partial accounts, but they are eye-witness accounts.

Initially, I devalued my reports from Chiapas or Cuba or Russia. I thought that the two ways of knowing were related to one's familiarity with the culture and languages of a given time and place, and that therefore my lack of an ethnographer's familiarity with these places made my accounts little more than tourist musings. Respect for cultural immersion as the only way to "insider" knowledge had been a lesson of my graduate studies in anthropology—remember that two years is regarded as the appropriate duration of fieldwork—but I now believe it to be something of a superstition. Although I claim to know only Haiti with an anthropologist's depth, I have found that I can hope for both ways of knowing across boundaries of culture, language, gender, and class. It came as a surprise to me that, on my visits to health projects in Chiapas, I could quite quickly break through the superficial silence that Dr. Plarr encountered in the barrio of the poor. I was also surprised to discover that in a Russian prison, after a fairly rapid and mutual sizing up, I could again hear a resounding silence be broken by an even louder stream of complaint.

The two ways of knowing are not about understanding the details of the history of any given place, as important as these may be to getting the story right. The two ways of knowing, I have come to believe, are not about linguistic competence. To get beyond the first silence requires compassion and solidarity—other sentiments discredited in many academic circles, where they are often in short supply. They are in short supply in general, and this is why you can go to any one of these so-called barrios and meet people who have lived or worked or conducted research in them for decades without ever breaking through the superficial silence. Furthermore, much of what is written by experts about AIDS in Cuba, tuberculosis in Russia, or the origins of violence in Haiti and Chiapas has the added disadvantage of being untrue.

"Bearing witness," like "solidarity" and "compassion," is a term worth rehabilitating. It captures both ways of knowing, both forms of silence. Bearing witness is done on behalf of others, for their sake (even if those others are dead and forgotten). It needs to be done, but there is no point exaggerating the importance of the deed. I would like to insist that the term as used here acknowledges that, no matter how great the pain of bearing witness, it will never be as great as the pain of those who endure, whether in silence or with cries, the indignities described in these pages.

It is my hope, of course, that *Pathologies of Power* is regarded as a contribution to a critical anthropology of structural violence. Nancy Scheper-Hughes has described the anthropology of suffering as "a new kind of theodicy, a cultural inquiry into the ways that people attempt to explain the presence of pain, affliction, and evil in the world."[4] I tried to contribute to this analytic project when, as a graduate student, I explored local interpretations of the rank suffering that was the lot of the people with whom I lived (and with whom I live to this day). In central Haiti, accusations of sorcery were central to the way in which much suffering was explained. It was in Haiti, too, that I learned about a different kind of sorcery, much more malignant in its impact—surely, structural violence damages and destroys more lives in a day than does a century's worth of sorcery—than the accusations I chronicled in my first book. And structural violence takes its toll in ways that seem to defy explanation. How else would we explain the intense focus on the actions and ideologies of its victims rather than those of its unseen perpetrators? Because this book is my own attempt to "explain the presence of pain, affliction, and evil," it remains an exercise in theodicy. Since all inquiries are cultural, I do not presume that this one is not.

CHAPTER 1

ON SUFFERING
AND STRUCTURAL
VIOLENCE

SOCIAL AND ECONOMIC RIGHTS
IN THE GLOBAL ERA

Growth of GNP or of industrial incomes can, of course, be
very important as *means* to expanding the freedoms enjoyed
by the members of the society. But freedoms depend also on
other determinants, such as social and economic arrangements (for example, facilities for education and health care)
as well as political and civil rights (for example, the liberty to
participate in public discussion and scrutiny).

Amartya Sen, *Development as Freedom*

Where do people earn the Per Capita Income? More than one
poor starving soul would like to know.

In our countries, numbers live better than people. How
many people prosper in times of prosperity? How many
people find their lives developed by development?

Eduardo Galeano, "Those Little Numbers and People"

Everyone knows that suffering, violence, and misery exist. How to define
them? Given that each person's pain has for him or her a degree of reality that the pain of others can surely never approach, is widespread agreement on the subject possible? And yet people do agree, as often as not,
on what constitutes extreme suffering: premature and painful illnesses,
say, as well as torture and rape. More insidious assaults on dignity, such
as institutionalized racism and gender inequality, are also acknowledged
by most to cause great and unjust injury.

So suffering is a fact. Now a number of corollary questions come to
the fore. Whenever we talk about medicine or policy, a "hierarchy of suf-

fering" begins to take shape, for it is impossible to relieve every case at once. Can we identify the worst assaults? Those most at risk of great suffering? Among persons whose suffering is not fatal, is it possible to identify those most at risk of sustaining permanent and disabling damage? Are certain "event" assaults, such as torture or rape, more likely to lead to later sequelae than is sustained and insidious suffering, such as the pain born of deep poverty or racism? Are certain forms of insidious discrimination demonstrably more noxious than others?

Anthropologists and others who take these as research questions study both individual experience and the larger social matrix in which it is embedded in order to see how various social processes and events come to be translated into personal distress and disease. By what mechanisms, precisely, do social forces ranging from poverty to racism become *embodied* as individual experience?[1] This has been the focus of most of my own research in Haiti, where political and economic forces have structured risk for AIDS, tuberculosis, and, indeed, most other infectious and parasitic diseases. Social forces at work there have also structured risk for most forms of extreme suffering, from hunger to torture and rape.

Working in contemporary Haiti, where in recent decades political violence has been added to the worst poverty in the hemisphere, one learns a great deal about suffering. In fact, the country has long constituted a sort of living laboratory for the study of affliction, no matter how it is defined.[2] "Life for the Haitian peasant of today," observed the anthropologist Jean Weise some thirty years ago, "is abject misery and a rank familiarity with death."[3] The biggest problem, of course, is unimaginable poverty, as a long succession of dictatorial governments has been more engaged in pillaging than in protecting the rights of workers, even on paper. As Eduardo Galeano noted in 1973, at the height of the Duvalier dictatorship, "The wages Haiti requires by law belong in the department of science fiction: actual wages on coffee plantations vary from $.07 to $.15 a day."[4]

In some senses, the situation has worsened since. When in 1991 international health and population experts devised a "human suffering index" by examining several measures of human welfare ranging from life expectancy to political freedom, 27 of 141 countries were characterized by "extreme human suffering."[5] Only one of them, Haiti, was located in the Western hemisphere. In only three countries on earth was suffering judged to be more extreme than that endured in Haiti; each of these three countries was in the midst of an internationally recognized civil war.

Suffering is certainly a recurrent and expected condition in Haiti's Central Plateau, where everyday life has felt, often enough, like war. "You get up in the morning," observed one young widow with four children, "and it's the fight for food and wood and water." If initially struck by the austere beauty of the region's steep mountains and clement weather, long-term visitors come to see the Central Plateau in much the same manner as its inhabitants do: a chalky and arid land hostile to the best efforts of the peasant farmers who live here. Landlessness is widespread and so, consequently, is hunger. All the standard measures reveal how tenuous is the peasantry's hold on survival. Life expectancy at birth is less than fifty years, in large part because as many as two of every ten infants die before their first birthday.[6] Tuberculosis and AIDS are the leading causes of death among adults; among children, diarrheal disease, measles, and tetanus ravage the undernourished.[7]

But the experience of suffering, it's often noted, is not effectively conveyed by statistics or graphs. In fact, the suffering of the world's poor intrudes only rarely into the consciousness of the affluent, even when our affluence may be shown to have direct relation to their suffering. This is true even when spectacular human rights violations are at issue, and it is even more true when the topic at hand is the everyday violation of social and economic rights.[8] Because the "texture" of dire affliction is better felt in the gritty details of biography, I introduce the stories of Acéphie Joseph and Chouchou Louis.[9] Since any example begs the question of its relevance, I will argue at the outset that the stories of Acéphie and Chouchou are anything but "anecdotal." In the eyes of the epidemiologist as well as the political analyst, they suffered and died in exemplary fashion. Millions of people living in similar circumstances can expect to meet similar fates. What these victims, past and present, share are not personal or psychological attributes. They do not share culture or language or a certain race. What they share, rather, is the experience of occupying the bottom rung of the social ladder in inegalitarian societies.

ACÉPHIE'S STORY

For the wound of the daughter of my people is my
        heart wounded,
I mourn, and dismay has taken hold of me.
Is there no balm in Gilead? Is there no physician there?
Why then has the health of the daughter of my people
        not been restored?

O that my head were waters, and my eyes a fountain of
      tears, that
I might weep day and night for the slain of the daughter
of my people!

Jeremiah 8:22–9:1

Kay, a community of fewer than three thousand people, stretches along
an unpaved road that cuts north and east into Haiti's Central Plateau.
Striking out from Port-au-Prince, the capital, it can take several hours
to reach Kay, especially if one travels during the rainy season, when the
chief thoroughfare through central Haiti turns into a muddy, snaking
path. But even in the dry season, the journey gives one an impression of
isolation, insularity. The impression is misleading, as the village owes its
existence to a project conceived in the Haitian capital and drafted in
Washington, D.C.: Kay is a settlement of refugees, substantially composed of peasant farmers displaced more than forty years ago by the construction of Haiti's largest dam.[10]

Before 1956, the village of Kay was situated in a fertile valley, and
through it ran the Rivière Artibonite, Haiti's largest river. For genera-
tions, thousands of families had farmed the broad and gently sloping
banks of the river, selling rice, bananas, millet, corn, and sugarcane in
regional markets. Harvests were, by all reports, bountiful; life there is
now recalled as idyllic. When the valley was flooded, the majority of the
local population was forced up into the stony hills on either side of the
new reservoir. By all the standard measures, the "water refugees" became exceedingly poor; the older people often blame their poverty on
the massive buttress dam a few miles away, bitterly noting that it brought
them neither electricity nor water.

In 1983, when I began working in the Central Plateau, AIDS was already afflicting an ever-increasing number of city dwellers but was unknown in areas as rural as Kay. Acéphie Joseph was one of the first villagers to die of the new syndrome. But her illness, which ended in 1991,
was merely the latest in a string of tragedies that she and her parents
readily linked together in a long lamentation, by now familiar to those
who tend the region's sick.

The litany begins, usually, down in the valley, now hidden under the
still surface of the lake. Both Acéphie's parents came from families who
had made a decent living by farming fertile tracts of land—their "ancestors' gardens"—and selling much of their produce. Her father tilled

the soil, and his wife, a tall and wearily elegant woman not nearly as old as she looks, was a "Madame Sarah," a market woman. "If it weren't for the dam," he once assured me, "we'd be just fine now. Acéphie, too." The Josephs' home was drowned, along with most of their belongings, their crops, and the graves of their ancestors.

Refugees from the rising water, the Josephs built a miserable lean-to on a knoll of high land jutting into the new reservoir. They remained poised on their knoll for some years; Acéphie and her twin brother were born there. I asked what had induced them to move higher up the hill, to build a house on the hard stone embankment of a dusty road. "Our hut was too near the water," replied their father. "I was afraid one of the children would fall into the lake and drown. Their mother had to be away selling; I was trying to make a garden in this terrible soil. There was no one to keep an eye on them."

Acéphie attended primary school in a banana-thatched and open shelter in which children and young adults received the rudiments of literacy in Kay. "She was the nicest of the Joseph sisters," recalled one of her classmates. "And she was as pretty as she was nice." Acéphie's beauty—she was tall and fine-featured, with enormous dark eyes—and her vulnerability may have sealed her fate as early as 1984. Though still in primary school then, she was already nineteen years old; it was time for her to help generate income for her family, which was sinking deeper and deeper into poverty. Acéphie began to help her mother by carrying produce to a local market on Friday mornings. On foot or with a donkey, it takes over an hour and a half to reach the market, and the road leads right through Péligre, site of the dam and a military barracks. The soldiers liked to watch the parade of women on Friday mornings. Sometimes they taxed them, literally, with haphazardly imposed fines; sometimes they levied a toll of flirtatious banter.

Such flirtation is seldom rejected, at least openly. In rural Haiti, entrenched poverty made the soldiers—the region's only salaried men—ever so much more attractive. Hunger was a near-daily occurrence for the Joseph family; the times were as bad as those right after the flooding of the valley. And so when Acéphie's good looks caught the eye of Captain Jacques Honorat, a native of Belladère formerly stationed in Port-au-Prince, she returned his gaze.

Acéphie knew, as did everyone in the area, that Honorat had a wife and children. He was known, in fact, to have more than one regular partner. But Acéphie was taken in by his persistence, and when he went to speak to her parents, a long-term liaison was, from the outset, a serious possibility:

> What would you have me do? I could tell that the old people were uncom-
> fortable, worried; but they didn't say no. They didn't tell me to stay away
> from him. I wish they had, but how could they have known?...I knew it
> was a bad idea then, but I just didn't know why. I never dreamed he would
> give me a bad illness, never! I looked around and saw how poor we all
> were, how the old people were finished....What would you have me do? It
> was a way out, that's how I saw it.

Acéphie and Honorat were sexual partners only briefly—for less than a month, according to Acéphie. Shortly thereafter, Honorat fell ill with unexplained fevers and kept to the company of his wife in Péligre. As Acéphie was looking for a *moun prensipal*—a "main man"—she tried to forget about the soldier. Still, it was shocking to hear, a few months after they parted, that he was dead.

Acéphie was at a crucial juncture in her life. Returning to school was out of the question. After some casting about, she went to Mirebalais, the nearest town, and began a course in what she euphemistically termed a "cooking school." The school—really just an ambitious woman's courtyard—prepared poor girls like Acéphie for their inevitable turn as servants in the city. Indeed, becoming a maid was fast developing into one of the rare growth industries in Haiti, and, as much as Acéphie's proud mother hated to think of her daughter reduced to servitude, she could offer no viable alternative.

And so Acéphie, twenty-two years old, went off to Port-au-Prince, where she found a job as a housekeeper for a middle-class Haitian woman who worked for the U.S. embassy. Acéphie's looks and manners kept her out of the backyard, the traditional milieu of Haitian servants. She was designated as the maid who, in addition to cleaning, answered the door and the phone. Although Acéphie was not paid well—she received thirty dollars each month—she recalled the gnawing hunger in her home village and managed to save a bit of money for her parents and siblings.

Still looking for a *moun prensipal*, Acéphie began seeing Blanco Nerette, a young man with origins similar to her own: Blanco's parents were also "water refugees," and Acéphie had known him when they were both attending the parochial school in Kay. Blanco had done well for himself, by Kay standards: he chauffeured a small bus between the Central Plateau and the capital. In a setting in which the unemployment rate was greater than 60 percent, he could command considerable respect, and he turned his attentions to Acéphie. They planned to marry, she later recalled, and started pooling their resources.

Acéphie remained at the "embassy woman's" house for more than three years, staying until she discovered that she was pregnant. As soon as she told Blanco, she could see him becoming skittish. Nor was her employer pleased: it is considered unsightly to have a pregnant servant. And so Acéphie returned to Kay, where she had a difficult pregnancy. Blanco came to see her once or twice. They had a disagreement, and then she heard nothing more from him. Following the birth of her daughter, Acéphie was sapped by repeated infections. A regular visitor to our clinic, she was soon diagnosed with AIDS.

Within months of her daughter's birth, Acéphie's life was consumed with managing her own drenching night sweats and debilitating diarrhea while attempting to care for the child. "We both need diapers now," she remarked bitterly, toward the end of her life. As political violence hampered her doctors' ability to open the clinic, Acéphie was faced each day not only with diarrhea but also with a persistent lassitude. As she became more and more gaunt, some villagers suggested that Acéphie was the victim of sorcery. Others recalled her liaison with the soldier and her work as a servant in the city, by then widely considered to be risk factors for AIDS. Acéphie herself knew that she had AIDS, although she was more apt to refer to herself as suffering from a disorder brought on by her work as a servant: "All that ironing, and then opening a refrigerator." She died far from refrigerators or other amenities as her family and caregivers stood by helplessly.

But this is not simply the story of Acéphie and her daughter, also infected with the virus. There is also Jacques Honorat's first wife, who each year grows thinner. After Honorat's death, she found herself desperate, with no means of feeding her five hungry children, two of whom were also ill. Her subsequent union was again with a soldier. Honorat had at least two other partners, both of them poor peasant women, in the Central Plateau. One is HIV-positive and has two sickly children. And there is Blanco, still a handsome young man, apparently in good health, plying the roads from Mirebalais to Port-au-Prince. Who knows if he carries the virus? As a chauffeur, he has plenty of girlfriends.

Nor is this simply the story of those infected with HIV. The pain of Acéphie's mother and twin brother was manifestly intense. But few understood her father's anguish. Shortly after Acéphie's death, he hanged himself with a length of rope.

CHOUCHOU'S STORY

I never found the order
I searched for
but always a sinister
and well-planned disorder
that increases in the hands
of those who hold power
while the others
who clamor for
a more kindly world
a world with less hunger
and more hopefulness
die of torture
in the prisons.
Don't come any closer
there's a stench of carrion
surrounding me.

Claribel Alegría,
"From the Bridge"

Chouchou Louis grew up not far from Kay, in another small village in the steep and infertile highlands of Haiti's Central Plateau. He attended primary school for a couple of years but was forced to drop out when his mother died. Then, in his early teens, Chouchou joined his father and an older sister in tending their hillside garden. In short, there was nothing remarkable about Chouchou's childhood. It was brief and harsh, like most in rural Haiti.

Throughout the 1980s, church activities formed Chouchou's sole distraction. These were hard years for the Haitian poor, beaten down by a family dictatorship well into its third decade. The Duvaliers, father and son, ruled through violence, largely directed at people whose conditions of existence were similar to those of Chouchou Louis. Although many tried to flee, often by boat, U.S. policy maintained that Haitian asylum-seekers were "economic refugees." As part of a 1981 agreement between the administrations of Ronald Reagan and Jean-Claude Duvalier (known as "Baby Doc"), refugees seized by the U.S. Coast Guard on the high seas were summarily returned to Haiti. During the first ten years of the accord, approximately twenty-three thousand Haitians applied for political asylum in the United States. Eight applications were approved.[11]

A growing Haitian pro-democracy movement led to the flight of Duvalier in February 1986. Chouchou Louis, who must have been about twenty years old when "Baby Doc" fell, shortly thereafter acquired a small radio. "All he did," recalled his wife, years later, "was work the land, listen to the radio, and go to church." On the radio, Chouchou heard about the people who took over after Duvalier fled. Like many in rural Haiti, Chouchou was distressed to hear that power had been handed to the military, led by hardened *duvaliéristes*. It was this army that the U.S. government termed "Haiti's best bet for democracy." (Hardly a disinterested judgment: the United States had created the modern Haitian army in 1916.) In the eighteen months following Duvalier's departure, more than $200 million in U.S. aid passed through the hands of the junta.[12]

In early 1989, Chouchou moved in with Chantal Brisé, who was pregnant. They were living together when Father Jean-Bertrand Aristide— by then considered the leader of the pro-democracy movement—declared his candidacy for the presidency in the internationally monitored elections of 1990. In December of that year, almost 70 percent of the voters chose Father Aristide from a field of almost a dozen presidential candidates. No run-off election was required—Aristide won this plurality in the first round.

Like most rural Haitians, Chouchou and Chantal welcomed Aristide's election with great joy. For the first time, the poor—Haiti's overwhelming majority, formerly silent—felt they had someone representing their interests in the presidential palace. This is why the subsequent military coup d'état of September 1991 stirred great anger in the countryside, where most Haitians live. Anger was soon followed by sadness, then fear, as the country's repressive machinery, which had been held at bay during the seven months of Aristide's tenure, was speedily reactivated under the patronage of the army.

One day during the month after the coup, Chouchou was sitting in a truck en route to the town of Hinche. Chouchou offered for the consideration of his fellow passengers what Haitians call a *pwen*, a pointed remark intended to say something other than what it literally means. As they bounced along, he began complaining about the condition of the roads, observing that, "if things were as they should be, these roads would have been repaired already." One eyewitness later told me that at no point in the commentary was Aristide's name invoked. But his fellow passengers recognized Chouchou's observations as veiled language deploring the coup. Unfortunately for Chouchou, one of the passengers was an out-of-uniform soldier. At the next checkpoint, the soldier had him seized and dragged from the truck. There, a group of soldiers and their lackeys—their *attachés,* to use the epithet then in favor—immediately began beating Chouchou, in front of the other passengers; they continued to beat him as they brought him to the military barracks in Hinche. A scar on his right temple was a souvenir of his stay in Hinche, which lasted several days.

Perhaps the worst after-effect of such episodes of brutality was that, in general, they marked the beginning of persecution, not the end. In rural Haiti, any scrape with the law (that is, the military) led to a certain blacklisting. For men like Chouchou, staying out of jail involved keeping the local *attachés* happy, and he did this by avoiding his home village. But Chouchou lived in fear of a second arrest, his wife later told me, and his fears proved to be well-founded.

On January 22, 1992, Chouchou was visiting his sister when he was arrested by two *attachés.* No reason was given for the arrest, and Chouchou's sister regarded as ominous the seizure of the young man's watch and radio. He was roughly marched to the nearest military checkpoint, where he was tortured by soldiers and the *attachés.* One area resident later told us that the prisoner's screams made her children weep with terror.

On January 25, Chouchou was dumped in a ditch to die. The army scarcely took the trouble to circulate the *canard* that he had stolen some bananas. (The Haitian press, by then thoroughly muzzled, did not even broadcast this false version of events; fatal beatings in the countryside did not count as news.) Relatives carried Chouchou back to Chantal and their daughter under the cover of night. By early on the morning of January 26, when I arrived, Chouchou was scarcely recognizable. His face, and especially his left temple, was deformed, swollen, and lacerated; his right temple was also scarred. His mouth was a coagulated pool of dark blood. Lower down, his neck was peculiarly swollen, his throat collared with bruises left by a gun butt. His chest and sides were badly bruised, and he had several fractured ribs. His genitals had been mutilated.

That was his front side; presumably, the brunt of the beatings had come from behind. Chouchou's back and thighs were striped with deep lash marks. His buttocks were macerated, the skin flayed down to the exposed gluteal muscles. Already some of these stigmata appeared to be infected.

Chouchou coughed up more than a liter of blood in his agonal moments. Although I am not a forensic pathologist, my guess is that the proximate cause of his death was pulmonary hemorrhage. Given his respiratory difficulties and the amount of blood he coughed up, it is likely that the beatings caused him to bleed, slowly at first, then catastrophically, into his lungs. His head injuries had not robbed him of his faculties, although it might have been better for him had they done so. It took Chouchou three days to die.

EXPLAINING VERSUS MAKING SENSE OF SUFFERING

When we come to you
Our rags are torn off us
And you listen all over our naked body.
As to the cause of our illness
One glance at our rags would
Tell you more. It is the same cause that wears out
Our bodies and our clothes.

The pain in our shoulder comes
You say, from the damp; and this is also the reason
For the stain on the wall of our flat.
So tell us:
Where does the damp come from?
> Bertolt Brecht, "A Worker's Speech to a Doctor"

Are these stories of suffering emblematic of something other than two tragic and premature deaths? If so, how representative is either of these experiences? Little about Acéphie's story is unique; I have told it in some detail because it brings into relief many of the forces restricting not only her options but those of most Haitian women. Such, in any case, is my opinion after caring for hundreds of poor women with AIDS. Their stories move with a deadly monotony: young women—or teenage girls— fled to Port-au-Prince in an attempt to escape from the harshest poverty; once in the city, each worked as a domestic; none managed to find the financial security that had proven so elusive in the countryside. The women I interviewed were straightforward about the nonvoluntary aspect of their sexual activity: in their opinions, poverty had forced them into unfavorable unions.[13] Under such conditions, one wonders what to make of the notion of "consensual sex."

What about the murder of Chouchou Louis? International human rights groups estimate that more than three thousand Haitians were killed in the year after the September 1991 coup that overthrew Haiti's first democratically elected government. Almost all were civilians who, like Chouchou, fell into the hands of the military or paramilitary forces. The vast majority of victims were poor peasants, like Chouchou, or urban slum dwellers. But note that the figures just cited are conservative estimates; I can testify that no journalist or human rights observer ever came to count the body of Chouchou Louis.[14]

Thus the agony of Acéphie and Chouchou was, in a sense, "modal" suffering. In Haiti, AIDS and political violence are two leading causes of death among young adults. These afflictions are not the result of accident or a *force majeure;* they are the consequence, direct or indirect, of human agency. When the Artibonite Valley was flooded, depriving families like the Josephs of their land, a human decision was behind it; when the Haitian army was endowed with money and unfettered power, human decisions were behind that, too. In fact, some of the same decision makers may have been involved in both cases.

If bureaucrats and soldiers seemed to have unconstrained sway over the lives of the rural poor, the agency of Acéphie and Chouchou was, correspondingly, curbed at every turn. These grim biographies suggest that the social and economic forces that have helped to shape the AIDS epidemic are, in every sense, the same forces that led to Chouchou's death and to the larger repression in which it was eclipsed. What's more, both of these individuals were "at risk" of such a fate long before they met the soldiers who altered their destinies. They were both, from the outset, victims of structural violence. The term is apt because such suffering is "structured" by historically given (and often economically driven) processes and forces that conspire—whether through routine, ritual, or, as is more commonly the case, the hard surfaces of life—to constrain agency.[15] For many, including most of my patients and informants, choices both large and small are limited by racism, sexism, political violence, *and* grinding poverty.

While certain kinds of suffering are readily observable—and the subject of countless films, novels, and poems—structural violence all too often defeats those who would describe it. There are at least three reasons. First, the "exoticization" of suffering as lurid as that endured by Acéphie and Chouchou distances it. The suffering of individuals whose lives and struggles recall our own tends to move us; the suffering of those who are "remote," whether because of geography or culture, is often less affecting.

Second, the sheer weight of the suffering makes it all the more difficult to render: "Knowledge of suffering cannot be conveyed in pure facts and figures, reportings that objectify the suffering of countless persons. The horror of suffering is not only its immensity but the faces of the anonymous victims who have little voice, let alone rights, in history."[16]

Third, the dynamics and distribution of suffering are still poorly understood. Physicians, when fortunate, can alleviate the suffering of the sick. But explaining its distribution requires many minds and resources. Case studies of individuals reveal suffering, they tell us what happens to one or many people; but to explain suffering, one must embed individual biography in the larger matrix of culture, history, and political economy.

In short, it is one thing to make sense of extreme suffering—a universal activity, surely—and quite another to explain it. Life experiences such as those of Acéphie and Chouchou, and of other Haitians living in poverty who shared similar social conditions, must be embedded in ethnography if their representativeness is to be understood. These local understandings must be embedded, in turn, in the historical system of which Haiti is a part.[17] The weakness of such analyses is, of course, their great distance from personal experience. But the social and economic forces that dictate life choices in Haiti's Central Plateau affect many millions of individuals, and it is in the context of these global forces that the suffering of individuals acquires its own appropriate context.

Similar insights are central to liberation theology, which preoccupies itself with the suffering of the poor. In *The Praxis of Suffering*, Rebecca Chopp notes, "In a variety of forms, liberation theology speaks with those who, through their suffering, call into question the meaning and truth of human history."[18] Unlike most previous theologies, unlike much modern philosophy, liberation theology attempts to use social analysis both to explain and to deplore human suffering. Its key texts draw our attention not merely to the suffering of the wretched of the earth but also to the forces that promote that suffering. The theologian Leonardo Boff, commenting on one of these texts, observes that it "moves immediately to the structural analysis of these forces and denounces the systems, structures, and mechanisms that 'create a situation where the rich get richer at the expense of the poor, who get even poorer.'"[19]

Put simply, few liberation theologians reflect on suffering without attempting to understand the mechanisms that produce it. Theirs is a theology that underlines connections. Robert McAfee Brown has these connections, and also the poor, in mind when, paraphrasing the Uruguayan Jesuit Juan Luis Segundo, he observes that "the world that is satisfying to us is the same world that is utterly devastating to them."[20]

MAKING SENSE OF STRUCTURAL VIOLENCE

Events of massive, public suffering defy quantitative
analysis. How can one really understand statistics
citing the death of six million Jews or graphs of third-
world starvation? Do numbers really reveal the agony,
the interruption, the questions that these victims put to
the meaning and nature of our individual lives and life
as a whole?

Rebecca Chopp, *The Praxis of Suffering*

My apologies to chance for calling it necessity.
My apologies to necessity if I'm mistaken, after all.
Please, don't be angry, happiness, that I take you as
     my due.
May my dead be patient with the way my memories
     fade.
My apologies to time for all the world I overlook
     each second.

Wisława Szymborska, "Under One Small Star"

How might we discern the nature of structural violence and explore its
contribution to human suffering? Can we devise an analytic model, one
with explanatory and predictive power, for understanding suffering in a
global context? This task, though daunting, is both urgent and feasible
if we are to protect and promote human rights.

Our cursory examination of AIDS and political violence in Haiti suggests that analysis must, first, be *geographically broad*. The world as we
know it is becoming increasingly interconnected. A corollary of this fact
is that extreme suffering—especially when on a grand scale, as in genocide—is seldom divorced from the actions of the powerful.[21] The analysis must also be *historically deep*: not merely deep enough to remind us
of events and decisions such as those that deprived Acéphie's parents of
their land and founded the Haitian military, but deep enough to recall
that modern-day Haitians are the descendants of a people kidnapped from
Africa in order to provide our forebears with sugar, coffee, and cotton.[22]

Social factors including gender, ethnicity ("race"), and socioeconomic
status may each play a role in rendering individuals and groups vulnerable to extreme human suffering. But in most settings these factors by
themselves have limited explanatory power. Rather, *simultaneous* con-

sideration of various social "axes" is imperative in efforts to discern a
political economy of brutality. Furthermore, such social factors are differentially weighted in different settings and in different times, as even
brief consideration of their contributions to extreme suffering suggests.
In an essay entitled "Mortality as an Indicator of Economic Success and
Failure," Amartya Sen reminds us of the need to move beyond "the cold
and often inarticulate statistics of low incomes" to look at the various
ways in which agency—what he terms the "capabilities of each person"—is constrained:

> There is, of course, plenty of [poverty] in the world in which we live. But
> more awful is the fact that so many people—including children from disad-
> vantaged backgrounds—are forced to lead miserable and precarious lives
> and to die prematurely. That predicament relates in general to low incomes,
> but not just to that. It also reflects inadequate public health provisions and
> nutritional support, deficiency of social security arrangements, and the
> absence of social responsibility and of caring governance.[23]

To understand the relationship between structural violence and human
rights, it is necessary to avoid reductionistic analyses. Sen is understand-
ably concerned to avoid economic reductionism, an occupational hazard
in his field. But numerous other analytic traps can also hinder the quest
for a sound analytic purchase on the dynamics of human suffering.

The Axis of Gender

Acéphie Joseph and Chouchou Louis shared a similar social status, and
each died after contact with the Haitian military. Gender helps to explain why Acéphie died of AIDS and Chouchou from torture. Gender
inequality helps to explain why the suffering of Acéphie is much more
commonplace than that of Chouchou. Throughout the world, women
are confronted with sexism, an ideology that situates them as inferior to
men. In 1974, when a group of feminist anthropologists surveyed the
status of women living in disparate settings, they could agree that, in
every society studied, men dominated political, legal, and economic institutions to varying degrees; in no culture was the status of women gen-
uinely equal, much less superior, to that of men.[24] This power differential has meant that women's rights are violated in innumerable ways.
Although male victims are clearly preponderant in studies of torture, females almost exclusively endure the much more common crimes of domestic violence and rape. In the United States alone, the number of such

aggressions is staggering. Taking into account sexual assaults by both intimates and strangers, "one in four women has been the victim of a completed rape and one in four women has been physically battered, according to the results of recent community-based studies."[25] In many societies, crimes of domestic violence and rape are not even discussed and are thus invisible.

In most settings, however, gender alone does not define risk for such assaults on dignity. It is *poor* women who are least well defended against these assaults.[26] This is true not only of domestic violence and rape but also of AIDS and its distribution, as anthropologist Martha Ward points out: "The collection of statistics by ethnicity rather than by socioeconomic status obscures the fact that the majority of women with AIDS in the United States are poor. Women are at risk for HIV not because they are African-American or speak Spanish; women are at risk because poverty is the primary and determining condition of their lives."[27]

Similarly, only women can experience maternal mortality, a cause of anguish around the world. More than half a million women die each year in childbirth, but not all women face a high risk of this fate. In fact, according to analyses of 1995 statistics, 99.8 percent of these deaths occurred in developing countries.[28] Recent reported maternal mortality rates for Haiti vary, depending on the source, with numbers ranging from 523 deaths per 100,000 live births to the much higher rates of 1,100 and even as high as 1,400 deaths per 100,000 live births. Needless to say, these deaths are almost entirely registered among the poor.[29] Gender bias, as Sen notes, "is a general problem that applies even in Europe and North America in a variety of fields (such as division of family chores, the provision of support for higher training, and so on), but in poorer countries, the disadvantage of women may even apply to the basic fields of health care, nutritional support, and elementary education."[30]

The Axis of "Race" or Ethnicity

The idea of "race," which most anthropologists and demographers consider to be a biologically insignificant term, has enormous social currency. Racial classifications have been used to deprive many groups of basic rights and therefore have an important place in considerations of human inequality and suffering. The history of Rwanda and Burundi shows that once-minor ethnic categories—Hutu and Tutsi share language and culture and kinship systems—were lent weight and social meaning

by colonial administrators who divided and conquered, deepening social inequalities and then fueling nascent ethnic rivalry. In South Africa,
one of the clearest examples of the long-term effects of racism, epidemiologists report that the infant mortality rate among blacks may be as
much as ten times higher than that of whites. For black people in South
Africa, the proximate cause of increased rates of morbidity and mortality is lack of access to resources: "*Poverty* remains the primary cause of
the prevalence of many diseases and widespread hunger and malnutrition among black South Africans."[31] The dismantling of the apartheid
regime has not yet brought the dismantling of the structures of oppression and inequality in South Africa, and persistent social inequality is no
doubt the primary reason that HIV has spread so rapidly in sub-Saharan
Africa's wealthiest nation.[32]

Significant mortality differentials between blacks and whites are also
registered in the United States, which shares with South Africa the distinction of being one of the two industrialized countries failing to record
mortality data by socioeconomic status. In 1988 in the United States,
life expectancy at birth was 75.5 years for whites, 69.5 years for blacks.
In the following decade, although U.S. life expectancies increased across
the board, the gap between whites and blacks widened by another 0.6
years.[33] While these racial differentials in mortality have provoked a
certain amount of discussion, public health expert Vicente Navarro recently pointed to the "deafening silence" on the topic of class differentials in mortality in the United States, where "race is used as a *substi-
tute* for class." But in 1986, on "one of the few occasions that the U.S.
government collected information on mortality rates (for heart and
cerebrovascular disease) by class, the results showed that, by whatever
indicators of class one might choose (level of education, income, or occupation), mortality rates are related to social class."[34]

Indeed, where the major causes of death (heart disease and cerebrovascular disease) are concerned, class standing is a clearer indicator than
racial classification. "The growing mortality differentials between whites
and blacks," Navarro concludes, "cannot be understood by looking only
at race; they are part and parcel of larger mortality differentials—class
differentials."[35] The sociologist William Julius Wilson makes a similar
point in his landmark study *The Declining Significance of Race*, where
he argues that "trained and educated blacks, like trained and educated
whites, will continue to enjoy the advantages and privileges of their class
status."[36] Although new studies, discussed in Chapters 5 and 6, show

that race differentials persist even among the privileged, it is important to insist that it is the African American poor—and an analysis of the mechanisms of their impoverishment—who are being left out. At the same time, U.S. national aggregate income data that do not consider differential mortality by race and place miss completely the fact that African American men in Harlem have shorter life expectancies than Bangladeshi men.[37] Again, as Sen remarks, race-based differences in life expectancy have policy implications, and these in turn are related to social and economic rights:

> If the relative deprivation of blacks transcends income differentials so robustly, the remedying of this inequality has to involve policy matters that go well beyond just creating income opportunities for the black population. It is necessary to address such matters as public health services, educational facilities, hazards of urban life, and other social and economic parameters that influence survival chances. The picture of mortality differentials presents an entry into the problem of racial inequality in the United States that would be wholly missed if our economic analysis were to be confined only to traditional economic variables.[38]

Other Axes of Oppression

Any distinguishing characteristic, whether social or biological, can serve as a pretext for discrimination and thus as a cause of suffering. Refugee or immigrant status is one that readily comes to mind, when thinking of the poor and the powerless. Sexual preference is another obvious example; homosexuality is stigmatized to varying degrees in many settings. "Gay bashing," like other forms of violent criminal victimization, is sure to have long-term effects. But crimes against gay men and women are again felt largely among the poor.

Questions about the relationship between homophobia and mortality patterns have come to the fore during the AIDS pandemic. In regard to HIV disease, homophobia may be said to lead to adverse outcomes if it "drives underground" people who would otherwise stand to benefit from preventive campaigns. But gay communities, at least middle-class ones in affluent nations, have been singularly effective in organizing a response to AIDS, and those most closely integrated into these communities are among the most informed consumers of AIDS-related messages in the world.[39]

Homophobia may be said to hasten the development of AIDS if it denies services to those already infected with HIV. But this phenomenon has not been widely observed in the United States, where an "AIDS deficit"—fewer cases than predicted—has been noted among gay men, though not in other groups disproportionately afflicted with HIV disease in the early years of the epidemic: injection drug users, inner-city people of color, and persons originally from poor countries in sub-Saharan Africa or the Caribbean.[40] Those engaged in sex work have not benefited from the AIDS deficit. However, males involved in prostitution are almost universally poor, and it may be their poverty, rather than their sexual preference, that puts them at risk of HIV infection. Many men involved in homosexual prostitution, particularly minority adolescents, do not necessarily identify themselves as gay.

None of this is to deny the ill effects of homophobia, even in a country as wealthy as the United States. The point is rather to call for more fine-grained, more systemic analyses of power and privilege in discussions about who is likely to have their rights violated and in what ways. We did not need the AIDS pandemic to teach us this. In *Maurice,* E. M. Forster explores English class politics as much as he does the affective experience of Maurice, an upper-middle-class man who falls in love with Clive, an aristocrat with the expected political ambitions. Maurice's liberation, it would seem, comes from his relationship with Alec, a servant on Clive's family estate. In a postscript to the book, Forster deplores the persecution of gays in England, noting that "police prosecutions will continue and Clive on the bench will continue to sentence Alec on the dock. Maurice may get off."[41]

The Conflation of Structural Violence and Cultural Difference

Awareness of cultural differences has long complicated discussion of human suffering. Some anthropologists have argued that what outside observers construe as obvious assaults on dignity may in fact be long-standing cultural institutions highly valued by a society. Often-cited examples range from female circumcision in the Sudan to headhunting in the Philippines. Such discussions invariably appeal to the concept of cultural relativism, which has a long and checkered history in anthropology. Is every culture a law unto itself and answerable to nothing other than itself? In recent decades, confidence in reflexive cultural relativism faltered as anthropologists turned their attention to "complex societies" characterized by extremely inegalitarian social structures. Many found themselves unwilling to condone social inequity merely because it was buttressed by cultural beliefs, no matter how ancient or picturesque. Citizens of the former colonies also questioned cultural relativism as part of a broader critique of anthropology: for them, it appeared to be a mechanism for rationalizing and perpetuating inequalities between First and Third Worlds.[42]

But this question has not yet eroded a tendency, evident in many of the social sciences but perhaps particularly in anthropology, to confuse structural violence with cultural difference. Far too many ethnographies have conflated poverty and inequality, the end results of a long process of impoverishment, with "otherness." Quite often, such myopia does not come down to motives but rather, as Talal Asad has suggested, to our "mode of perceiving and objectifying alien societies."[43] Part of the problem may be the ways in which the term "culture" is used. "The idea of culture," explains Roy Wagner approvingly in a book on the subject, "places the researcher in a position of equality with his subjects: each 'belongs to a culture.' "[44] The tragedy, of course, is that this equality, however comforting to the researcher, is entirely illusory. Anthropology has usually "studied down" steep gradients of power.

Such illusions suggest an important means of sustaining other misreadings—most notably, the conflation of poverty and cultural difference—for they suggest that the anthropologist and "his" subject, being *from* different cultures, are *of* different worlds and *of* different times.[45] These sorts of misreadings, innocent enough when kept among scholars, are finding a more insidious utility within elite culture as it becomes increasingly *transnational*. Concepts of cultural relativism, and even arguments to reinstate the dignity of different cultures and "races," have been easily adopted and turned to profit by some of the very agencies that perpetuate extreme suffering.[46] The abuse of the concept of cultural specificity is particularly insidious in discussions of suffering in general and of human rights abuses specifically: cultural difference, verging on a cultural determinism, is one of several forms of essentialism used to explain away assaults on dignity and suffering. Practices including torture are said to be "part of their culture" or "in their nature"—"their" designating either the victims, or the perpetrators, or both, as may be expedient.[47]

Such analytic vices are rarely questioned, even though systemic studies of extreme suffering suggest that the concept of culture should enjoy only an exceedingly limited role in explaining the *distribution* of misery. The role of cultural boundary lines in enabling, perpetuating, justifying, and interpreting suffering is subordinate to (though well integrated with) the national and international mechanisms that create and deepen inequalities. "Culture" does not explain suffering; it may at worst furnish an alibi.[48]

STRUCTURAL VIOLENCE AND EXTREME SUFFERING

At night I listen to their phantoms
shouting in my ear
shaking me out of lethargy
issuing me commands
I think of their tattered lives
of their feverish hands
reaching out to seize ours.
It's not that they're begging
they're demanding
they've earned the right to order us
to break up our sleep
to come awake
to shake off once and for all
this lassitude.
    Claribel Alegría, "Nocturnal Visits"

Clearly, no single axis can fully define increased risk for extreme human suffering. Efforts to attribute explanatory efficacy to one variable lead to immodest claims of causality, for wealth and power have often protected individual women, gays, and ethnic minorities from the suffering and adverse outcomes associated with assaults on dignity. Similarly, poverty can often efface the "protective" effects of status based on gender, race, or sexual orientation. Leonardo Boff and Clodovis Boff, liberation theologians writing from Brazil, insist on the primacy of the economic:

> We have to observe that the socioeconomically oppressed (the poor) do not simply exist alongside other oppressed groups, such as blacks, indigenous peoples, women—to take the three major categories in the Third World. No, the "class-oppressed"—the socioeconomically poor—are the infrastructural expression of the process of oppression. The other groups represent "superstructural" expressions of oppression and because of this are deeply conditioned by the infrastructural. It is one thing to be a black taxi-driver, quite another to be a black football idol; it is one thing to be a

woman working as a domestic servant, quite another to be the first lady of the land; it is one thing to be an Amerindian thrown off your land, quite another to be an Amerindian owning your own farm.[49]

This is not to deny that sexism or racism has serious negative consequences, even in the wealthy countries of North America and Europe. The point is simply to call for more honest discussions of who is likely to suffer and in what ways.

The capacity to suffer is, clearly, a part of being human. But not all suffering is equivalent, in spite of pernicious and often self-serving identity politics that suggest otherwise. Physicians practice triage and referral daily. What suffering needs to be taken care of first and with what resources? It *is* possible to speak of extreme human suffering, and an inordinate share of this sort of pain is currently endured by those living in poverty. Take, for example, illness and premature death, the leading cause of extreme suffering in many places in the world. In a striking departure from previous, staid reports, the World Health Organization now acknowledges that poverty is the world's greatest killer: "Poverty wields its destructive influence at every stage of human life, from the moment of conception to the grave. It conspires with the most deadly and painful diseases to bring a wretched existence to all those who suffer from it."[50]

Today, the world's poor are the chief victims of structural violence—a violence that has thus far defied the analysis of many who seek to understand the nature and distribution of extreme suffering. Why might this be so? One answer is that the poor are not only more likely to suffer; they are also less likely to have their suffering noticed, as Chilean theologian Pablo Richard, noting the fall of the Berlin Wall, has warned: "We are aware that another gigantic wall is being constructed in the Third World, to hide the reality of the poor majorities. A wall between the rich and poor is being built, so that poverty does not annoy the powerful and the poor are obliged to die in the silence of history."[51]

The task at hand, if this silence is to be broken, is to identify the forces conspiring to promote suffering, with the understanding that these are differentially weighted in different settings. If we do this, we stand a chance of discerning the causes of extreme suffering and also the forces that put some at risk for human rights abuses, while others are shielded from risk. No honest assessment of the current state of human rights can omit an analysis of structural violence, as the following chapters attempt to show.

CHAPTER 2

PESTILENCE
AND RESTRAINT

GUANTÁNAMO, AIDS, AND THE
LOGIC OF QUARANTINE

The awkward fact with which U.S. policy wrestles is that
people flee the world's Haitis for a combination of motives.
All are deserving of some compassion, but how much?

Newsweek, December 2, 1991

Haitians are the immigrants that Americans love to fear
and hate.

Robert Lawless, *Haiti's Bad Press*

The U.S. travel ban and the distorted portrayal of Cuba in
both popular and scholarly media ensure that the majority of
North Americans do not learn that a poor, Third World
country, gripped by economic crisis, and under constant
attack from the most powerful nation in the world, is still
able to achieve health standards higher than those in the
capital of that powerful nation, Washington, D.C.

Aviva Chomsky, " 'The Threat of a Good Example':
Health and Revolution in Cuba"

Haiti, it is well known, is a country long wracked by political turmoil.
But the coup d'état of September 1991 was unique in many respects.
Most significantly, it represented the overthrow of Haiti's first democratically elected president, Jean-Bertrand Aristide, whose popular support was so strong that he had won 67 percent of the vote while running
against almost a dozen candidates. By any criteria, Aristide was more
popular in his country than any other sitting president in the hemisphere.
Thus when he was overthrown, a great deal of military force was required to silence Haitians' angry opposition to the coup. More so than

any of the scores of convulsions preceding it, the push against Aristide's government generated refugees, many of them young people who had been active in the pro-democracy movement.

Once outside Haiti, these refugees collided with a series of structures and opinions long in the making. Those who fled Haiti by sea collided with U.S. immigration policy. These "boat people" would also come up against a host of preexisting notions about Haiti and Haitians—a widely held U.S. "folk model" of Haiti that has been clearly reflected in American popular commentary on Haiti from its independence in 1804 to the days of the current political and economic crisis.[1]

Perhaps nowhere has this model had greater effect than in the lives of a few hundred HIV-positive Haitian refugees who were detained for as long as two years on the U.S. naval base at Guantánamo Bay, Cuba. "U.S. Base Is an Oasis to Haitians" read the headline of an article published on November 28, 1991, in the New York Times, often termed our national paper of record.[2] The perspective of Yolande Jean, interned on the base for eleven months, is somewhat different from that of the Times:

> We were in a space cordoned off with barbed wire. Wherever they put you, you were meant to stay right there; there was no place to move. The latrines were brimming over. There was never any cool water to drink, to wet our lips. There was only water in a cistern, boiling in the hot sun. When you drank it, it gave you diarrhea.... Rats crawled over us at night.... When we saw all these things, we thought, it's not possible, it can't go on like this. We're humans, just like everyone else.[3]

Guantánamo, this "oasis" without cool drinking water, is an otherwise fully equipped U.S. military base, located roughly a third of the way between Haiti and Florida on the island of Cuba. In 1903, Guantánamo was leased "indefinitely" to the United States for two thousand dollars per year; and, by the terms of the lease, the base is not subject to Cuban laws.[4] Had Yolande Jean been on the other side of the fence that separates the base from Cuba, she would not have been expelled, as Cuba does not restrict immigration or entry to only those who are HIV-negative. Instead, she might have been placed in an AIDS sanatorium. An article from the New England Journal of Medicine (which might be termed medicine's journal of record) describes Santiago de las Vegas, one of the sanatoriums:

> Located in a suburb of Havana, Cuba's main quarantine facility is largely fenced in and is composed of barracks housing hundreds of people. Since inspectors from other nations have not been permitted to report on condi-

tions in the quarantine facility, it is impossible to know how much better or worse they are than those at Guantánamo.[5]

In reality, it is not "impossible to know how much better or worse [conditions] are than those at Guantánamo." Indeed, it *has* been possible to visit these "quarantine facilities" and to interview HIV-positive persons living there. I have done so. The Cuban AIDS program has in fact hosted hundreds of visitors from North America and elsewhere. Some have been highly critical of the sanatoriums, but none of their reports have described situations as awful as those depicted by the Haitians on Guantánamo. Since I did not visit a "quarantine facility" during the time that the Haitians were detained on Guantánamo, I will save my comments on Santiago de las Vegas for the close of this chapter, relying instead on the impressions of those better placed to make contemporaneous comparisons.

In 1991, the same year that Yolande's troubles began, anthropologist Nancy Scheper-Hughes interviewed a number of internees in the Santiago de las Vegas sanatorium. Here is how she described the facility:

> Today Santiago de las Vegas is a suburban community of several acres dotted with modern, one- and two-story apartment duplexes surrounded by lush vegetation, palm trees, and small gardens. The community resembles many of the suburban, middle class housing developments one finds almost anywhere in Mexico or Brazil. (During a recent visit in March 1994 to two Israeli [kibbutzim] I noted an immediate similarity in the organization and the "feel" of social relations between the kibbutz and the sanatorium as collectivist, residential institutions. However, the Havana sanatorium was more attractive and the housing was more comfortable.)[6]

The comments of Patricia, the wife of a soldier who had contracted HIV during military service in Africa, were not atypical of those Scheper-Hughes interviewed. Like Yolande Jean, Patricia was asymptomatic; her HIV infection had been detected through mass screening. Like Yolande Jean, Patricia was separated from her children. But the tenor of her comments is strikingly different:

> Naturally, one feels homesick. You miss your children a great deal. But our needs and the needs of our children are taken care of and we have to accept our situation with as much good will as we can.
> We celebrate Mother's Day, we go out on excursions to the movies, to the beach, to watch baseball games. And, of course, those of us who are responsible may go home on the weekends or, if you live far away as we do, on a longer visit. Now I feel like I am a stranger when I am away from the sanatorium and walk down the street in my own community.[7]

These scenarios—one on Guantánamo and one on the outskirts of Havana—would seem to describe settings that are phenomenologically quite distinct. Both, of course, are found on the same Caribbean island. In both cases, individuals found themselves restrained by a state using force in the name of public health. The architects of these policies cannot look to the historical record to support these approaches, for quarantine has not been shown to be an effective measure in containing sexually transmitted diseases.[8] In short, both Guantánamo and the Cuban AIDS program, in its early incarnation, could be termed misguided public health initiatives in this regard.

But the similarities evaporate quickly on closer examination. One quarantine facility is sun-baked asphalt surrounded by barbed wire; the other, a verdant and shady campus that resembles an affluent Latin American residential neighborhood. One is peopled by soldiers and detainees; the other, by doctors, nurses, patients, and a single security guard. One was a military facility housing the sick, staffed by only one physician with infectious-disease training; the other, though briefly a military facility during its history, has for years been a medical center with a large staff of specialist physicians, nurses, and social workers.

If these two settings are so different, what forces would lead commentators to suggest that they are similar? What symbolic work do these forced comparisons perform? In what cultural and political contexts are these commentaries embedded? Moreover, how are the events on Guantánamo linked to the logic of quarantine that underlies such responses to HIV infection?

Most of the rest of this chapter attempts to answer these questions by examining the experience of Yolande Jean and other Haitians detained on Guantánamo. Accounts of what happened there conflict, even when offered by eyewitnesses. The version offered here—that of the detainees, many of whom I interviewed in 1993—differs significantly from the accounts offered by journalists, U.S. government officials, and even the Haitians' lawyers.

CLOSING THE DOOR ON HAITIAN REFUGEES

Although Cuba is the stage on which the contrapuntal dramas of Yolande and Patricia were played out, Haiti and the United States are the nations most centrally concerned in the intersection of events and processes that led to Yolande Jean's detention.

The U.S. Immigration and Naturalization Service (INS) has long argued that Haitians are "economic refugees," fleeing poverty. For ten years, including the last four of the Duvalier dictatorship and six years of military juntas, the United States, in defiance of international law, forcibly returned Haitian refugees to their country. This was the result of an arrangement, brokered in 1981, by which the government of Jean-Claude Duvalier permitted U.S. authorities to board Haitian vessels and to return to Haiti any passengers determined to have violated the laws of Haiti. The United States granted asylum to exactly eight of 24,559 Haitian refugees applying for political asylum during that period.[9]

In the two weeks after the coup of 1991, with the attention of the world press fixed on Haiti, the United States suspended the practice of seizing and repatriating Haitians. As the Haitian military continued to arrest and execute partisans of the overthrown President Aristide, refugees streamed out of Haiti, both by sea, to the United States, and by land, to the Dominican Republic. A quarter of a million Haitians were displaced in the first three months after the coup, by conservative estimates.[10]

On November 18, 1991, with an estimated fifteen hundred Haitians already dead and military repression churning full throttle, the administration of U.S. President George Bush announced that it was resuming forced repatriation; those intercepted would be returned to Haiti without being interviewed by the INS. The following day, the United Nations High Commissioner for Refugees announced his "regrets that the U.S. Government has decided to proceed unilaterally and return a number of asylum-seekers to Haiti."[11] Human rights organizations also denounced the decision, and several sued the Bush administration when the first groups of refugees were returned to Haiti. The case eventually ended up before the U.S. Supreme Court, which ruled in favor of the U.S. government. Professor Kevin Johnson of the University of California writes of the High Court's "shameful acquiescence" to the Bush administration:

> The courts were the last constitutionally viable means by which to halt the Executive Branch's unlawful treatment of the Haitians. As the constitution mandates, the Judiciary must check the excesses of the Executive. The Rehnquist Court, however, consistently deferred to the Executive Branch on immigration matters and refused to assert the Judiciary's constitutional role in reviewing challenges to the interdiction program. The Haitians, in this instance, suffered from that abdication.[12]

Although little public outcry about the matter arose, certain human rights advocates were able to force a compromise: the refugees would be brought to the naval base at Guantánamo rather than being returned immediately to Haiti. Shortly thereafter, scores of canvas tents were erected within the confines of the base. "The military and Coast Guard emphasize that theirs is a humanitarian mission," explained the *New York Times*.[13]

In the eight months following the coup, the U.S. Coast Guard intercepted thirty-four thousand Haitians on the high seas; the majority of these refugees were transported to Guantánamo. By all accounts, conditions in the camp were grim: the inmates lived in tents and other makeshift shelters on a landing strip, surrounded by barbed wire. These shelters, according to the Haitians, were infested with rats, scorpions, and snakes. The lodgings were permeable to rain, and sanitary facilities were unavailable. Yet, despite these deplorable conditions, the detainees' chief complaint was of mistreatment by their American hosts.

Shortly after the arrival of the first refugees, rumors of mistreatment, including beatings and arbitrary detention, began to filter through the Haitian advocacy organizations based in the United States. It was difficult to verify the rumors because the U.S. military restricted access to the base. As uncritical stories based on military briefings continued to appear in the mainstream press, a group of journalists sued the U.S. government for access to the base. Ingrid Arnesen of *The Nation* filed one of the first stories of visiting Guantánamo. One of the detainees, who had been on the base for more than a year, spoke to Arnesen in no uncertain terms:

> Since we left Haiti last December we've been treated like animals. When we protested about the camp back then, the military beat us up. I was beaten, handcuffed, and they spat in my face. I was chained, made to sleep on the ground. July, that was the worst time. We were treated like animals, like dogs, not like humans.[14]

In short, the Haitians and their advocates failed to see the humane aspect of this "humanitarian mission." By the middle of 1992, events on the base were subject to the usual divergent readings. Stories in the mainstream U.S. media continued to portray Guantánamo as a haven for refugees. Haitians, including the Haitian American print and radio media, tended to refer to the base as a "concentration camp," a "prison," or, at best, "a detention facility."

Curiously enough, the Bush administration seems to have adopted a reading close to the one popular among Haitians. They realized that refugees were being detained on the base for long periods of time—some would remain there almost two years—without a meaningful hearing. In response, the administration gathered some of the nation's leading legal talent to justify this practice. Since Guantánamo is not technically on U.S. soil, the Bush administration lawyers developed a torturous rationale:

> While conceding that the Haitians are treated differently from other national groups who seek asylum in the U.S., the Government claimed that the U.S. Constitution and other sources of U.S. and international law do not apply to Guantánamo—this despite the fact that the U.S. military base at Guantánamo is under the exclusive jurisdiction and control of the U.S. Government.[15]

Guantánamo thus became a place where non-U.S. nationals could be stowed away in a sort of lawless limbo, out of reach of U.S. or international law. Officials charged with upholding U.S. law could intercept refugees, take them to a U.S. military base, and openly declare any actions taken there above the law. Neither the hypocrisy nor the irony was lost on the Haitians.

Most Haitians listen to radio; anyone who did so in the early months of 1992 came to know Guantánamo as a place best avoided. But in Haiti, military and paramilitary repression of the popular movement continued apace: those associated with community organizing or the democratic movement were hunted down as subversive. Since that included the majority of the population, these were dangerous times for many. Yolande Jean's case is instructive.

Both Yolande and her husband, Athenor, were members of Komite Inite Demokratik, a democratic organization founded shortly after Duvalier's departure; Yolande was heavily involved in adult literacy projects. After the coup, both Yolande and Athenor were subjected to many threats. On April 27, 1992, Yolande was arrested and taken to Recherches Criminelles, the police station that served as the headquarters of Colonel Michel François, the alleged boss of Haiti's death squads. The interview was more than perfunctory; during the course of her torture, Yolande, visibly pregnant with her third child, began to bleed. On her second day in prison, she miscarried. She did not receive medical attention.

Yolande decided at that moment that if she survived detention, she would flee the country. Perhaps because at the time the Haitian business elite was anxious to resume negotiations to end the already porous U.S. trade embargo, internal pressure was being exerted on the military police to release political detainees.[16] Yolande was released from prison the following day. Shortly thereafter, she entrusted her sons to a kinswoman and headed for northern Haiti. Her husband remained in hiding. She would not see him again.

> I took the boat on May twelfth, and on the fourteenth they came to get us. They did not say where they were taking us. We were still in Haitian waters at the time.... We hadn't even reached the Windward Passage when American soldiers came for us. But we thought they might be coming to help us... there were sick children on board. On the fourteenth, we reached the base at Guantánamo.

Yolande's initial instinct—that the U.S. soldiers "might be coming to help us"—was soon revised: "They burned all of our clothes, everything we had, the boat, our luggage, all the documents we were carrying." U.S. television had displayed images of Haitian boats burning, but both the Coast Guard and the media described the fires as the destruction of unseaworthy vessels—with no mention of personal items. When asked what reasons the U.S. soldiers gave for burning the refugees' effects, Yolande replied,

> They gave us none. They just started towing our belongings, and the next thing we know, the boat was in flames. Photos, documents. If you didn't have pockets in which to put things, you lost them. The reason that I came through with some of my documents is because I had a backpack and was wearing pants with pockets. They went through my bag and took some of my documents. Even my important papers they took. American soldiers did this. Fortunately, I had hidden some papers in my pockets.

Haiti was full to overflowing with people just like Yolande Jean. Soon Guantánamo was full to overflowing as well. On May 24, 1992, President Bush issued Executive Order 12,807 from his summer home in Kennebunkport. Referring to the Haitian boats, he ordered the Coast Guard "to return the vessel and its passengers to the country from which it came... provided, however, that the Attorney General, in his unreviewable discretion, may decide that a person who is a refugee will not be returned without his consent."

As attorney Andrew Schoenholtz of the Lawyers Committee for Human Rights wryly observed, "Grace did not abound; all Haitians have been returned under the new order."[17]

The bottom line: all Haitians leaving Haiti by sea would be intercepted and returned to Haiti without being processed by the INS. The Voice of America affiliates in Haiti broadcast this policy, in Creole. By the summer of 1992, Haitians under the gun understood that they would find no safe haven outside the country. Haiti more and more resembled a burning building from which there was no exit. The Bush administration's actions—denying the refugees legal counsel or a hearing, preventing press coverage of the conditions of the detainees—reinforced widely held beliefs that Haitians were being singled out for racist and exclusionary treatment. Furthermore, Haitians were well aware that Cubans who made it to the United States were automatically declared political refugees—regardless of whether they had any evidence of persecution.

In spite of the odds against all Haitians seeking asylum, Yolande Jean's case for refugee status should have been airtight. She was a longstanding member of an organization targeted for political repression; she and her husband had been arrested and tortured; and she had managed to preserve key documents proving this. In fact, Yolande Jean was indeed one of those few refugees who passed scrutiny; U.S. law provided her safe haven as a bona fide political refugee. One problem remained, however: Yolande, like all the refugees, had been tested for HIV. Unlike most, her test was positive.

THE VIRUS AND THE "OASIS": YOLANDE'S STORY

It was inevitable, really, that AIDS—or fear of it—would surface in the course of the Haitian refugee crisis. In the 1990s, HIV was certain to be present in any group of more than thirty thousand young adults from almost anywhere in the Caribbean (with the exception of Cuba). U.S. legislators at state and federal levels had introduced enormous numbers of bills regarding HIV, most of them punitive, restrictive, and directed at infected persons. Although immigration law is in principle strictly separated from laws regarding political refugees, anyone familiar with INS policies toward Haitians could have predicted mandatory HIV screening.

By the time mass screening of all refugees was completed, the U.S. government had identified 268 HIV-positive refugees. Although Yolande and many others had already passed the stringent requirements for refugee status and were thus guaranteed asylum, authorities invoked U.S. immigration law to keep these Haitians out. In contrast, Cubans who hijacked planes to Miami or who arrived on U.S. soil by other means were not even tested for HIV, as Haitians were quick to point out.

Immigration legislation regarding HIV has a short and undistinguished history. Although legislation to exclude or otherwise punish those with

AIDS was introduced shortly after the syndrome was recognized, it was not until 1986 that the Department of Health and Human Services (HHS) began to draft laws requiring immigrants to be tested for and found free of HIV. This legislation was sponsored in the Senate by Senator Jesse Helms and was approved—unanimously—in June 1987. "This Senate action was extraordinary," notes a legal opinion, "in that it assumed a responsibility, previously entrusted exclusively to the HHS, to determine which communicable diseases would be grounds for excluding aliens."[18]

Public health specialists spoke out against this policy, which they regarded as unwarranted. Debate around this issue led, in fact, to a reconsideration of several other disorders on the list. By 1990, the U.S. Centers for Disease Control came to argue that HIV and all other sexually transmitted pathogens should not be grounds for exclusion. They recommended that only active pulmonary tuberculosis should remain on the list, and a second bill, reflecting their expert opinion, was introduced in Congress. As lawyer Elizabeth McCormick describes:

> Opposition to the [second] bill was led by Sen. Jesse Helms, who considered the proposal an attempt to appease the AIDS lobby and the "homosexual rights movement which fuels it." Sen. Helms claimed that HHS was not acting in the interest of the public health but was "promoting an agenda skewed to placate the appetite of a radical and repugnant political movement."[19]

These debates played themselves out on Guantánamo. Again, the experience of Yolande Jean is instructive, for it reveals the repercussions of both arbitrary laws and arbitrary proceedings:

> They sent me to Camp Number 3, to have a blood test. They didn't specify what test they were doing, but everyone had one. The others [who had been classed as bona fide political refugees] were authorized to leave for the United States. There I was, and they didn't call me…I was the last person left in the camp.
>
> After three days of waiting, they called me. They told me, "You have a little problem." They asked my age, they asked for a photo ID. They told me I had a little problem, but they'd send me to see a doctor…and he'd resolve everything for me. They said, after twenty-two days you'll be fine, you'll go to the United States. I asked what sort of problem they were referring to. They said, "It's a little virus you have." I replied, "There's no such thing as a 'little virus'; speak clearly so that I can understand."
>
> They put me in a small room, and eight soldiers surrounded me….I told them not to touch me. Don't worry, they said, you'll be cured. I told them to speak clearly so that I could understand. Even the interpreter couldn't explain. Tell me! I see what you're saying—that I have AIDS. Fine, I have

AIDS. Don't tell me, then, that you'll cure me. That in twenty-two days I'll be fine!

At that point, two military police turned me around, grabbed me by both arms in order to put me on the bus for [Camp] Bulkeley.

Out of encounters such as this was born the "HIV detention camp" on Guantánamo, known as Camp Bulkeley. Inmates received new bracelets identifying them as HIV-positive. Yolande Jean insisted, "They were even harsher with us than with the others," and a group of American lawyers concurred: "[Starting] in February 1992 those testing positive were interviewed and required to meet a higher standard to establish that they had a 'well-founded fear' of persecution. The Immigration and Naturalization Service denied requests by the refugees' attorneys to be present at these interviews."[20]

In the spring of 1993, Judge Sterling Johnson, a Bush appointee who years earlier had himself been an officer on Guantánamo, heard the case brought against the U.S. government by the Haitians and their advocates. The more depositions he heard, the more convinced he became that the detention of the HIV-positive Haitians represented "cruel and unusual punishment" in violation of the Eighth Amendment of the U.S. Constitution. In his 1993 ruling on the case, he described Haitians detained in Camp Bulkeley as follows:

They live in camps surrounded by razor barbed wire. They tie plastic garbage bags to the sides of the building to keep the rain out. They sleep on cots and hang sheets to create some semblance of privacy. They are guarded by the military and are not permitted to leave the camp, except under military escort. The Haitian detainees have been subjected to pre-dawn military sweeps as they sleep by as many as 400 soldiers dressed in full riot gear. They are confined like prisoners and are subject to detention in the brig without hearing for camp rule infractions.[21]

As terrible as this sounds, the stories told by the Haitians interned there are even worse. While the U.S. press wrote of the detainees as unfortunates caught in a bureaucratic limbo, the Haitians spoke of far more malicious mistreatment. Yolande Jean recalled the events of July 17, 1992:

We had been asking them to remove the barbed wire; the children were playing near it, they were falling and injuring themselves. The food they were serving us, including canned chicken, had maggots in it. And yet they insisted that we eat it. "Because you've got no choice." And it was for these reasons that we started holding demonstrations.

In response, they began to beat us. On July eighteenth, they surrounded us, arrested some of us, and put us in prison, in Camp Number 7...Camp 7 was a little space on a hill. They put up a tent, but when it rained, you got wet. The sun came up, we were baking in it. We slept on the rocks; there were no beds. And each little space was separated by barbed wire. We couldn't even turn around without being injured by the barbed wire.

For the Haitian refugees, then, Guantánamo represented a health hazard rather than an oasis. Even without subjecting the detainees to such privations, it was unsafe to keep more than two hundred HIV-positive persons, many of them co-infected with the organism that causes tuberculosis, cramped together in such close quarters. This brings to the fore the question of medical care for the HIV-positive refugees and their dependents: who was providing it, and how?

The camp was served by a battalion aid station clinic staffed by two military physicians, one specializing in infectious disease and another in family practice. Again, commentary on this version of the doctor-patient relationship resembles positioned rhetoric. To quote the *New England Journal of Medicine*:

> That the military physicians worked hard to treat the Haitians at the camp was not in dispute. Nonetheless, Judge Johnson concluded that "the doctor-patient relationship has been frustrated." The Haitians believed that the military physicians were involved in their continued detention, and there were also great cultural differences between the physicians and the Haitian patients. As a result, the patients did not trust either their diagnosis or the medications prescribed for them.[22]

In all that regards Haiti, attributing diverging interpretations of a situation to "great cultural differences" has been a recurrent theme. But Yolande Jean did not refer, even once, to cultural differences as an explanation of the substandard medical care:

> They gave me two pills and an injection. I asked them, why the injection? Because you have a little cold, they replied. But it wasn't a vaccine, it was an injection in the buttocks. And if you didn't want it, you had no choice: they simply said, it's for your own good. You have to accept it, or they call soldiers to come and hold you, force you to take it, or they put you in the brig and bring your pills to you there. There were people who refused to have their blood drawn; soldiers came to handcuff them, tie them up in order to draw their blood.
>
> I learned that the injection the doctor had given me was Depo-Provera. I began having heavy bleeding. I bled for three months, lost weight. There

were other women who'd had the injection before me, but I didn't know that. If I'd learned of this ahead of time, I would've tried to warn the others and prevent their receiving it.... When I learned this, I tried to stop them. No, I said, you will not commit this crime.

Depo-Provera, an analog of the hormone progesterone, is prescribed as a long-acting contraceptive. The *forced* use of such an agent has been discussed—theoretically—by several medical ethicists and adamantly rejected on moral grounds. In legal terms, the forced injection of any substance represents the felony crime of assault. This is true even across settings marked by "great cultural differences."[23]

The degree to which commentators invoke cultural differences serves as a marker, it seems, for the degree to which these commentators are uncomfortable with full exposure of what happened on Guantánamo. Even though the concept of cultural distinctness is widespread in Haiti, it never figured in the commentaries of the Haitian detainees. The refugees I interviewed spoke of forced blood draws and forced medication; they spoke of the brig, of solitary confinement, of barbed wire. And yet, even the Haitians' advocates—their lawyers—failed to capture the refugees' outrage over this treatment. To quote one of the lawyers:

> The military doctors are probably moved by humanitarian and population control objectives. On the one hand, the doctors may be concerned that HIV+ refugee women who get pregnant pose a serious health risk to themselves and their babies. On the other hand, the doctors are also undoubtedly eager to limit the growth rate of the refugee population on Guantánamo, particularly because it is a population which has a high prevalence of HIV infection.[24]

The prisoners, organized by, among others, Yolande Jean, began holding peaceful demonstrations in June 1992. These were met, according to those interviewed, with intimidation, open threats, and detention in the brig. In July, the prisoners rioted, responding to the soldiers' dogs and aluminum batons with rocks. About twenty inmates were arrested and placed in Camp 7, in near-solitary confinement.

Outcry over Guantánamo came late, but it eventually became an issue in the 1992 U.S. presidential election. Prior to the adoption of the cynical *realpolitik* of Bill Clinton's presidency, the official platform of the Clinton-Gore ticket described George Bush's treatment of the Haitian refugees as "inhuman." One of the platform's planks, called simply "Stop the Forced Repatriation of Haitian Refugees," read as follows:

· Reverse Bush Administration policy, and oppose repatriation.
· Give fleeing Haitians refuge and consideration for political asylum until democracy is restored to Haiti. Provide them with safe haven, and encourage other nations to do the same.[25]

The platform also quite specifically promised to "stop the cynical politicization of federal immigration policies" and to "direct the Justice Department to follow the Department of Health and Human Services' recommendation that HIV be removed from the immigration restrictions list."[26]

As the presidential campaign heated up, it became clear that Clinton's proposed policy toward Haitian refugees would not be popular. The cover of the September 1992 edition of USA Today carried a photograph of a huddled mass of Haitian refugees, some of them children, on the decks of a Coast Guard cutter. "As compassionate as Americans try to be," asked the caption, "can we realistically afford an open border policy?"[27] One read, in some newspapers, of "the outrage over treatment of the Haitian refugees,"[28] but this outrage was strangely absent from most expressions of public opinion, which was perhaps more accurately reflected in the comments of immigration officials. One Associated Press reporter interviewed Duke Austin, special assistant to the director of congressional and public affairs at the INS. Mr. Austin could not understand all the fuss about the HIV-positive internees: "They're gonna die anyway, right?"[29]

In the same edition that announced, "Boat with 396 Haitians Missing; Cuba Reports 8 Survivors," the Orlando Sentinel wrote of "what could be a huge problem for the state: An explosion of Haitian migrants to South Florida." The story, which ran on the front page, continued by noting, "Many fear that tens of thousands of refugees could sail for Miami around Inauguration Day, Jan. 20, because of President-elect Bill Clinton's pledge to give Haitians a fair hearing for political asylum in the United States."[30] On January 28, however, Clinton began backpedaling, stating that he would continue his predecessor's policies.

Hearing of this, a number of refugees detained on Guantánamo began a hunger strike. Yolande Jean was widely recognized as the leader of this movement:

Before the strike, I'd been in prison, a tiny little cell, but crammed in with many others, men, women, and children. There was no privacy. Snakes would come in; we were lying on the ground, and lizards were climbing over us. One of us was bitten by a scorpion...there were spiders. Bees were stinging the children, and there were flies everywhere: whenever you tried to eat something, flies would fly into your mouth. Because of all this, I just got to the point, sometime in January, I said to myself, come what may, I might well die, but we can't continue in this fashion.

We called together the committee and decided to have a hunger strike. Children, pregnant women, everyone was lying outside, rain or shine, day and night. After fifteen days without food, people began to faint. The colonel called us together and warned us, and me particularly, to call off the strike. We said no.

At four in the morning, as we were lying on the ground, the colonel came with many soldiers. They began to beat us—I still bear a scar from this—and to strike us with nightsticks.... True, we threw rocks back at them, but they outnumbered us and they were armed. They then used big tractors to back us against the shelter, and they barred our escape with barbed wire.

Yolande Jean was arrested and placed in solitary confinement. Her version did not make it into the *New York Times,* which reported only that "at least seven Haitian refugees protesting their detention here by refusing food have lost consciousness."[31] No mention was made of any retribution by the strikers' wardens.

Even the lawyers for the Haitian detainees, who reached the base in the middle of the strike, seemed a bit annoyed by their clients' actions: "The hunger strike took us all by surprise, especially given the fact that the litigation team is in the middle of settlement negotiations with the Department of Justice."[32] The Haitians, it seems, were no longer impressed by bureaucratic efforts to have them released. They continued what they termed "active, nonviolent resistance." On March 11, eleven prisoners attempted to escape to Cuba but were recaptured. Two of the detainees tried to commit suicide, one by hanging.

A letter from Yolande Jean to her family was widely circulated in the community of concern taking shape in response to the situation on Guantánamo:

> To my family:
> Don't count on me anymore, because I have lost in the struggle for life. Thus, there is nothing left of me. Take care of my children, so they have strength to continue my struggle, because it is our duty.
> As for me, my obligation ends here. Hill and Jeff, you have to continue with the struggle so that you may become men of the future. I have lost hope; I am alone in my distress. I know you will understand my situation, but do not worry about me because I have made my own decision. I am alone in life and will remain so. Life is no longer worth living to me.

Hill and Jeff, you no longer have a mother. Understand that you
don't have a bad mother, it is simply that circumstances have taken
me to where I am at this moment. I am sending you two pictures so
you could look at me for a last time. Goodbye my children. Goodbye
my family. We will meet again in another world.

The Haitians' advocates, including Haitian refugee groups in the eastern United States, stepped up their pressure. On March 26, 1993, Judge
Johnson of New York again ruled against the administration. He ordered
that all detainees with fewer than 200 total T-lymphocytes be transferred
to the United States. It was the first time that T-cell subsets had been mentioned in a judicial order. A Justice Department spokesperson complained
that "there are aspects of Judge Johnson's decision that we would find it
difficult to live with." The first of these, he noted, "would be the judge's
very expansive view of the rights of aliens, who came into American hands
purely out of our own humanitarian impulses to rescue them at sea."[33]

Finally released from internment by the direct order of a federal judge,
the refugees came to the United States in small groups, Yolande almost
directly from solitary confinement. They arrived on the American main-
land before dawn on April 8, 1993. At the beginning of the summer,
however, more than 150 Haitians still remained on the base, and some
of them initiated a second hunger strike. Eventually, these actions, in
concert with the legal and moral pressures brought to bear on the U.S.
government, led to the closing of what Judge Johnson would call "the
only known refugee camp in the world composed entirely of HIV-
positive refugees." Like its predecessor, the Clinton administration had
failed to prove that Haitians like Yolande Jean warranted "the kind of
indefinite detention usually reserved for spies and murderers."[34]

HAITIANS AND HIV: BIASED PRESS, PUBLIC MYTHS

The detention of HIV-positive Haitian refugees raises a host of questions
regarding a complex symbolic web linking xenophobia, racism, and a
surprisingly coherent "folk model" of Haitians to which many North
Americans subscribe. The persistent notion of Haitians as infected and,
more important, as *infecting,* clearly underpinned much of the American response.[35] One legal scholar acutely observed, "The exclusion of
HIV-infected Haitian refugees flows from the once firmly held percep-
tions that Haiti is the birthplace and primary source of the HIV virus
and that most Haitian refugees are fleeing economic hardship rather than
political persecution."[36]

In analyzing these issues, it is important to examine how the U.S. legal system was used to buttress an illegal policy toward Haitians. The policies elaborated by the Bush administration invoked the rule of law rather than any moral principles, but the forced repatriation of self-proclaimed refugees in fact violated a number of preexisting laws, including the Immigration and Nationality Act and the United Nations Convention Relating to the Status of Refugees. A human rights lawyer summarizes the legal case that can be made against his own government's policy:

> The U.S. policy of forced repatriation violated international legal obligations of the United States under Article 33 of the Protocol relating to the status of Refugees and undermines the credibility of the U.S. commitment to international law in the eyes of the rest of the world. The United States correctly condemned the forced repatriation of Vietnamese asylum-seekers from Hong Kong following flawed screening procedures and also criticized the Malaysian and Thai governments for pushing back boats filled with Vietnamese asylum-seekers. The horrific human rights violations since the September 1991 coup render especially cruel the U.S. practice of forcibly repatriating all Haitians without even attempting to determine who among them might fear persecution at the very hands of the Haitian armed forces waiting for them at the dock in Port-au-Prince.[37]

Another lawyer put it succinctly: "By treating Haitians differently than any other refugee group, the U.S. government has created a two-track asylum process—one for Haitians and one for everyone else."[38]

With legal opinions such as these, how, precisely, did two consecutive U.S. administrations manage to detain people like Yolande Jean? Certainly U.S. lawmakers seem to support the exclusion of HIV-positive entrants: a February 1993 vote on a proposal to remove HIV infection from the list of diseases that would exclude an immigrant from the country failed in the Senate by a vote of 76 to 23. To no one's surprise, Senator Jesse Helms again led the opposition to the bill.

But popular support for these policies is also disturbingly strong. When public health officials, led by HHS Secretary Louis Sullivan, recommended removing HIV from the list of diseases for which entrants could be excluded, the response was brisk: "During a thirty day public comment period following the issuance of Dr. Sullivan's proposal, the HHS received 40,000 letters in opposition to the elimination of HIV infection as a ground for exclusion of aliens."[39]

With or without HIV, Haitians are not welcome, it would seem. As mentioned earlier, South Florida newspapers were full of alarmist headlines, such as the *Orlando Sentinel*'s "South Florida Braces for Haitian

Time Bomb." The August 9, 1993, edition of *Newsweek* dedicated its cover story to the "immigration backlash," headlining its polling results: "60% of Americans Say Immigration Is 'Bad for the Country.' " Haitians fared especially poorly in the sympathy sweepstakes. *Newsweek* pollsters asked, "Should it be easier or more difficult for people from the following places to immigrate to the U.S.?" In the responses, only Haiti and China were singled out by name. Contrary to the rumor of a "groundswell of revulsion" over ill-begotten policy toward Haitians, only 20 percent of those polled said immigration should be easier for Haitians, while 55 percent said it should be more difficult.[40] After a decade during which less than 0.5 percent of Haitian applicants were granted asylum, one wonders how much more difficult it could be.

The data certainly call into question such constructions as the narrative of public outrage mentioned earlier. The trickle of public outrage against the U.S.-sponsored violation of Haitian detainees' rights paled in comparison to the forty thousand postage stamps' worth of outrage against liberal lawmakers who wished to allow HIV-positive refugees into the country.

Discordant stories of Guantánamo pose questions of representation and interpretation of the events and processes that have marked the lives of Yolande Jean and many other Haitians. That there will be dominant and oppositional accounts of what happened on Guantánamo is self-evident; that the accounts of the powerful will be undergirded by solid institutional supports, including those who control the mainstream media, is equally predictable. But we also find interesting and unexpected twists. On Guantánamo, the so-called oppositional voices that came from the advocates of the Haitians—lawyers, sympathetic academics, and those from several human rights organizations—were often similar to the dominant voices more intimately linked to state power. Unless one listens to the detainees themselves, much of the oppositional criticism of Guantánamo leaves the impression that the U.S. military authorities, including doctors, were themselves frustrated victims of bureaucratic snarls. The image offered is of unfortunates languishing on a base—not that of active, malicious harassment.

For example, medicolegal specialist George Annas offers the following assessment in the *New England Journal of Medicine:* "That the military physicians worked hard to treat the Haitians at the camp was not in dispute."[41] But in fact this *was* in dispute, as Yolande's account reveals. The detainees' version of events, and their outrage, is all too often lost in journalistic and scholarly accounts.

In light of the strong forces constraining candid discussion of Guantánamo, the conclusion of one of the lawyers for the Haitians is less surprising: "We need to convince the Clinton people that what we want is
reasonable and cost-effective."[42] No need, apparently, to convince the
Clinton people that the events on Guantánamo were an abomination
and a crime: "cost-effectiveness" is what matters. Journalists know this;
lawyers know this.

In their earnest efforts to convince the empowered that their solution
was "reasonable and cost-effective," the Haitians' advocates misrepre-
sented Guantánamo. They made the naval base resemble a sanatorium—
a misguided public health intervention—when in fact it resembled a dun-
geon, a malignant expression of longstanding U.S. policies toward
Haitians.

PUBLIC HEALTH AND PRIVATE CONCERNS: JESÚS'S VERSION

What of Santiago de las Vegas, the Cuban "quarantine facility"? It seems
fitting to close with a reconsideration of Cuba's AIDS program after examining the great discrepancies between three versions of what went on
at Guantánamo: the official versions (and their echoes in the mainstream
press); the version offered by the Haitians' advocates; and the story told
by the detainees themselves. Granted that in this postmodern moment,
when we are told that only willfully naïve positivists seek something
called the truth, it is important to acknowledge that more than one discrepant version may be true in some important sense. But some versions,
surely, must have more points of contact with external reality and actual
events than others.

So it is with Santiago de las Vegas and the Cuban AIDS program. The
discrepancies in reporting on the Cuban facility are no less great than
those encountered in considering the forced detention of HIV-positive
Haitians, and it has been even more difficult for the Cubans, banned by
their powerful neighbor to the north from much international dialogue,
to respond in public forums. It is true that the first AIDS residential program was initially a military operation. Why? Because most of the first
Cubans diagnosed with HIV were young soldiers, social workers, and
health professionals serving as *internacionalistas* in Africa.

Take, for example, the case of Jesús Valle. "I was only eighteen when
I went to the Congo," he recalled many years later. "I was not involved
in any armed conflict; we did not even carry weapons. We were more involved in projects, and there was a lot of free time. So we had a lot of

time to drink beer and flirt with girls. That's how it all started for me, in 1985."[43]

Cuba began its HIV screening program early, compared to many other countries. Cuba's policies to protect its population from transfusion-associated HIV compare favorably to almost any other country's, including those of (notoriously) France and (less notoriously) the United States.[44] In 1983, the etiologic agent of AIDS had not been identified, but blood-borne infection was suspected. Cuba therefore banned the importation of factor VIII and other hemo-derivatives, and the Ministry of Public Health ordered the destruction of twenty thousand units of blood product. As of December 31, 2000, Cuba continued to have the lowest HIV incidence in the hemisphere and has registered only ten cases of transfusion-associated HIV—only two of those among Cuba's hemophiliacs.[45]

The first case of HIV disease was diagnosed in late 1985 by Dr. Jorge Pérez Ávila, an infectious-disease specialist who was asked to evaluate a Cuban *internacionalista* returning from Mozambique. Well before the term "AIDS" had been coined, the Ministry of Public Health had been charged with ensuring that diseases virtually eradicated in Cuba, such as malaria, were not reintroduced by returning *internacionalistas* and physicians. At about the time that HIV was thought to be endemic in Central Africa, Cuba began systematically testing all returning residents for this and other infectious diseases—a program very much in keeping with established medical practice in Cuba.[46]

That's how Jesús Valle, who felt "just fine" on returning from the Congo, was diagnosed with HIV infection. "I was diagnosed on February twenty-seventh, 1986," he recalled more than a decade later. "That day was the most uncertain moment of my life. It seemed that my very light was being extinguished—the light born of all the ideas and dreams fostered from the time of my childhood."

Jesús was sent, along with a score of others (including some from his brigade) to Santiago de las Vegas, an old hacienda about half an hour from Havana—and five minutes away from a famous leprosarium that, now almost empty, has remained a site of religious pilgrimage in Cuba. The idea was to create a similar facility for Cubans infected with HIV. At the same time the *internacionalistas* began showing up there, serosurveys began to turn up scores of cases of HIV infection among gay and bisexual men, many of them with links to Europe or North America.

The population of Santiago de las Vegas soon grew to include an eclectic collection of Cubans. It was a volatile mix. On the one hand, the soldiers (and their *machista* culture), their wives, families, and girlfriends. On the other, gay and bisexual men.[47] Subjecting such a disparate group, some of them sick, to military discipline was "an experiment that more or less failed," recalled Eduardo Campo, also an *internacionalista*, who was diagnosed at the same time as Jesús. Gay residents of the sanatorium complained of homophobia not among the staff but among the soldiers. The military doctors felt overwhelmed as much by the cultural clashes as by the unusual infections that plagued some of those interned. They argued to their superiors that the facility would best be managed by the public health and infectious-disease specialists rather than by the armed forces.

By 1988, the military was anxious to turn the matter over to the Ministry of Public Health. Vice-Minister Héctor Terry Molinert turned to infectious-disease specialists at the Pedro Kourí Institute of Tropical Medicine, a well-known referral center in Havana. Its director tapped Jorge Pérez, who had recently been named medical director of the institute's in-patient unit. Since Pérez was a civilian, he agreed to accept the responsibility of running the facility only if he could have liberty to create as he saw fit a program to meet the needs of a small but growing epidemic. As Pérez explained in a 1997 interview, "I saw that Cuba had a chance that many other countries did not: a small number of cases, and the public health capacity to intervene definitively in order to prevent a major epidemic." Pérez also noted that he did not want to relinquish his duties at the Pedro Kourí Institute, and he suggested that the sanatorium become the responsibility of the institute. Dr. Terry accepted his proposal and in 1989 named Pérez director of Cuba's national AIDS program and of the sanatorium.

One of Pérez's first acts was to order the fences around the hacienda-turned-military-facility torn down. He then began the more delicate task of building bridges between splintered groups of people bound together only by a shared lab result. (Most of the HIV-positive residents were asymptomatic.) He kept the focus medical but also instituted a number of initiatives designed to create respect and harmony within the sanatorium and the other facilities that were being created. Initially the Cuban program called for those living with HIV to "prove they were responsible" before they were allowed to leave the sanatorium, even when accompanied by chaperones. Somewhat defensively, perhaps, Jorge Pérez recalled what was meant by the term "responsible":

> Of course we meant that safe sex had to be practiced. Of course we wanted people who knew they were infected to be responsible in protecting others.

But we also meant that they needed to eat responsibly, to care for themselves, to take medications that would prevent opportunistic infections.
Even though we have very much changed the structure of the sanatorium, I
think we were justified in making demands of the people living here, living
with HIV. They know so much more about the disease than others, and this
was especially true more than a decade ago.

Among Pérez's many innovations was to encourage occupational
therapy by having residents practice their professions within the facility.
Thus several physicians and nurses living with HIV came to run the
infirmary there; several were involved in work at the infectious-disease
institute. He also sent residents to study at Havana University and sent
others back to their workplaces.

Cuba screened millions of its citizens and diagnosed a very small number of cases compared to other countries in the Caribbean. While the
sanatorium approach was being denounced abroad, the demand for facilities was growing within Cuba—even the program's most hardened
detractors acknowledge widespread local support for the sanatoriums.
"Cubans in general—gays as well as heterosexuals—expressed strong
support for the government AIDS program which they see as protecting
them," wrote Scheper-Hughes after visits in 1991 and 1993. "But there
are also sanatorium dissidents who are bitter and refuse to acquiesce to
the surveillance requirements of the sanatorium."[48]

Just as sanatoriums were being established in each of Cuba's
provinces, the Soviet Union came unhinged. In the space of less than a
year, Cuba lost 85 percent of its foreign trade.[49] Despite this huge blow
to the economy, which in 1990 led Fidel Castro to declare a "Special Period in the Time of Peace," the government did not reduce outlays to the
national AIDS program. On the contrary, funding increased; and the program's goals, including the establishment of sanatoriums, were preserved.
Many specialists argued that, in a time of economic upheaval, they could
do a better job of protecting the health of AIDS patients through prompt
diagnosis of opportunistic infections and through nutritional supple-
mentation if the patients were in residential facilities such as that run by
Dr. Pérez.

As those in charge of the Cuban AIDS program deliberated the merits of various approaches to AIDS education, they built new residential
units—air-conditioned, with color televisions—on the grounds. They
left the old hacienda intact. Interestingly enough, the ranch had been
owned before the Cuban revolution by a wealthy man who liked to
cross-dress. His portrait in drag remains prominently displayed in the

reception area of the older building. "Our patron saint," remarked Pérez, chuckling.[50] He no longer bristles over accusations of homophobia, most of which came from abroad. "I always saw myself as open-minded about matters of the heart, and although it would be some years before I made my slide saying 'All forms of love are valid' "—he referred here to a staple image from his traveling slide show—"I always knew that the job was to open up the facilities even as we opened up prejudiced minds."

Little did Pérez imagine that he would be branded as a violator of human rights and as the director of a series of "prison camps." "The U.S. media," notes historian Aviva Chomsky, "seized upon words like 'involuntary'; 'quarantine'; 'human rights violation'; 'totalitarian'; 'prison'; and 'rigid surveillance.' "[51] Pérez responded to these accusations with good humor, diligence, and ongoing commitment to the care of the patients. As one Cuban AIDS activist, himself gay and quite active in international AIDS organizing, remarked, "Jorge wins people over simply by being open and warm. They can see he cares about people living with HIV."

But the accusations rankled, especially when it seemed as if, in the Caribbean region, Cuba alone was having success in containing HIV and in protecting the social and economic rights of the vulnerable.[52] Cuban health officials fought back, sometimes underlining the hypocrisy inherent in these critiques. In 1989, for example, Vice-Minister of Public Health Héctor Terry Molinert emphasized the differences between the Cuban AIDS situation and the one in the United States:

> In Cuba, nobody lacks economic resources because of being an AIDS carrier. In Cuba, no one dies abandoned on the streets for lack of access to a hospital. In Cuba, we haven't had to open hospices so that patients who have been abandoned have a place to die in peace. In Cuba, no one's house has been set on fire because its inhabitants are people with AIDS. In Cuba, no homosexual has been persecuted because he's assumed to be likely to spread the virus. In Cuba, we don't have the problem of national minorities or drug addicts with high rates of AIDS.[53]

Although Jorge Pérez immediately went about transforming the sanatorium approach to one in which a patient could choose ambulatory versus residential treatment, he is quick to point out that there was little reason for sanctimony regarding the system he dismantled. "Those who accuse us of having had bad AIDS prevention policies lack humility," he remarked in 1997, when I interviewed him. "It's not as if it is clear which way is most effective. As far as I can see, we have done a pretty good job of educating the population and in containing HIV. We have done it while taking good care of people living with HIV. This is more than most countries can say."

By 1993, Pérez had made residential treatment optional. Initially, most people living in the sanatoriums chose to remain there. Living conditions were better, certainly, than the situation faced by most of the Cuban poor, who could not count on access to many of the amenities available in facilities like Santiago de las Vegas. Jesús Valle was still there in 1997, deploring the U.S. embargo, which he knew was making it difficult for his doctors to acquire medicines that might help him: "Even if the U.S. government rails against the Cuban government for political reasons, it's not as if we're guilty. We're only people. We're sick, and we want to live, to have access to medicines. We want to die knowing that our efforts were not in vain."

By January 2001, when I last visited, more modern housing had gone up within the facility. As in previous years, the chief problem remained the irregular supply of antiretroviral medications, a problem that both patients and staff blamed on the U.S. embargo. "There's a long waiting list to get in here," said Pérez, as we walked through the well-tended grounds. Eduardo Campo had chosen to remain at Santiago, and his wife was there with him. "It's easier here," he said. "If they find better drugs, I'll be close by." Jesús was no longer living in Santiago de las Vegas, Eduardo reported, but was in another facility run by the AIDS program.

AIDS AND THE POLITICS OF EMBARGO, QUARANTINE, AND DETENTION

In the end, Santiago de las Vegas was no more a "prison camp" than Guantánamo was an "oasis" for Haitian refugees. The whole sorry tale could be summed up several ways, but here's one reading: in 1991, on a military base beyond the rule of law, the world's only remaining superpower simultaneously engaged in and denied officially sanctioned violations of the rights of HIV-positive Haitian refugees. The same newspaper that termed this U.S. military base an "oasis" for Haitians readily printed highly critical assessments of Cuba's sanatoriums.[54]

Is such hypocrisy rare? Stories about Cuban medicine and human rights are often difficult to decipher, regardless of provenance. When Cuban health officials approached recrudescent dengue with the same fervor they used in attacking HIV, they engaged the military and the national guard in an effort to exterminate the mosquitoes involved in transmitting dengue. The effort was praised by the World Health Organization—whose Director General declared that the "strategy defined by the

Cuban government is highly valid, and I am sure that it will be crowned by success"[55]—but excoriated in the U.S. press. I happened to be in Havana when *Science* ran a blurb quoting an official from the U.S. Centers for Disease Control: "The problem with the Cuban program and those that rely on a paramilitary type of organizational structure is they have no sustainability."[56] When the Bolivian military engaged in a similar effort some years later, the *Lancet* hailed it as innovative: the Ministry of National Defense was offering "a valuable complement to the assistance offered by the national health services." The article praised "a novel methodology which relies on the association of medical-to-military terminology. Thus, the terms 'frontier,' 'enemy,' 'territory,' 'defences,' 'attack,' 'ammunition,' 'offensive,' and so on are adapted to health problems....Role-playing and practical work are important teaching approaches."[57]

The point is that understanding the complexities of AIDS and quarantine requires wading through a swamp of ideology. Just as U.S. detention of HIV-positive Haitian refugees was in keeping with longstanding and discriminatory policies toward Haitians, so too was Cuba's AIDS program completely in keeping with Cuban approaches to infectious diseases, as more scholarly assessments invariably agreed. But although U.S. treatment of Haitian detainees occurred in defiance of both U.S. and international laws, no Cuban or international laws were violated by Cuba's Ministry of Public Health when it advanced its controversial AIDS program. Whether or not Cuba's program stands the test of time remains to be seen, but such policies—including mandatory testing and any sort of sanatorium placement—should not be advocated in the United States, because of the great potential for abuses. This, in turn, stems from lack of a true commitment to equity, allowing people to be readily and officially "discriminated against" along lines of race, class, nationality, gender, and sexual preference. Simply put, *America Needs Human Rights,* as the title of a book by Anuradha Mittal and Peter Rosset notes:

> It is a systematic and widespread violation of the most basic of human rights for so many to go without, amid so much plenty. Human rights are the birthright of everyone: no one has the right to deny them, and everyone has the right to fight for their own rights. A human rights perspective builds on the civil and women's rights struggles that came before, and extends them into the "food, shelter, and jobs" arena of economics.[58]

The promotion of equity—and thus of social and economic rights—is the central ingredient for respecting human rights in health care. At the close of June 2000, the World Health Organization released an assessment of the health care systems of all member states. The evaluation relied on several indicators, including quality of health services; overall level of health; health disparities; and the nature of health system financing. Of all 191 member states, the United States spent the highest portion of its gross domestic product (GDP) on health—but ranked only thirty-seventh in terms of overall performance. Tiny Cuba, spending a smaller portion of its GDP, was ranked at roughly the same level as the United States and was one of the four highest-ranked countries in Latin America. (It is notable that the other countries with high indicators are either industrialized or have long histories of social-democratic government and universal health care.) As for "fairest mechanism of health system financing," Cuba was the number one nation in Latin America; the United States did not even figure in the top fifty in this category.[59] Clearly, it has been hard to see this from within the United States, where there is an embargo on honest assessment of Cuba's health programs.

Perhaps the best place from which to view Cuba is within the borders of its other neighbor, where I sit as I write this. Although popular conceptions in the United States sometimes underscore similarities between Haiti and Cuba—one generates boat people, the other *balseros*—a starker contrast could not be found within this hemisphere. The countries have some similarities: less than one hundred miles apart, the two islands have identical climates and topography. From the end of the fifteenth to the early nineteenth century, these two countries had a great deal in common: both were colonized (and later struggled over) by European powers; both constituted the final port of call for large numbers of African slaves; both were plantation economies during these centuries. But their histories diverged sharply in more recent times. Like Haiti, Cuba has known major economic disruption in the past decade. The impact on Cuba of the breakup of the Soviet Union, which contained its major trading partners, has been much commented upon. The Miami papers were full of predictions of the imminent fall of Castro and the end of communism in Cuba. But in fact Cuba, unlike Haiti or Chiapas or Peru, has not experienced significant unrest or political violence in decades.

The Cuban economy, however, did sustain major blows. I'm no economist—and it is even more difficult to wade through the reigning ideology in economics than it is in public health—but reports suggest a net loss, between 1989 and 1994, of the majority of all Cuba's foreign trade. This was as severe a contraction as that faced by any Latin American economy. What impact did this have on the health of the

Cuban poor? Was the story the same as in Haiti (or Peru or Chiapas), where economic turmoil led to immediate and adverse effects on the health of the population? The short answer: no.[60] In fact, although much is made of the U.S. embargo's adverse impact on Cuban health, the Cuban people remain healthy. Even epidemic optic neuropathy, locally and internationally attributed to vitamin deficiency, was more likely caused by an as yet unidentified viral pathogen.[61] The hemisphere is full of "mineshaft canaries"—populations far more vulnerable to nutritional deficiencies than even the poorest Cubans—and they would have presented with optic neuropathy well before the Cubans, if indeed vitamin deficiencies had been the cause. That much seemed obvious from Haiti.

In fact, overall morbidity and mortality trends showed little if any change during what was termed locally the "special period." One reason—and there are no doubt several—is that in Cuba health spending increased during the "special period," in order to buffer the vulnerable from adverse health outcomes. Between 1990 and 1997, health spending increased in both absolute and relative terms, growing from 6.6 to 10.9 percent of government outlays.[62]

Some years ago I turned, with fascination and a bit of dread, to comparing these two neighbors. Haiti has the highest rate of maternal mortality in the hemisphere; Cuba, one of the lowest. Haiti has the highest infant mortality rate in the hemisphere; Cuba, the lowest. In fact, infant mortality in the Mission Hill neighborhood, merely yards from the front door of the Brigham and Women's Hospital in Boston, compares unfavorably to rates in Cuba.[63] The leading killers of young adults in Haiti are HIV and tuberculosis; Cuba has the lowest prevalence of HIV in the hemisphere and remarkably little tuberculosis. Typhoid, measles, diphtheria, dysentery, polio, malaria, and most other parasitic infestations—all are common in Haiti and almost unknown in Cuba. And so on. There's a saying in Cuba: "We live like poor people, but we die like rich people."

In Haiti, as in Chiapas and the slums of Lima, poor people live and die like poor people. They die of preventable or treatable infections, and of violence. Why, then, do Cubans leave Cuba? One reason is probably that poor people not only want to die like rich people, they want to live like them, too. This is for me a philosophical question rather than a medical one. I have not interviewed poor people who die of the diseases that end affluent lives in their eighth decade. The people who crowd our waiting rooms here in Haiti do not have such expectations; they do not have such life expectancies.

Thinking of Haiti's boat people and of their miserable experience on Guantánamo brings back more recent memories of Elián González—the story of the decade, as far as immigration cases go. I have only to close my eyes to see the iconic photo of the boy in a striped shirt emblazoned on billboards in both Miami and Havana. The newspapers of both countries ran countless stories. The U.S. presidential candidates, goaded by the curiously influential Cuban American lobby in south Florida, were forced to comment on the case.

I was in Havana in January 2000. Huge demonstrations assembled in front of the U.S. consulate—rather cheerful-looking matrons seemed to dominate the crowds. In the Cuban press, caricaturists made direct references to Haitian refugees. One cartoon caught my attention: in it, a boy wearing Elián González's shirt and about his size is standing on a dock. Unlike Elián, this boy is black. On the horizon, an unseaworthy vessel with tattered sails is arriving from Haiti. The boy has been brought before an INS official, who is obese and mean-looking. Inspecting the boy, the official is speaking to two companions: one is a famous anti-Castro Cuban American, and the other looks a lot like the Statue of Liberty. "Let's throw that one back in," says the INS official. "He's Haitian: can't make any money off of him."

Even certain U.S. officials had to concede that the ironies of the differential treatment accorded Haitians and Cubans were painful. Speaking of six-year-old Sophonie Telcy, an orphan subject to deportation at any time, one U.S. representative observed that her "situation is far worse than Elián's. She has no family in Haiti, and the government there has no policy for dealing with orphans. She could end up living on the street if she has to go back."[64] In an editorial entitled "Haitian Orphan's Story Draws No Crowds," Adrian Walker writes that "Sophonie Telcy has no cheering sections outside the home of her guardians, no television crews, and no celebrities forming a human chain on her behalf. No one has suggested that her presence on these shores constitutes a miracle."[65]

Perhaps the Elián González story will help to expose some of the hypocrisy surrounding both our policies toward Cuba and our attitudes and policies regarding Haitians. The idea that the González child would have his rights violated by returning to Cuba with his father is laughable, especially if one regards social and economic rights as important to child welfare. Harvard historian John Coatsworth put it trenchantly:

In Cuba, Elián will have his father and the rest of his immediate family, a decent standard of living, free public education through university, cradle to grave medical care, and a relatively crime-free environment. His life expectancy will be about what he could expect in Miami (73 years). His chances of getting into college will be a bit lower. The likelihood of being assaulted, robbed, or murdered substantially less.

In short, Elián's chances in Fidel Castro's Cuba appear to be infinitely better than in most of the developing world. Better than in most places—like Haiti, for example—to which U.S. authorities routinely deport undocumented immigrants and their children. In Haiti, one out of eight children dies before the age of 5 and nearly half have no school to go to. Malnutrition and violence are endemic and male life expectancy at birth is 51 years.[66]

Is a U.S. blockade against Cuba legitimate on human rights grounds?[67] The experience of Haitian refugees on Guantánamo reminds us that the U.S. government's actions against people living with HIV have been far less honorable than the actions of the Cubans. Although the human rights community recognizes this, it is always slow to denounce the actions of the United States. At the height of the Haitian refugee crisis, the United Nations High Commissioner for Refugees could make feeble protests but was not about to take the UN's most powerful pot to task for calling the outcast kettle black. As the Haitians say, *ravet p'ap ka gen rezon devan poul:* a cockroach can never be right when in the presence of a hungry chicken.

—January 2001

POSTSCRIPT: MAY 23, 2002

Of all the chapters in this book, this one proves the most painful to update. Not that there isn't news: the events chronicled here have their own impetus, as they're fueled by powerful interests and structures long in place. Painful, rather, because I write about Haiti, my home, and consider all that might have been good. So much is reduced, like Haiti's once-verdant hillsides, to ash and dust.

But not all the news is bad in considering the fates of those whose stories were told here. Jesús and Eduardo and most other Cuban patients are faring well, and now all have access to antiretroviral therapy. Dr. Jorge Pérez remains director of Cuba's national AIDS program and medical director of Havana's leading infectious-disease facility, although he has passed on supervision of Santiago de las Vegas to one of his younger colleagues. Yolande Jean, having escaped the "oasis" that was Guantánamo, is faring well almost a decade after the awful events she reported. She was eventually reunited with her sons: they are now sturdy teenagers and live in the New York area with their mother. Their father was never heard from again. Guantánamo itself, however, is once again teeming with prisoners: this time, with men captured in Afghanistan and alleged to be al-Qaeda terrorists. Journalists' access to the U.S. base is again sharply restricted.[68]

Some of the authors of the crimes committed against Yolande and her family, and against thousands of others, have been brought to justice in Haiti. Although a biased U.S. press and even certain human rights organizations are beginning to say, with great and unwarranted authority, that Haitians live with a government that operates with the same impunity they knew during the Duvalier and military dictatorships, this is simply not true. Horrible poverty is difficult to police. Underpaid and undertrained police are themselves difficult to police. But it is no longer the government itself that persecutes the poor and vulnerable.

Indeed, landmark human rights trials have taken place recently in Haiti, a first. The most important of these occurred in Gonaïves, once famous as the place where Haiti's declaration of independence was signed, after the slaves' decisive 1803 victory over Napoléon's forces. The decrepit seaport later became famous—during the same military dictatorship that persecuted Yolande Jean—for accepting a shipload of toxic waste that had originated in Philadelphia. The City of Brotherly Love had a hard time ridding itself of its glowing dreck, and so the garbage sailed the high seas for over a year, until the right combination of bribes and lawlessness brought it to port not far from a dusty Haitian slum called Raboteau.

Raboteau, being a poor neighborhood of fishermen and scrap dealers, was of course a stronghold of Aristide supporters. Shortly after the coup of September 30, 1991—the event that led Yolande Jean and hundreds of thousands to flee their homes—the citizenry of Raboteau organized peaceful protests. Thousands marched in the unpaved streets. The marchers were not happy about the toxic refuse from Philadelphia, not a bit. But their greatest grievance was the overthrow of their country's first democratically elected government.

During the first years of military rule, groups organized themselves as best they could against the growing power of paramilitary bands. By 1994, much of this resistance had been pushed underground, but activists in Raboteau continued to confront the dictatorship publicly. As Colin Granderson, then head of the United Nations/Organization of American States human rights mission to Haiti testified, Raboteau kept the flame of democracy burning for the rest of Haiti. The army, aware of the practical and symbolic importance of the flame, was determined to extinguish it.

On April 18, 1994, the army sought to arrest the young leadership of the Raboteau resistance. Others got in the way and paid the price: one elderly blind man was badly beaten and died the next day. This, however, was said to be but a "rehearsal" for the real strike that was to come. The massacre perpetrated in the ensuing days was orchestrated by high-ranking officers in the Haitian army:

> The main attack started before dawn on April 22. Army troops and para-militaries approached Raboteau from several angles and started shooting. They charged into houses, breaking down doors, stealing and destroying possessions. They terrorized the occupants. Young and old, men, women, and children were threatened, beaten, forced to lie in open sewers and arrested. The onslaught forced many to take the familiar route to the harbor, but this time an armed ambush awaited them. Many were killed; some were wounded, on the beach, in the water, and in boats. Some were arrested, imprisoned, and tortured. One girl shot in the leg had to flee the hospital the next day, and another hospital a few days later when soldiers came looking for her.[69]

The death toll is hard to ascertain, for many of the bodies were washed out to sea; others, buried in shallow graves, were disinterred and consumed by pigs and dogs. But local estimates went no lower than dozens.

Finding evidence was impossible until well after the military high command left Haiti in October 1994. The Aristide government—following the examples of South Africa, Chile, and Argentina—then formed a "truth commission," and Raboteau was one of its major investigations. Even given the lost year between crime and investigation, the prosecution was able to prepare dossiers—"sufficiently documented to present to the jury"[70]—on eight of the people killed that day. The prosecution brought these charges not only against the local perpetrators—twenty-two soldiers and paramilitary—but also against their commanders. Thirty-seven, including the entire high command of the Haitian army, were tried *in absentia*.

In a surprising and unprecedented example of comeuppance, the members of the military and paramilitary who had conducted the raid were brought to trial in the city of Gonaïves itself. It took five years of pre-trial proceedings before the trial commenced. The problem was not that people were afraid to testify. Indeed, thirty-four eyewitnesses offered, during the course of the trial, "highly consistent [accounts], corroborated by expert testimony."[71] Rather, the problem was that the Haitian judicial system had all but collapsed, as had its physical infrastructure, during the course of the Duvalier and military dictatorships. "The old Gonaïves courthouse had no electricity, telephone, or toilet. During slow trials one could observe the appeals court through the floorboards."[72]

The trial took six weeks, from September 28 to November 10, 2000, and was covered by the local radio and television. There was enormous interest because nothing of the sort had ever happened before in Haiti. The jury delivered guilty verdicts for sixteen of the twenty-two accused and convicted, *in absentia,* all members of the Haitian high command, including many who had benefited from training in the United States. From their hiding places in the United States, Panama, and the Dominican Republic, the self-promoted generals and colonels were nonetheless a palpable presence in Gonaïves, like the rank dust that hangs over the city most of the time.[73]

The process of collecting evidence was slow, certainly, and the trial was at times raucous; but local and international jurisprudence experts agreed that it was a marvelously successful strike against impunity. All agreed that the trial rose to international standards and was fundamentally fair to victims and defendants alike. Lawyer Brian Concannon, one of the leading figures at the trial, argued that "the Raboteau trial should also serve as a model, and an inspiration, for efforts to combat impunity around the world. The dedication of the victims, and the Haitian government's persistence and innovation in trying new approaches, are transferable to many situations."[74]

In convicting the high command, the trial also inculpated by association their benefactors abroad. The transnational mechanisms of structural violence were exposed clearly. Perhaps for this reason, as much as any other, the Raboteau trial went largely unnoticed in the U.S. and foreign press, which instead ran story after story about how hopeless Haiti's judicial and police systems were—as if decades of corruption and U.S. pressure to incorporate former soldiers into the police force could be erased in a few years. (At the same time, serious reform efforts were implemented: one of Aristide's first moves on returning to Haiti was to disband the army and to integrate the police force with women.)

And another note of caution was sounded by the United Nations Independent Expert on Haiti. Adama Dieng noted that the "Haitian justice system must continue to pursue those convicted in absentia" and called on "countries where the fugitives may be found, especially Panama, the United States, Honduras, and the Dominican Republic, [to] cooperate with Haitian authorities to arrest and extradite them."[75]

Alas, these countries did not cooperate willingly with Haitian authorities. Haiti was increasingly isolated from other Latin American countries that were harboring the coup-prone generals, sometimes at the behest of the United States. The United States refused to release a large cache of 160,000 pages of relevant information, even though the Haitian government, a host of human rights groups, and members of the U.S. Congress had called on the United States to see these documents returned to Haiti. After a decade spent studying twenty "truth commissions" around the world, Priscilla Hayner observes that "the Haitian case is perhaps the worst example of a foreign power blocking a state's access to its own truth."[76] Her study is worth citing at length:

> When U.S. forces invaded Haiti in the fall of 1994, they drove trucks straight to the offices of the armed forces and the brutal paramilitary group, the Front for Haitian Advancement and Progress (FRAPH), hauling away documents, photos, videos, and other material that contained extensive evidence of the egregious abuses of these forces, including gruesome "trophy photos" of FRAPH victims. Some foreign rights advocates in Haiti who came into possession of some of this material also handed it over to U.S. troops, relieved that it would be in safer hands. "There wasn't a photocopier working in the entire country, so you couldn't make copies of things, and in the chaos of the moment nowhere else was secure," one person told me. But everyone assumed the material would be returned to Haiti when things settled down. On the contrary, none of these approximately 160,000 pages of documents, photographs, videotapes, or audiotapes have been released by the United States back to the country to which they belong. They remain in U.S. government hands, under the control of the Department of Defense. The assumed reason for this intransigence is not flattering: the United States provided direct support to some of those directly implicated in abuses, paying key FRAPH leaders as intelligence sources, and these documents would almost certainly reveal these connections and the complicity of the U.S. government in supporting known thugs. The United States eventually offered to return the documents only if the Haitian government would agree to restrictions on the use of the material, and after certain portions were blacked out, but the Haitians refused these conditions. Despite formal requests to the U.S. government for access to the documents, the Haitian truth commission completed its work, and a number of important trials have gone forward, without the benefit of any of this damning documentary evidence.[77]

The Haitian government was anxious to obtain these files and also to prevent the generals and colonels from preparing coups from abroad. A long legal struggle, with broad international grassroots support, led to recovery of the documents in January 2001. In addition, as the result of pressure from Haiti and others, including Amnesty International–U.S.A., two members of the high command have been ordered deported from the United States and are in INS custody. Colonels Hebert Valmond, the head of intelligence in the high command, and Carl Dorélien, head of personnel, were both convicted of murder in the Raboteau case. They fled to Florida, apparently a haven from democracy, when constitutional rule was restored in Haiti. Both are appealing recent deportation orders.[78] Emmanuel "Toto" Constant, the founder of FRAPH, is still living as a free man in Queens, New York, despite a 1995 deportation order. U.S. officials admit that Constant was paid by the CIA and discussed his paramilitary activities with the agency. He now remains under an order of deportation, although it has been delayed under State Department advisement.[79]

The Haitian government is concerned about such individuals, and with good reason. In the past several months, former Haitian military officers have staged coup attempts from the Dominican Republic and perhaps from other countries. In July 2001, five police officers were killed in the line of duty in the town closest to our clinic. On December 17, 2001, a more ambitious effort succeeded in penetrating the presidential palace and in assaulting Aristide's residence. And even when they fall short of their mission, such attempts are not wholly unsuccessful, since their goal is to complement "political" efforts to discredit and destabilize the elected government.[80]

The main political opposition is a motley group called, without irony, the "Convergence Démocratique." Although it consists mostly of right-wingers, its leadership is all over the map politically.[81] The Convergence is, however, united in its unswerving opposition to Aristide and to the right of the poor majority to have a say in Haiti's affairs. The level of support for those who came to constitute the Convergence, as gauged by polls, has run between 4 and 12 percent.[82] (Remember, Aristide won 93 percent of the vote in the November 2000 elections.) It is the "intelligentsia" of the Convergence who come up with cockamamie stories about how each coup against Aristide is really a sham authored by himself, accusations that echo their comments (the *classe politique* includes the same cast of characters as in previous decades) regarding the attempts on Aristide's life in the 1980s.[83]

Although the Convergence has scant popular support within Haiti, it clearly has support in Washington. The Convergence is funded, at least in part, by the U.S. International Republican Institute, which is associated, to no one's surprise, with the U.S. Republican Party[84] and obtains funding from Congress through the National Endowment for

Democracy.[85] In this sense, then, Haitians do experience impunity, but it comes from the U.S. government, not from their own.

The Haitian government has recently joined Cuba as one of the only republics in the hemisphere under a U.S. aid embargo. Trumped-up charges regarding the proper methods of tallying ballots during the May 2000 legislative elections are the avowed reason for this embargo, which extends even to loans already approved for improving health care and education. Ironically, charges of election irregularities were being leveled against the Haitian government at the same time as serious allegations concerning the U.S. electoral process, most notably in Florida, were being investigated.

Are there credible claims, for example, that Aristide didn't win fair and square? No, the complaints this time are about the legislative elections that took place in May 2000, months before Aristide was reelected by yet another landslide. Critics seeking to impugn the elections that delivered a massive victory for the party associated with Aristide argued that vote counting was not performed correctly for eight senatorial seats. So, presto, official foreign aid to Haiti—necessary to rebuild the ravaged infrastructure—was frozen by fiat.

The Haitian government then followed all the stipulations of a series of accords advanced by the Organization of American States in June 2001: the seven senators involved (one of the seats had already expired, and that election was rerun) not only agreed to run-offs with their second-place challengers but also resigned so that new elections could be held. Nevertheless, the aid embargo remains, suggesting that perhaps the actual reason it was imposed was not really U.S. concern over local elections.

Those who study patterns of U.S. giving to Haiti and to other countries would be a bit suspicious. In the past, the U.S. government had little trouble running hundreds of millions of dollars through the Duvalier dictatorship. The United States was unstintingly generous to the post-Duvalier military, whose spectacular exploits included the torching of Aristide's church during mass. And even during the leaky, half-hearted embargo against the military regime that ousted Aristide (and was eventually found guilty of war crimes), the United States was providing training, on U.S. soil, to the officers of that very regime.

Suspicions about the real reasons behind the U.S. aid embargo against Haiti are only fanned when one looks elsewhere for examples of whether adherence to certain electoral procedures determines the flow of U.S. aid. Take Pakistan, which until recently was under a similar embargo, with some justification, since General Pervez Musharraf came to power in a military coup. "My personal objective when I got here in August," U.S.

Ambassador Chamberlin said in a November 2001 interview, "was to work very hard to improve Pakistani-American relations, with the aim that at the end of my three years here we could lift American sanctions on Pakistan. I could never have dreamed that we'd have accomplished so much in my first three months."[86] The reason for the "accomplishments," of course, is clear: all the unpleasantries were quickly forgotten as of September 11, 2001, when new uses for Pakistan were found.[87]

The hypocrisy behind trade and aid sanctions has been noted by almost all neutral observers.[88] How does this hypocrisy play itself out among the poor? The impact of this aid embargo is far greater in Haiti than on the neighboring island of Cuba, with its healthy population. Cuban health indices are better than ever, in spite of the embargo; it's the Cuban economy that suffers. The current U.S.-sponsored embargo against Haiti, however, is targeting the most vulnerable population in the hemisphere. Its impact has been profound, as a report from the Inter-American Development Bank (IDB) is quick to note. In a recent report on Haiti, IDB officials write that "overall, the major factor behind economic stagnation is the withholding of both foreign grants and loans, associated with the international community's response to the critical political impasse. These funds are estimated at over US$500 million."[89]

The IDB should know, for it is among the institutions punishing Haiti. U.S. Congresswoman Barbara Lee made the following statement in recent weeks:

> The U.S. has used its veto powers on the IDB's Board of Directors to stop all loans designated to Haiti and has chilled funding opportunities at the other financial institutions, like the World Bank and IMF, pending a resolution of the political situation in Haiti. This situation is unique because the loans in question have been approved by the bank's board of executive directors, and the Haitian Government has ratified the debt and signed contractual documents.
>   This veto is particularly disturbing since the charter of the IDB specifically states that the Bank shall not intervene in the politics of its member states. The Bush Administration has decided to leverage political change in a member country by embargoing loans that the Bank has a contractual obligation to disburse.[90]

Take as a specific example Inter-American Development Bank Loan no. 1009/SF-HA, "Reorganization of the National Health System." On July 21, 1998, the Haitian government and the IDB signed a $22.5 million loan for Phase I of a project to "decentralize and reorganize" the Haitian health care system. The need to improve the health care system then, as now, was urgent: there are 1.2 doctors, 1.3 nurses, and 0.04 dentists per 10,000 Haitians; 40 percent of the population is without access to any form of primary health care; HIV and tuberculosis rates are by far the highest in the hemisphere, as are rates of infant, juvenile, and maternal mortality. To use its own jargon, the IDB project would target 80 percent of the population for access to primary health care through the construction of low-cost clinics and local health dispensaries. The funds would be used to train community health agents and to purchase medical equipment and essential medicines. To be judged successful by its own criteria, the project must lead to a drop in the infant mortality rate from 74 to 50 deaths per 1,000 live births; a drop in the juvenile mortality rate from 131 to 110 deaths per 1,000 births: a drop in the birth rate from 4.6 to 4; and a drop in the general mortality rate attributable to the lack of proper health care from 10.7 per 1,000 to 9.7 per 1,000. These were not overly ambitious goals. Most who evaluated the project thought it feasible and well designed.

So what's the holdup? In order for funds to be disbursed by the IDB, the loan agreement had to be ratified by the Haitian parliament. In October 1998, the Haitian Minister of Health presented the project to Haiti's famously obstructionist 46th Legislature, which included many people currently in the Democratic Convergence, soon to be voted out of office. For weeks, the parliament simply failed to meet. When it did meet, it failed to obtain a quorum. The goal was clear enough within Haiti: paralyze all social services, including health care, in order to undermine every effort of the executive branch, even then associated with Aristide, to improve the living conditions of the poor majority that had elected him by a landslide in 1990 and would do so again in November 2000. The Haitian people were well aware of the parliamentary gridlock, which is why they voted a straight ticket that supported the party associated with Aristide in the May 2000 parliamentary elections.

In October 2000, after the installation of the more representative 47th Legislature, the new parliament voted immediately to ratify the health project along with the three other vital IDB loan agreements. Still no money—but it was on the way, the Haitians were told. An official decree saying as much was published in the government's newspaper on January 8, 2001.

By early March 2001, the IDB had not yet disbursed the loan, but it announced that it intended to work with the new Aristide government, reelected a few months previously, and intended to finance projects already in the pipeline. It demanded, however, that a number of conditions be met, including a requirement that the government pay $5 million in arrears to the IDB. On May 15, 2001, notwithstanding the fact that not one penny of this or any other IDB loan had been disbursed, the IDB advised the Haitians that the government would be required to pay what it called a "credit commission" of 0.5 percent on the entire balance of undisbursed funds effective twelve months after the date on which the loans had been approved. As of March 31, 2001, then, Haiti already owed the IDB a $185,239.75 "commission fee" on a loan never received. The total amount of such fees owed on five development loans from the IDB, all taken out in previous decades, was $2,311,422. The IDB advised the government that payment must begin on September 15, 2001, with the balance due on October 5, 2001. In mid-May, amid rumors that the IDB was shutting down its offices in Haiti, the bank announced that the country representatives and top staff were being recalled to Washington "for consultations."

As of May 2002, the health loan has still not been disbursed. Even more disturbing is a recent Associated Press wire story titled "Haiti Clamors for Release of Blocked Loans That Might Take Years to Disburse." The chief IDB officer in Haiti called for the payment of "$20 million in loan arrears and reform [of government] economic practices" prior to access to credit. Many of the loans on which arrears are "owed" were, of course, made to the dictatorships and military juntas of past years. One educational loan may go through, but the IDB officer allowed that "if other new loans are not added, Haiti will probably be paying out more than it is getting."[91]

The loan details may seem pedestrian to an academic audience. They certainly would hold no great interest for me were it not for their direct and profound impact on the bodies of the vulnerable. Trust me, the details are of life-and-death significance.

The courtyard around our hospital remains overflowing. Over the past year, our general ambulatory clinic has seen an enormous increase in demand. We are staffed to receive about 35,000 visits per year but will this year see an estimated 160,000 patients. Meanwhile, visits to most neighboring facilities show them to have very few patients, because the services are too expensive for the destitute sick. We have registered a rise in trauma cases, in large part a result of road accidents. The sequelae of accidents are more serious, because patients are required to travel farther to receive care and because many require, but do not receive, the care of orthopedic and trauma surgeons. Malaria remains a major contributor to anemia and death and is, in our facility, the leading single diagnosis during the rainy season. Malaria deaths continue to occur, even though Haiti has not yet registered chloroquine-resistant cases: lack of access to care remains the primary problem, as noted in the initial IDB proposal, drafted years ago.

Polio, previously thought to have been eradicated from the Western hemisphere, has again resurfaced on the island.[92] Whether wild type or vaccine-related strain, polio virus will continue to spread if national vaccination efforts are not supported through Ministry of Health programs; national coverage is imperative. And we have documented outbreaks of anthrax, meningococcus, and drug-resistant tuberculosis. The degree to which these pathogens spread will be determined largely by the capacity of the public health system, rather than nongovernmental organizations, to respond. The Haitian Ministry of Health is anxious to serve the destitute sick, but, as in any other setting, funds are required to rebuild a shattered public health infrastructure.

Of course, claims of causality are always difficult to prove. But whether or not these conditions are caused by international policies, it is clear that aggressive humanitarian aid could have an immediate and salutary impact if it could be channeled through institutions with national reach. Increasingly, however, aid has been decreased or funneled to nongovernmental organizations that make largely local contributions. That our own hospital is overwhelmed is the "ethnographically visible" result of the embargo—and of a history of applying a much more generous line of credit to Haiti's dictatorships.

Many of the rural poor whom we see in our clinic are bitter about the current embargo, which they seem to regard as an attempt to bring down "their" government. One patient observed that "every time the Haitians try to organize our country so that everyone can eat, there is an embargo from the United States." When I asked which other embargos she had in mind, she replied, "From 1804 until the end of slavery in the United States. That's over fifty years, no?" She was right: the United States refused to recognize Haiti diplomatically until 1862. To quote a U.S. senator from South Carolina, speaking on the Senate floor in 1824, "The peace and safety of a large portion of our union forbids us even to discuss [it]."[93]

In a setting of enormous poverty, the funds invested in an anti-Aristide opposition have had significant impact. Most Haitians are surprised neither by the embargo nor by U.S. support for the opposition. These offenses square neatly with almost two centuries of foreign and local disdain for the Haitian poor. This is the view from central Haiti, a view almost never acknowledged by Haiti's elite, much less beyond the country's borders. But there were echoes of this view, finally, in an editorial in the *Miami Herald*:

Where else in the world does [the United States] deny sending crucial aid to a famished neighbor in spite of its underdeveloped political system? Haitians are well aware of Washington's game and are likening its freezing of desperately needed funds to the U.S. embargo imposed on Haiti after their 1804 revolution made the island the world's first black republic. Haiti needs help, not unmerited manipulation.[94]

Have Haiti's successes in persecuting human rights abusers and war criminals been obliterated by recent events? Certainly so, to judge by inches of type.[95] The epoch-making Raboteau trial went largely unnoticed outside Haiti. And the situation here continues to worsen. But the Haitian people have always managed to stand for something, even in the most difficult moments. I'll close with the words of human rights lawyer Brian Concannon:

This insistence on justice by the Haitian people and government is a lesson to the rest of the world, which almost always has more resources and less justice. Efforts by Chile to prosecute Pinochet are laudable, but come twenty-eight years after his crimes. The resources committed for the International Criminal Tribunal for Former Yugoslavia are impressive, but have produced half the convictions of the Raboteau trial. The key to Haiti's relative success, and its lesson to the rest of the world, is the government's acting on what the victims of Haiti, and of Chile and the Balkans, have always known: there is no reconciliation, there is no democracy, without justice.[96]

CHAPTER 3

LESSONS FROM CHIAPAS

As hard as concerned Americans have had to strain to understand the Zapatista revolt and its confusing and sorrowful aftermath, we will have to work harder to understand Mexican issues in the future. Our problem is not merely the media, or our notorious inability to learn another language. It is our entire evasive and mendacious culture, which (to the enormous profit of the megacompanies that feed it) makes our selfish decadence entertaining to us, sells us headsets that deafen us to crying injustices in our own country, and changes every real, complicated, painful struggle into a brief sensation of stars, or meteors, gloriously noble or wicked, always somehow erotically intriguing today, dead boring tomorrow. If in this culture we have to hide or fight to comprehend reality right here, we have to leave all that is familiar and comfortable to comprehend reality in Mexico.

John Womack Jr., *Rebellion in Chiapas*

I want there to be democracy, no more inequality—I am looking for a life worth living, liberation, just like God says.

José Pérez, twenty-four years old, Zapatista,
captured at Oxchuc, January 4, 1994

We have to shift our attention from an exclusive concentration on incomes and commodities (often used in economic analyses) to things that people have reason to value intrinsically. Incomes and commodities are valued mainly as "instruments"—as means to other ends. We desire them for what we can do with them; possessing commodities or income is not valuable in itself. Indeed, we seek income primarily for the help it might provide in leading a good life—a life we have reason to value.

Amartya Sen, 1995 Innocenti Lecture of UNICEF

On January 1, 1994, the world's attention was drawn to the Mexican state of Chiapas. Before dawn, masked rebels took over the administrative offices in San Cristóbal de las Casas, a small city nestled in the high limestone mesas of southern Mexico. The city takes its name from the famous "Protector of the Indians," Fray Bartolomé de Las Casas, who condemned the Spanish colonists for their brutal treatment of the native population. Las Casas accompanied Columbus on his third voyage to the New World, not as a priest but as an aspiring colonist. His experience on the island of Hispaniola, where he saw countless indigenous people die of imported infection, mistreatment, and outright slavery, led to his change of heart.[1] Although Las Casas is remembered less fondly in Haiti—some say he advised that Africans would be hardier slaves than the manifestly frail *indios*—the cleric is remembered in most of Latin America as an ardent defender of the rights of the hemisphere's indigenous population.[2]

After leaving Hispaniola, Las Casas the priest made his way from the Royal Court, where he petitioned Spain's rulers to recognize the "full humanity" of the Indians, to southern Mexico. In 1544, he was named bishop of San Cristóbal, at the time the chief administrative outpost of the Spanish Crown.

But, it would seem, his influence has faded: the ensuing centuries have not been kind to the indigenous people of Chiapas. Any visitor to the lovely city of San Cristóbal de las Casas is struck by the deep divide—manifest in speech, dress, and station—between the poorer *indígenas* and the European-featured elite. The 1994 uprising nonetheless took the latter group by surprise:

> Even in their most fretful nightmares of being overrun by the "Indiada" (the Indian hordes), the good burghers of San Cristóbal never believed this day would come. Now, at dawn in the center of their fortress city, the rebels raised their black flag with the red star and the letters "E," "Z," "L," "N," emblazoned upon the standard.[3]

Ejército Zapatista de Liberación Nacional. The Zapatista rebels—in large part both "Indian" and poor—took their name from Emiliano Zapata, the revolutionary who at the beginning of the twentieth century fought for the land rights of Mexico's poor *campesinos* and was executed for his trouble in 1919.[4]

The opening salvo of the modern Zapatistas' war of words was the Declaración de la Selva Lacandona (Declaration from the Lacandón Jungle), launched the night before the uprising from the dense highland forests of eastern Chiapas. On the radio station XOECH in Ocosingo, to the east of San Cristóbal and closer to the jungle, the Zapatistas declared:

> *¡Hoy decimos basta!* Today we say enough is enough! To the people of Mexico, Mexican brothers and sisters: We are a product of 500 years of struggle—first against slavery, then during the War of Independence against Spain led by insurgents, then to promulgate our constitution and expel the French empire from our soil, and later [when] the dictatorship of Porfirio Díaz denied us the just application of the Reform laws and the people rebelled and leaders like Villa and Zapata emerged, poor men just like us. We have been denied the most elemental education so that others can use us as cannon fodder and pillage the wealth of our country. They don't care that we have nothing, absolutely nothing, not even a roof over our heads, no land, no work, no health care, no food, and no education. Nor are we able freely and democratically to elect our political representatives, nor is there independence from foreigners, nor is there peace or justice for ourselves and our children.[5]

The Zapatista offensive, which targeted the town halls of San Cristóbal and six other cities and also an army barracks, was launched on the very day that the North American Free Trade Agreement (NAFTA) was signed.[6] The Mexican government responded, as one might expect, with fire: within days, clashes between army units and Zapatistas had left scores dead. But the rebellion was not so easily suppressed. First, the rebels' campaign had been years in the planning.[7] Second, the Zapatistas had generated considerable sympathy elsewhere in Mexico and, indeed, around the world. Their supporters had access to electronic mail, and their mysterious and mediagenic spokesman, Subcomandante Marcos, issued volley after volley of trenchant communiqués.[8]

I heard about the Zapatista uprising while in central Haiti. My own interest in Chiapas was intense, since Partners In Health had for many years supported a community health project there. Partners In Health, a nongovernmental organization, was created to remediate inequalities in access to modern medical care. With deep roots in Haiti, our group had no choice but to learn about the importance of social and economic rights—not simply access to health care but to education, housing, and clean water—as we watched the peasants we sought to serve struggle for these rights. From the mid-1980s on, Partners In Health has made common cause with poor communities in the United States, Siberia, Peru, Chiapas, and most of all in Haiti.

Haitians were also following the developments in southern Mexico with great interest, but for other reasons: the Caribbean nation was then trapped in the third year of a debilitating military coup. News from Chiapas was hard to come by in rural Haiti. The Haitian army had put all the independent radio stations out of commission—resorting, on one spectacular occasion, to a rocket launcher. And yet those Haitians who did learn of the Mexican rebellion seemed to take heart from it. A young Haitian in hiding declared that the Zapatistas "are just like us, except they have weapons." What U.S. press reports portrayed as yet more "ethnic strife" many Haitians recognized as a movement for social justice. Shortly after the rebellion began, I went to a mass in which the officiating Haitian priest described the Chiapas rebels as standing "at the forefront of the struggle for social justice."

Armed rebels were not part of the picture that a newly modernizing and globalizing Mexico, dominated for seventy years by the Institutional Revolutionary Party (PRI), wished to project. Subsequent investigation would show that the Mexican government had been aware of the planned rebellion for at least a year before the attack on the town halls.[9] Washington, it would seem, was also in the know.[10] Advisers to President Salinas de Gortari counseled against spectacular reprisals, arguing that a bloodbath would weaken confidence in NAFTA. But overt conflict in Chiapas continued until peace talks were initiated, on February 21, through the mediation of the Catholic Church. The Zapatistas designated the local bishop—Samuel Ruíz García, already regarded with suspicion by the Salinas government for his espousal of liberation theology—as an intermediary worthy of their trust. An uneasy truce was called.

But with so many just demands unmet, the Zapatistas refused to declare their campaign over. When Salinas promised a "conditional pardon" if the Zapatistas agreed to surrender, the rebels responded to the government's offer by suggesting that the government ask them for pardon instead. They added:

> Or should we ask pardon from the dead, our dead, those who die "natural" deaths of "natural causes" like measles, whooping cough, breakbone fever, cholera, typhoid, mononucleosis, tetanus, pneumonia, malaria, and other lovely gastrointestinal and lung diseases? Our dead, the majority dead, the democratically dead, dying from sorrow because no one did anything, because the dead, our dead, went just like that, without anyone even counting them, without anyone saying, "ENOUGH!" which would have at least given some meaning to their deaths, a meaning which no one ever sought for them, the forever dead, who are now dying again, but this time in order to live.[11]

Since the uprising, the Mexican government has greatly increased its military presence in Chiapas: up to seventy thousand troops have been stationed there, and new fortifications have been built. Human rights organizations have documented the effects not only of the militarization of the region but also of its "paramilitarization."[12] Armed groups known as *guardias blancas,* with close ties to the PRI and the police, have harassed peasant groups thought to be sympathetic to the Zapatistas and have also engaged in persistent persecution of the church and its local representatives.[13]

Anyone who knows Haiti would see a familiar pattern here. Years of struggle and dashed hopes exacted a great toll on the poor of Haiti. The chronic violence of Haiti in the 1990s wore people down. Although their spirits were lifted by the dissolution of the Haitian army in 1995 and the return of Haiti's democratically elected president, these victories were paid for dearly. By 1997, the popular movement that had brought to power a liberation theologian preaching justice for the poor seemed at its ebb.

Had three years of conflict in Chiapas been as hard for its most impoverished residents, the ones we'd been working with through Partners In Health? I hadn't been to Chiapas in almost four years. In mid-November 1997, I traveled there from central Haiti with this and other questions on my mind. In addition to the usual anxiety about our own friends' safety, I worried about reports of renewed violence in the regions where they were working. How had the violence affected our sister organization? What was the scale of this violence? Who was orchestrating it, and against whom was it directed?

MOISÉS GANDHI AND THE STRUGGLE FOR SOCIAL JUSTICE

The road to Moisés Gandhi leads through a heavily militarized zone; to reach the village, one must pass through a newly created army post, and then a buffer "peace camp" staffed by a couple of Europeans. Just beyond these two encampments is a small chapel named for Saint Francis of Assisi. Inside the church, you see some signs of the times: statues of Saint Francis, clippings about a recent Zapatista march, and posters decrying neoliberal economic policy. Our co-workers, all of them community health workers and most of them native Tzeltal speakers, were gathered here at the church to conduct a training session. The health workers had recently formed the Organización de Promotores de Salud Autónomos, Pluriétnicos Mayas de Chiapas (the Organization of Autonomous, Multiethnic Mayan Health Workers of Chiapas).

We had supported our sister organization's work in Chiapas well before the uprising, and we had not been surprised to learn that many of our friends were sympathetic to—or involved in—the rebellion. Indigenous and poor, they were landless and frequently sick. Two months earlier, Moisés Gandhi and the surrounding communities had declared themselves part of a new "autonomous zone"—El Municipio Rebelde Ernesto Che Guevara.[14]

I was traveling with Jody Heymann, a pediatrician long committed to the health of the region's poor and a board member of Partners In Health. When Jody and I arrived with Julio Quiñones Hernández, himself a health worker and community organizer, the training session at the church was well under way. Julio introduced us to about twenty health workers, who hailed from communities throughout the newly proclaimed *municipio*. In spite of the tensions (an army post stood intimidatingly near), they welcomed us warmly and with confidence: people knew and trusted Julio. He, in turn, had a deep, almost tender respect for what the health workers were trying to do. Like most village health workers in the poorer reaches of Chiapas, those gathered in the courtyard of St. Francis were also peasant farmers, men and women who worked the land in order to feed their families a meager harvest of corn and beans. I was thinking, of course, of the community health workers I knew in Haiti, who labored under similar conditions.

Soon we began participating actively in the training discussions. At first, our exchanges were focused on the material at hand. The subject of the session was "the use and abuse of medicines," and the health workers were interested in my and Jody's vision of the proper role of antibiotics and other medications.

Julio proved to be an energetic, talented teacher and facilitator. He and his co-workers in San Cristóbal, for example, had developed innovative and "culturally appropriate" training materials for a community in rebellion. Someone passed one of the illustrated workbooks to me. In the section on "Prices of Medicines," cartoons depicted sacks of money marked with the names of large pharmaceutical companies and the countries in which they were based—in most cases, the United States. We discussed the topic of generic medications in detail, along with the impact of drug-company advertising on prescribing practices. Because the autonomous community had just built a new "autonomous clinic," people evinced great interest in learning how to identify and acquire essential drugs.

Later, the talk turned informal. Over a meal of rice, beans, potatoes, and tortillas—since 1994, noted one of the participants, the men have to cook, too—the health workers told us their stories. Tomás was compact and hale, and his hands and arms bore the marks of hard labor. Unlike most of the men, he was bearded. He was unsure of his age—"I think I'm about fifty"—and was already a grandfather. He explained quietly that he, his father, and his grandfather had all "worked like slaves" on land that had been appropriated from his forebears. From the way Tomás spoke, it was clear that local interpretations of current events emerged directly from the region's troubled history. Past wounds were not forgotten; in Tomás's telling, even tribute obligations to the Spanish Crown still chafed (note that Mexico declared its independence from Spain in 1821). The anthropologist George Collier, who has spent three decades studying agrarian change in Chiapas and to whose understanding of these processes I am much indebted, underlines the need to "look at the bitter history of the indigenous people and their subjugation under the Spanish *conquistadores,* a legacy of injustice that continues to taint present-day relations between indigenous and non-indigenous Mexicans."[15]

But was the 1994 revolt only about respect for indigenous people? Our hosts spoke mostly about land, food, and social services, as had the Declaración de la Selva Lacandona, which, strikingly, mentioned health care even before food and education. Whether the oppressors were representatives of the Spanish Crown, the local elite, the ruling party of independent Mexico, or wealthy *indígenas,* the poor had always fared poorly. This account may sound ahistorical. But in reality Tomás was reminding us of the continuity of forces that had kept his people in poverty. Students of indigenous Maya "folklore"—and anthropology, certainly, has no shortage of them—have shown that many local stories of subjugation, epiphany, and liberation are, in fact, related to real events in the post-conquest period.[16] That history becomes paradigmatic of the long subjection of the local poor, regardless of ethnicity.

Their resentment of subjection had reached a boiling point, it would seem. The people of Moisés Gandhi spoke with spleen of the local landlords, many of whom, they said, lived in the nearby town of Ocosingo. "They treated us like animals," Tomás continued. "But since 1994, we have refused to work like that. We are still suffering, but we will no longer be treated like animals."

On many occasions, our hosts made the distinction between what life was like before 1994 and what it was like after the uprising, making it clear that the Zapatistas had opened up a new era in their own largely patient and long-suffering quest for dignity. The people of the *municipio* Che Guevara helped me make sense of the movement. They were calling their group of health workers "multiethnic" (*pluriétnicos*) to mark a departure from a past of ethnic strife, which had trammeled efforts to organize the rural poor. And they were speaking out more now than they had in decades.[17] "The government creates and foments divisions," they explained, taking particular advantage of an "unorganized peasantry." The only option, argued the health workers, was to organize their communities, to forge a new identity as full citizens. Said Tomás: "*Somos chiapanecos, somos mexicanos.*" And Juan, another leader, added: "*Estamos organizados.*"[18]

The Promotores de Salud Autónomos took organizing seriously, and their organization reached across boundaries of gender, ethnicity, and language. What bound them together was the experience of poverty and a lack of access to decent health care; they were bound, too, by their rejection of the government. In February 1997, ninety-one health workers from throughout Chiapas had gathered in the presence of fifteen organizations, including our own sister organization (represented by Julio and others) and the Diocese of San Cristóbal, to consider prospects for improving the health of the region's poor. At the end of the meeting, they issued the Declaration of Moisés Gandhi, which called for resistance to the Mexican government's plans for "normalizing" Chiapas. The "state of war," according to the declaration, made health work nearly impossible:

> Living and working conditions, already terrible, only become worse in this state of war. This war, which is not a public war declared by the government, is something very real in our communities, something permanent, and of "high intensity." Because every day, we have more dead and more bloodshed. Before, it was low intensity, but not now. They are killing community leaders and threatening priests: this is high intensity.[19]

Tomás, Juan, and others explained that they had repeatedly petitioned the federal government for basic public services and for an end to the militarization of their region, but their requests had gone unheard. In September 1997, they had joined other communities in declaring an autonomous government. A month later, paramilitary forces loyal to the PRI—*guardias blancas*—sacked and burned the administrative offices of the autonomy movement.

"CHIAPAS IS RICH, ITS PEOPLE ARE POOR"

During these conversations, a steady rain fell, turning the courtyard of St. Francis into mud. Darkness came quickly. Some of us bedded down in the church, stretching out on the floor or on the rough-hewn planks that constituted the pews. I asked some of the men about their families and heard more stories similar to Tomás's. The youngest of the men, eighteen-year-old Diego, had not said a word all day. (Most of the women had been quiet too.) Teasingly, I asked Diego why he was so silent. "He doesn't speak Spanish," explained another of the men. "He understands a good deal, but doesn't really speak it."

Chiapas is the only Mexican state in which more than 50 percent of the people identify themselves as indigenous.[20] Many of its people—the great majority in the eastern reaches of the state—are of Mayan descent. Like our Tzeltal hosts in Moisés Gandhi, their first languages are other than Spanish; like Diego, many of them, especially the women, don't speak Mexico's official tongue. Linguistic divides are just one index of the inequalities that characterize the state; it trails the rest of Mexico in almost every indicator. Its health indices are discouraging, as the Zapatistas repeatedly assert:

> Health? Capitalism leaves its mark: 1.5 million Chiapans have no medical services whatsoever. There are .2 clinics for every 1,000 people, five times less than the national average; there are .3 hospital beds for every 1,000 Chiapans, three times less than the rest of Mexico; there is one operating room for every 100,000 people, two times less than the rest of the country; there are .5 doctors and .4 nurses for every 1,000 population, two times less than the national average.[21]

Chiapans are also less likely to have access to clean water, electricity, and education than are Mexicans in general.[22] But, as one of the health workers in Moisés Gandhi observed, "It is not true that Chiapas is poor. Chiapas is rich in natural resources. It is the *people* of Chiapas who are poor."

This observation—Chiapas is rich; its people, poor—has become something of a slogan among the Zapatistas and their supporters. In a declaration made at the outset of the revolt, the Zapatistas observed that the region's poor bore a grotesque burden of treatable pathologies, many of them infectious diseases. They further argued that the government ignored these pathologies because such illnesses had ceased to afflict Mexicans who did not live in poverty—the sort of Mexicans for whom policy was designed and whose existence the media recognized. Other declarations noted that all of this misery was expanding right under the noses of tourists and other visitors to the region:

> The peace that some are now seeking was always war for us; it seems that the great lords of land, business, industry, and money are bothered that the Indians are going to die in the cities and stain the streets that until now

were dirtied only by the wrappings of imported products. They prefer that
the Indians continue to die in the mountains, far away from the good con-
sciences and tourists. It will not be like that anymore: the prosperity of the
few cannot be based on the poverty of the many. Now the comfortable will
have to share our fate, for better or worse. They had the chance before to
open their eyes and do something to stop the enormous historic injustice
that the country imposed on its original inhabitants, but they didn't see the
Indian as anything other than an anthropological object, a curiosity for
tourists, part of a "Jurassic Park" (is that how it's spelled?), which, luckily,
would disappear with a NAFTA that includes them only as disposable
waste, because the death of those in the mountains doesn't matter much.[23]

In addition to serving as picturesque natives for visitors to one of
Mexico's most beautiful regions, the people of Chiapas tilled the land
and tended livestock, again largely for the benefit of others. The Zapatistas denounced in no uncertain terms the use of locals as chattel.
Speaking of their relations with the landowners in Ocosingo and San
Cristóbal—"all *priistas*" (members of the PRI), according to our hosts—
Juan observed, "We are thought of as more lowly than oxen, but at least
they make sure that their livestock have basic medical care from a vet-
erinarian. They take better care of their pets." The people of the autonomous zones were tired of being Galeano's "nobodies"—people with
arms for working but no faces, people with "folklore" rather than culture. They were tired of playing the role of Mexico's chattel.

Scholars concur with this perception of exploitation. "Today," observes Collier, "Chiapas is almost an internal colony for the rest of Mexico, providing oil, electricity, timber, cattle, corn, sugar, coffee, and beans,
but receiving very little in return."[24] As our hosts in Moisés Gandhi had
explained, this internal colony had a long history, one they had not forgotten. When the Spanish arrived in the early sixteenth century, they
sniffed out and played on longstanding local enmities in order to advance
the conquest. In highland Chiapas, the Europeans found several indigenous groups. The largest of these were Tzotzils, living in towns such as
Zinacantán, close to present-day San Cristóbal, and Tzeltals, living closer
to Ocosingo. In part because of epidemics of imported disease, this first
contact with the Spanish ended in defeat for the indigenous population,
helpless against Europeans' hunger for gold and domination. But in 1524
uprisings against the Spanish began, and in 1527 a group of indigenous
people laid siege to the town of San Cristóbal. They failed, of course,
and the region's history has since been notable for the almost ceaseless

movements of its indigenous population. "Migration," notes historian John Womack, "is Chiapas's oldest story."[25]

Subsequent centuries were also marred by "Indian revolts," many ending in massacres of the natives, and the early twentieth century also had its rebellions, many of them launched in the name of land. But it was the Mexican Revolution that led to significant land reform. In his 1918 Manifesto to the Mexican People, Zapata—himself of Nahua descent—called for the revolution "to redeem the indigenous race, giving it back its lands and thereby its liberty; to convert the laborer in the fields, the present slave of the haciendas, into a man free and in control of his destiny through small property." The reforms of the Mexican Revolution, as codified in the constitution of 1917, were welcomed by the indigenous *campesinos* of Chiapas. Some received *ejido* lands, which were communally held; others—indigenous people toiling on ranches—benefited from constitutional reforms that abolished debt servitude.[26] This is one reason that the ruling party had been able to count on votes in Chiapas.[27]

The promise of land redistribution was welcome, certainly, but it is clear that in practice reforms most benefited certain strata of indigenous society, tightening relations between the ruling party and local *caciques*, or strongmen. Analysts of the Zapatista rebellion who assert that the "Mexican Revolution never reached Chiapas," or that it "came late," make a mistake, observes Womack: "The Revolution got to Chiapas about the same time, and about the same way, and with about the same limited results as in many other states."[28] The expected benefits did not reach the poor of Chiapas—that much is uncontested.

Many of the ranches the people of Moisés Gandhi described to us were holdovers from haciendas of colonial days. But as wheat and corn cultivation gave way to cattle, there was less need for labor, and the ranchers sought to push the indigenous *campesinos* off the more fertile land.[29] Many were forced into the highland canyons that became the bedrock communities of Zapatista support. But in most of these regions, even the most intensive subsistence farming could not support a growing peasant population.[30] Increasingly, indigenous people were forced to leave their communities to work coffee *fincas* on the fertile slopes of the Sierra Madre. Some continued to work as "debt slaves" on larger ranches. The term "slavery" and the expression "treated like animals" came up again and again in my visits to the autonomous zones. In the area referred to by Tomás, highland villagers were effectively peons and migrant laborers. Although the nature of labor arrangements has changed over the centuries—as tropical produce gave way to cattle, within ensuing displacements—the inequalities have remained constant. Of the landowners and burghers in question, Womack sums it up well:

> The new roads and the deal between the land-rich and labor-rich ladinos ruined many highland villagers. Soon most of them no longer had enough land to support themselves and owed the equivalent of 40 days' labor a year in taxes alone. The men had a choice: revolt with predictable consequences; migrate to try and farm elsewhere, but on any return to their communities risk jail or fines or overdue debt on unpaid taxes; or accept contracts from village elders that sanctioned advancing loans for a term of work in a logging camp or on the new plantations and farms in Soconusco or the central valley. A few went down to the jungle; fewer returned. Reasonably, most chose the migrant term down on the Pacific, an eight-day walk away. Migrant wages there then fell to the level of subsistence, which made a migrant's net income, after deductions, flimflam, and robbery along the way home, usually very little if anything, so that most migrants had to resubmit to exploitation year after year. Occasionally a critic complained of slavery. Ladinos would fly into righteous denials. They were right. There was no slavery (constitutionally forbidden), only annually recontracted debt peonage.[31]

By the middle of the twentieth century, a few thousand cattle-ranching families held more than three million hectares of land—about half the entire state. With the help of the *caciques,* the local landowners could readily raise small armed groups to keep unwanted Indians off "their" land. For decades, such *guardias blancas* have been a persistent feature of modern Chiapan society.

Whether these indigenous populations have "resisted Mexicanization" or whether they have been "left out of progress" remains a subject of debate. Though it is clear that conditions for the poor of Chiapas have always been miserable, a number of recent changes have conspired to make these conditions even less bearable—and also to permit the poor to bring their cause before a larger audience. The 1972 OPEC crisis ushered in Mexico's oil boom, and some of the oil came from Chiapas. Oil-led development was showy but fundamentally unstable, however, and left little money in the modernizing regions. When petroleum prices dropped in 1982, federal subsidies for both corn and coffee—already called into question during the talks leading to neoliberal trade agreements such as NAFTA—were dropped. These "adjustments" were demanded by Mexico's chief creditor and trading partner, the United States. Cheap corn from the U.S. heartlands poured into Mexico; Chiapas, home to only 3 percent of the nation's population but supplier of 13 percent of its corn, felt this shift keenly. In 1989, the bottom fell out of the world coffee market, with devastating effects on the small producers in the highlands.[32] Although the most vulnerable Chiapans were rendered even more vulnerable by many of these changes, others benefited from them, leading to rising social inequality on a local level. Observes Collier:

> Among the indigenous peasants I know, I saw a gap grow ever wider between the wealthy, who were able to infuse their farming with cash derived from wage work near oil fields, on dam projects, and in urban construction projects, and the poor, who are finding it increasingly impossible to be able to afford to farm even their own land.[33]

Some believe that the coup de grâce came in 1992, when President Salinas de Gortari officially halted land reform. Chiapas, with 25 percent of the country's pending land reform cases, headed the list of states awaiting distribution of land: fully 78 percent of designated *ejido* lands had not yet been divided into parcels. Subcomandante Marcos put it this way: "Salinas de Gortari arrived on the scene with his lackeys and his groups, and in a flash they destroyed [land reform]. We and our families have been sold down the river."[34] At the same time, the Mexican stock market boomed, and television and tourism brought conspicuous displays of wealth deeper into Chiapas. Although one hears much talk about the "Mexican bailout" by the United States, Mexico is not purely a poor country: rather, it has become one of the world's largest producers of new billionaires—mainly as a consequence of upward redistribution.[35] The declining fortunes of the indigenous peoples led to work migration—people going to Cancún, for example, in search of work building condos and hotels—and a growing resentment of longstanding and ever more visible inequalities.

All these national developments reflected shifts in the global economy. As Mexico was integrated into the modern world economy, a substantial segment of its population was excluded from the benefits of development, while they continued to pay development's price—not only through taxes and labor but also through an erosion of their own cultures. The ensuing loss of social solidarity has been much commented upon by the anthropologists and others who work in highland Chiapas.[36]

This is the situation into which news of the North American Free Trade agreement came. Was the Zapatista insurrection a rebellion against neoliberal trade policies, or was it a rebellion dominated by Mayan ethnic consciousness, pitting itself against wholesale Mexicanization? NAFTA is only one of the forces at work shaping the many intersecting and shifting identities available to the region's poor. They could see themselves as in-

digenous Chiapans, as Mayas (or other "Indians"), or as Mexican
campesinos.[37] Thus out of the confused swirl of *indigenismo* came a growing identification as the poor of Chiapas—the heirs of Zapata. Collier, who
has lived among the Zinacantecos for thirty years, is skeptical of those who
see the uprising as a Mayan movement: "Indigenous people who have responded to the Zapatista calling have done so primarily because they see
justice in the Zapatistas' political and economic demands on behalf of the
countryside's poor."[38] Like the villagers and health care workers cited here,
Collier sees the Zapatistas primarily as a movement for social justice:

> In contrast to some analysts, I posit that it is primarily a peasant rebellion,
> not an exclusively Indian rebellion, because although the Zapatistas are
> demanding rights for indigenous peoples, they are first and foremost calling
> attention to the plight of Mexico's rural poor and peasants, both indige-
> nous and non-indigenous.[39]

FROM OPTION FOR THE RICH TO OPTION FOR THE POOR

Liberation theology has clearly played a role in shaping identity in the context of the Chiapas uprisings. For decades, many Catholic catechists have
argued that although the region's poor were originally from many different groups, what they now had in common was their poverty. It was this
identification Tomás had in mind when he observed, *Somos chiapanecos,
somos mexicanos.* As we were meeting on parish property but also right
behind a sign that named the region El Municipio Rebelde Ernesto Che
Guevara, I asked our hosts about the role of the church in their struggle.

Blanca, who had said little during our discussion of land reform, grew
animated. "At least here," she said, referring to the diocese, "the church
is much more supportive of our struggle than any branch of government.
Some of the priests and nuns have been persecuted for our sake." The
other *promotores* nodded their agreement, sharing with us a news release, written a few days earlier, that denounced the persecution of
church activists in towns such as Tila, in the northern zone of Chiapas.
Their bottom line: "The church is on our side."

It has not always been so. During his tenure as bishop, Las Casas
worked to curb the murderous excesses of the *conquistadores,* but his
and subsequent centuries each had their ways of extracting wealth from
this "rich but poor" area. Sometimes the church provided a buffer for
the Indians against the worst depredations of the ruling groups, protecting, for example, indigenous land rights. But, as elsewhere in Latin
America, the colonizing church did not always seek to disturb the status

quo. As one early (and exceptional) bishop of Michoacán put it, "It would seem that the Spanish brought Christ to America in order to crucify the Indian."[40] After the Mexican Revolution, the Catholic Church was the target of state persecution because of its "reactionary, anti-progressive" stance and also for sponsoring an armed rebellion.[41]

Although the Catholic Church does not have a particularly distinguished history in Chiapas, it would seem to be making amends in recent times. Whereas in the 1930s the church was persecuted by the Mexican government for its reactionary positions, it is persecuted now in the era of financial globalization for its advocacy in making a preferential option for the poor.[42] This sea change for the institutional church in Chiapas has largely been attributed to Bishop Samuel Ruíz, who has not curried favor with the local elites. As one of my friends in Chiapas noted, "He did not do as he was expected—drink chocolate with the ladies and support the status quo. He came here over thirty years ago, declared he knew nothing of the indigenous people, and set out to learn and to help them."

As Ruíz is quick to point out, however, he earned his progressive stripes on the job. Consecrated as a bishop at the age of thirty-five, he was considered meek and conservative, unlikely to upset the longstanding alliance between the church and the state's hierarchies. But his pastoral work with the indigenous poor wrought a deep change in Samuel Ruíz: "On his hikes into the villages and new colonies and communities, among the plainest and simplest people he had ever known, he would often speak of 'the Indians' and 'the poor' as if they were the same, and the strength grew in him to stand up to the rich. 'I came to San Cristóbal to convert the poor,' he would later say, 'but they ended up converting me.' "[43]

Some refer to Ruíz as another Las Casas, but the Latin American church itself has also changed. Ruíz was concerned not only with the suffering of the indigenous poor but also with the mechanisms of their impoverishment. By the seventies, Bishop Ruíz was known as "Uncle Samuel" to the indigenous people, and as trouble to the landowners. Many date the beginnings of a radical peasant movement to 1974, when Ruíz organized a massive Indigenous Congress, marking the first time that indigenous Mexicans had been summoned by a nongovernmental agency without a hidden agenda.[44] Church support for the peasant movement was, of course, not the work of one man but of hundreds of priests and religious, working with thousands of lay catechists who had mastered the various indigenous languages or who were themselves indigenous people. Long before 1994, the local gentry had already labeled Ruíz a communist, accusing him of fomenting revolution and even of arming the *campesinos*.[45]

When the Zapatista uprising captured the consciousness of Mexico, the local elite claimed that Ruíz had organized the entire affair. Subcomandante Marcos, it was said, was clearly schooled in theology, and many further insisted that he was one of Ruíz's priests. Diocesan offices were bombed; priests, including at least four who were accused of being Marcos himself, were arrested by government agents.[46] Several expatriate priests sympathetic to the indigenous poor were expelled from Mexico, and a Canadian-born nun who had been a Zapatista partisan died in an attack on one of the towns. In an early communiqué, the rebels were at pains to deny official ties to the church:

> Our EZLN does not have any connection to authorities of the Catholic church, nor to those of any other creed. We have not received orientation or direction or ecclesiastical structural support, either from the Diocese of the state of Chiapas, or from any papal representative, or from the Vatican, or from anyone. Those who fight in our ranks are primarily Catholics, but we are also people of other beliefs and religions.[47]

Although the Zapatistas denied any church involvement in the rebellion, it is clear that, given the institutional landscape in Chiapas, they count on significant sympathy among the region's progressive Catholics. It had been Ruíz's position all along that the Zapatistas represent a sector of the population with legitimate grievances and that the rebels could not be excluded from negotiations. More important, Ruíz continued to press for an end to all forms of violence—he had recently rebaptized San Cristóbal's sixteenth-century cathedral as the Catedral de la Paz—including the structural violence endured by the poor.[48]

But peace is not easily achieved as long as structural violence persists. Many assume that tension has lessened in recent years. In fact, the attacks had been more frequent in the few months preceding our visit, in part because of the reorganization of the *guardias blancas* and other paramilitary groups. Although there is a confusing plethora of such groups—one of them goes, in sinister fashion, under the name "Paz y Justicia"—their unifying characteristic would seem to be ties with power, either local or federal. Only the federal government takes the trouble to deny such links. For the priests and religious who work with the organized poor, the *guardias* are self-evidently paid hit squads. Like the people of Moisés Gandhi, local clerics tend to speak of a "low-intensity war" or a *guerra sucia*—a "dirty war"—against the poor. Tellingly, paramilitary attacks are most likely to occur in precisely those regions where the Zapatistas are weak or absent. In the view of many here, these communities are more easily intimidated by the *guardias* and by the troops.

Human rights organizations, including the Diocesan Fray Bartolomé de Las Casas Human Rights Center and Human Rights Watch/Americas, have documented scores of attacks, many of them mortal and most of them aimed at members or perceived supporters of the Zapatistas.[49] Catholic catechists have been targeted, along with human rights monitors. The violence has led to scores of deaths and to the displacement of thousands in northern Chiapas.

On November 4, 1997, Bishop Ruíz, Bishop Raúl Vera, and several catechists were attacked in broad daylight by a heavily armed paramilitary group identified by locals as members of Paz y Justicia. Three members of the entourage sustained gunshot wounds. Months later, there had been no prosecution of those responsible for the attack.

In light of this renewed and rather spectacular persecution of the church, it was startling for me to see, in front of the Catedral de la Paz, a banner covered with the familiar image of the hooded Zapatista. Next to the image was written, in large letters, *"Bienvenidos, dignos forjadores de la libertad"* (Welcome, worthy forgers of freedom). Against this backdrop, I met Padre Eliberto, one of the priests harassed by the paramilitary groups; with him was a young doctor, Demóstenes. They were en route back to the parish in Tila and recounted in some detail the situation emerging in northern Chiapas.

Father Eliberto, bearded and with a piercing gaze, was an imposing figure: serious, to the point, and committed to the poor of his parish. The recent violence had in no way dampened his conviction. Dr. Demóstenes, a native of the Tila region, had worked with Father Eliberto for five years. As a physician sympathetic to the rural poor, he had also attended the February meeting in Moisés Gandhi. "It was an important gathering not only for the *promotores,*" he said passionately, "but also for all of us concerned about the health of the poor. We should be organizing around social justice themes and against those forces keeping the people so sick. That is why the counterstrike has been violent."

Together, the priest and the doctor mapped out the battle lines of a "dirty war" carried out, they said, by *guardias blancas* in the pay of local landowners or the ruling party. The maps made it clear that the parish was hemmed in by armed groups hostile to the social justice work that the priest and the doctor embraced. Both scoffed at the notion that the paramilitary groups were in any way "mysterious." Rather, the *guardias blancas* operated openly and with complete impunity, as every serious investigation has revealed.

Writing of the violence in Father Eliberto's parish, Human Rights Watch/Americas put it this way: "The government has shown through action and inaction that it is more than just permissive of the violent actions of [Paz y Justicia]. Human Rights Watch/Americas must conclude that authorities actively acquiesce to the abuses committed by armed civilians in Tila. Authorities frequently know about abuses but fail to act to prevent or punish them."[50] Bishop Ruíz was less delicate than the human rights group: the problems in northern Chiapas were "created intentionally," he observed in a radio broadcast prior to the attack on his entourage, "to make it look as though it is the communities alone who are involved in these confrontations, and that there are no outsiders provoking these conflicts. The Federal Army will then be needed as a saviour to impose law and order in this territory."

Father Eliberto and Demóstenes confront—and are exposed to—both the attacks on the poor and the official lies told about these attacks. As they left for Tila, it struck me that a priest and a doctor could together constitute a formidable resource, even though they had little more than conviction at their disposal. This was enough for them to take on their work with passion and resolve, sentiments not yet quenched—and perhaps fueled?—by threats and ongoing violence. I left the diocesan offices humbled by their determination. Foremost on their minds, they said, was food and shelter for the displaced. "A microscope would be helpful," added Dr. Demóstenes. "We're seeing a lot more tuberculosis than before."

THE STRUGGLE FOR HEALTH

In the morning of our second day in Moisés Gandhi, we went to visit the two clinics built by the people of the Municipio Rebelde Ernesto Che Guevara. They were small, clean, and square. One of them gleamed on the forested hillside of a settlement called Sacrificio. It was, repeated the health workers, a *trabajo de gente*—a work of the people. Sacrificio had formerly been a big ranch. Before that, they explained, it had been the land of their forebears. After 1994, the peasants simply reclaimed Sacrificio. From the city of Ocosingo—"the door to the Lacandón jungle"—the former landowners continue to push for either compensation or expulsion of the peasants from the homes they have built. Although the ranchers mustered a small *guardia blanca,* the squatters refused to budge. Speaking of the land, one of the health workers put it this way: "It doesn't matter to us what the government and the ranchers say. It's ours." Their comments reminded me of what I'd read about the original Zapatistas: they were "country people who did not want to move and therefore got into a revolution. They did not figure on so odd a fate. Come hell, come high water, agitators from the outside, or report of greener pastures elsewhere, they insisted only on staying in their little villages and little towns where they had grown up, and where before them their ancestors for hundreds of years had lived and died—in the small state of Morelos, in south-central Mexico."[51]

The people who had reclaimed Sacrificio were interested not only in their own history but also in the plight of poor people elsewhere. While they showed us the clinic, several of the health workers asked about the conditions of the Haitian poor and the U.S. poor. Was there much poverty in these places? And, if so, what was being done to address it? In what ways was poverty in a rich country different from poverty in a poor country? One of the women, Manuela, announced that her devout wish was to travel to Haiti and meet the health workers there. "I know we would have much to share," she said.

As we talked, they eagerly showed us every little room. We were moved, and impressed, but I felt an unspoken dread. Two clinics, built with little more than sheer force of will, now needed to be stocked and maintained. I thought about our clinic in Haiti; our experience there had taught us that the physical plant is only the beginning. Maintaining a steady flow of medicines and supplies causes far more headaches than constructing a clinic. "We have the clinics," the president of the *comisión municipal* observed wearily, as if reading my mind, "but we have no medicines other than the plants we grow. And some of that knowledge is lost."

The municipal president had escaped my notice, in large part because he blended in with the health workers: he was slight of frame, wore muddied and threadbare clothes, and had a backpack. He had no distinguishing garb, no badge of office. The autonomous government, he explained, consisted of several commissions—he spoke of commissions on health, human rights, agriculture, ecology and reforestation, education, and women's issues. When pressed for details, the president provided them, and they sounded very much like the points laid out in the Declaration of Moisés Gandhi, which were, in turn, nearly identical to those made by the Zapatistas.

My admiration for the people I met in Moisés Gandhi was tempered only by anxiety: how would this fragile shoot of popular democracy flourish in a setting notable for low-flying military planes and the other unsubtle reminders that Mexican officialdom was not hospitable to any moves toward autonomy? And there was irony, too: Mexico's progressive constitution of 1921, founded on the struggles of the first Zapatistas, guaranteed the people of Moisés Gandhi precisely what they didn't have: land, health care, and freedom from the peonage that had marked their lives for centuries. It promised them social and economic rights.

.   .   .   .   .

We rode to Ocosingo with Julio and the president of the autonomous government. Ocosingo, they explained, was the site of the bloodiest battle of January 1994. We saw little sign of this conflict: the sun gleamed through the thick clouds that had for two days drenched the highlands. Julio was dropping us off at a bus station so that we could take a truck back to San Cristóbal. As we wound our way into the cloud forests, we passed a large compound, clearly military in nature. Guard towers marked every corner, and it was hemmed by barbed wire. We asked the bus driver what it was. "It's the place the government built to hold the Zapatistas," he replied, keeping his eyes on the road. His reluctance to say more reminded me of Marcos's comments on the same building:

> You decide that it is better to go to Ocosingo, as ecology and other nonsense is all the fashion these days. Look at the trees, take a deep breath... now do you feel better? Yes? Then keep on looking to your left because if you don't, at the 7-kilometer mark you will see a magnificent edifice with the noble SOLIDARITY logo on the front. Don't look, I tell you, turn your head away, you don't want to know that this new building is a...jail.[52]

What will come of the noble efforts of the women and men of Municipio Rebelde Ernesto Che Guevara? What price will they pay for autonomy from the government, given that they desperately need the public services that are, according to Mexican law, their due? What hope can the *promotores* offer to the destitute sick of their highland hamlets? What ancient lore will help them when a young woman faces arrested labor and needs the assistance of a skilled obstetrician? What will come of Father Eliberto and Dr. Demóstenes and of the people they seek to serve? Will there be still more killings, displacements, malnutrition, and tuberculosis? If they are to respond to the needs of their people, Eliberto and Demóstenes need more than sacraments and solidarity.

Riding from Ocosingo to San Cristóbal, I thought of the people I'd met, but also of Haiti, ecologically devastated and now mired in chronic food shortfalls. Chiapas—with its lushly forested mountains, its waterfalls, its priceless cultural heritage—seems worlds away from Haiti. The mantra of our hosts ran through my mind: "Chiapas isn't poor. Its people are poor."

Although we're often told that we live in a time of limited resources, the numbers suggest that, to the contrary, we live in a time of unprecedented wealth. If Chiapas has a lesson for the rest of the world, it's that the world's resources must be more evenly shared. Human rights are respected when everyone has food, shelter, education, and health care— and the poor of Chiapas were claiming these rights. I'd left a Haiti marked by continued degradation, frustrated hopes, and new levels of hunger; I returned to a Chiapas marked by tension and violence but also, I found, by a persistent, hopeful resistance.

—December 1, 1997

POSTSCRIPT: AUGUST 7, 2000

There is abundant evidence that Acteal was a crime perpetrated by the Mexican state.

John Ross, *The War Against Oblivion*

The slaughter at Acteal was so awful that for a while many Mexicans believed some good must come of it, as if by divine justice, some compromise, some reconciliation, some peace.... But as usual the innocents died in vain. Since the massacre...the government has practically (nothing virtual about its military force) run the state as if it were under siege.

John Womack Jr., *Rebellion in Chiapas*

Civilians have become tyrants in what was once the province of the military, and in these wars there can never be victory, only ashes and a sea of tears.

Marjorie Agosin, *An Absence of Shadows*

I have been uncomfortable leaving this essay perched as if on the edge of a cliff. A few days after I originally finished writing it, paramilitary forces murdered forty-five civilians—mostly women and children—in the village of Acteal. Chiapas was again on the front pages of the international newspapers.[53]

In Mexico City, the government denied any responsibility for the bloodletting and vowed to bring its authors to justice. The federal officials promised an "exhaustive search" for the perpetrators, a promise echoed by local authorities. This made it sound as if there were doubts about who had carried out the Acteal massacre. Some officials insinuated that the Zapatistas were responsible for the killings, and this allegation, known to be groundless, was echoed dutifully in the press. Others were quick to echo the claims that local ethnic rivalry was to blame.[54] But as is so often the case in Latin America, there was never any mystery about who was to blame. First, there was no lack of witnesses to these murders, the largest massacre since the conflict began in 1994.[55] Second, for the massacre to have its intended effect, it was imperative that all concerned understand precisely who ordered and who executed the killings.

As in Tila, Moisés Gandhi, and the other communities discussed earlier, the perpetrators took few pains to hide their tracks and fewer still to hide their loyalties. After all, their point was to intimidate the population. To do that, they had to leave a signature that all could read. *Guardias blancas* in the service of local landowners, almost all with close ties to the ruling party, openly celebrated their "victory against Zapatista sympathizers." Arrests were few. Impunity was the language in which both threat and deed were delivered, and impunity is why, almost three years after the violent suppression, we can read that the attacks are still signed in blood. On June 7, 1998, Samuel Ruíz—who, a month earlier, had been stripped of much of his authority by church officials—resigned as chief mediator between the Zapatistas and the government, accusing President Ernesto Zedillo of "a constant and growing governmental aggression" against both the peace process itself and the negotiators and civilians judged sympathetic to the EZLN. Ruíz repeatedly underlined the government's failure to punish those responsible for Acteal and other civilian killings.

A 1998 investigative report by Global Exchange highlighted the intensified militarization since Acteal and also the impunity with which the *guardias* operated: "All the paramilitary groups so far identified [in Chiapas] (up to 12, according to Attorney General of the Republic Jorge Madrazo) are self-confessed supporters of the Institutional Revolutionary Party (PRI), Mexico's ruling party. Despite the heavy military presence in these areas, none of the groups, including Paz y Justicia (which has reportedly received close to half a million U.S. dollars from the PRI-controlled state government) has so far been disarmed."[56]

The 1999 Physicians for Human Rights report on health care in Chiapas observed that, "to date, the Government's investigations have not implicated any paramilitary groups in the Acteal massacre. Nor has the Mexican Army been charged with complicity in the training or arming of these shadowy groups. The lack of progress in the Acteal investigation was tacitly acknowledged by U.S. Secretary of State Madeleine Albright when she reported to a Congressional Subcommittee, 'We are following the investigation very closely, and we have communicated to the Mexican Government that we will be doing so,' she reported to Senator Patrick Leahy. 'I believe, Senator, that we are pressuring them to resolve the situation in Chiapas.'"[57]

It's always perilous, of course, to forecast the future. But the travails of the poor of Chiapas seem to be endless and predictable. In August 1998, Womack, one of Mexico's most astute observers, acknowledging the biblical proportions of the struggle there, hazarded the following prediction and analogy: "The prospect over the next two years in Chiapas is therefore grim—continued, dangerous, confounding struggles among the poor themselves to develop an effective strategy for their common, crucial struggle, no longer to reach the Promised Land (even without milk and honey), but just to stay in the Wilderness, out of Egypt."[58]

Womack was right, of course. The poor of Chiapas remain unprotected from military and paramilitary aggression.

> Paramilitaries continue to occupy territory in the municipality of Yajalón they seized in an attack on August 3rd. The attack occurred at 10:30 a.m. in the community of "Tierra y Libertad" (formerly two communities: Paraíso and Progreso). The paramilitaries, from the group Paz y Justicia, arrived in a group of about 70—30 dressed as state public security forces, 40 in civilian clothing, three in masks—armed with pistols, R-15's, and .22 caliber rifles. They proceeded to loot farms, fire in the air and behind fleeing townspeople, burn six houses, and drive 48 families into the mountains.[59]

Whether or not there will be another Acteal remains to be seen. But the signs all point to a recurrence. The year 2000 has seen armed forces violently enter many villages in the region. On February 12, the army entered at least three communities in Ocosingo, detaining several alleged Zapatista sympathizers; on March 17, a group of heavily armed Federal Prevention Police threatened residents of La Candelaria with forced evacuation; on May 8, three Tzotzil Indians were killed and three others injured in an ambush.[60] On August 7, paramilitary groups burned homes and forcibly expelled civilians from the village of Yajalón.[61] The structural violence that generates such atrocities remains unaddressed by the superficial palliatives of the Mexican government. Militarization has only exacerbated violence in Chiapas.[62]

The newly elected Vicente Fox has pledged to reduce dramatically the military presence there. Whether the end of single-party rule, after seventy years, will spell an end to the dirty war remains to be seen. But as Womack warned, unless "national elections deliver a government able and willing to liberate the poor (at least a little) from violence, indignity, and poverty, or 'civil society' moves the government firmly in that direction, the poor in Chiapas will have to struggle more grievously than ever to stay out of Egypt."[63] Many whose voices are cited here—health workers, priests, doctors—predict that the latest elections will do little to improve the lot of the poor of Chiapas. This week's harvest of shame undermines optimism. The struggle, grievous, continues.

CHAPTER 4

A PLAGUE ON
ALL OUR HOUSES?

RESURGENT TUBERCULOSIS
INSIDE RUSSIA'S PRISONS

Today's prisons mirror our catastrophic society. The evils that
plague us, plague them: no health care, no education, no
fairness, no rule of law.

>   Sergei Kovalyov, former political prisoner; quoted by Peter Juviler,
>   in *Human Rights: New Perspectives, New Realities,* 2000

I'm really sorry for what I did, but I don't want to die here in
prison. It would kill my parents.

>   Mischa Chukanov, twenty-two years old, tuberculosis patient
>   in the Matrosskaya Tishina Prison Infirmary, Moscow

In the days of the Soviet Union, the powerful Sanitation and
Epidemiology Service, or "SanEp," sought out infectious
diseases and stamped them out with compulsory vaccinations
and annual disease screenings: chest X-rays for tuberculosis,
blood tests for syphilis.... The SanEp tactics were brutal—
people were often taken from their families and hometowns
for months to years—but they were effective.

"Now, instead, we have human rights," said Alla Loseva,
the Voronezh tuberculosis hospital's deputy chief doctor,
rolling her eyes.

>   *New York Times,* December 5, 2000

SERGEI AND THE "NATURAL" HISTORY
OF MULTIDRUG-RESISTANT TUBERCULOSIS

Sergei was tall and thin, with black horn-rim glasses that gave him more
the look of an owlish accountant than a felon. His fellow prisoners and
their guards were silent as he told me his story. The only other sound aside
from his soft voice was that of coughing: like him, all the other young convicts who crowded the cell were sick with pulmonary tuberculosis. At

times, Sergei seemed bored with the tale; at times, intimidated by the hush. He punctuated his sentences with a rattling cough of his own, raising, as an afterthought, a long pale hand to his mouth.

Shortly after the breakup of the Soviet Union in 1991, Sergei explained, he became involved in a complicated scam—something to do with fake checks. Arrested in the Siberian city of Kemerovo, he was held in pre-trial detention for more than a year. Although Russian law prohibits such prolonged detention without trial, and the Ministry of Justice issues statements deploring the delays, the courts have been, by all accounts, overwhelmed by ever-growing caseloads: rates of imprisonment in Russia have doubled since the collapse of the Soviet Union.[1] And so the jail in Kemerovo was dank and crammed with other young men awaiting trial, most accused of nonviolent crimes like the one Sergei readily admits committing. Food and sanitary conditions were wretched, and Sergei began to cough and lose weight well before his case came to trial.

"I knew I had tuberculosis," he said simply, "because that's what everybody else had." After his trial, prison health authorities confirmed the diagnosis, and Sergei was transferred to a "TB colony"—a prison facility dedicated to the detention and care of convicts ill with tuberculosis. Since Colony 33, in the nearby town of Mariinsk—once notorious for its especially grim conditions—was already overflowing, Sergei was sent instead to a colony at Vladimir, about sixty miles east of Moscow. He began his therapy at precisely the time that Russia's massive TB infrastructure began to crumble. The political and economic upheavals associated with the dissolution of the Soviet Union meant drug stockouts, failure to pay prison officials, and a dramatic weakening of the civilian TB services.[2] Sergei completed a year of erratic treatment about seven years ago.

For about two years after his initial treatment, Sergei felt, he says, "just fine." Rather than moving him back to a regular prison, however, authorities offered him the chance to stay on at Vladimir and complete his sentence as a medical orderly assisting the nursing staff of the Vladimir colony. Three years later, he recalled in a low voice, his symptoms returned.

At this point in his narrative, Sergei paused, looking at the prison doctor. "He's due to be released soon," interjected the young doctor grimly, "but he's not responding to therapy." She had already informed me that the prison hospital under her direction had in recent months continued to face drug stockouts, a lack of X-ray film, and even food shortages. She did not add, as had the warden earlier, that her own pay had been in arrears for months; her worries were solely about her patients, to judge by her comments to me.

The doctor handed me Sergei's chest films, and I placed them in a view box affixed to the examining room wall. I tried not to wince. In recent months, in fact, there had been a marked enlargement of the cavities in Sergei's right upper lobe. Spreading inexorably, the recrudescent tubercle bacilli had already reduced the top half of that lung to Swiss cheese. The disease clearly had also spread to his left lung, which only a few months previously had been without radiographic abnormality.

Long and erratic treatment had done Sergei little good. Indeed, haphazard therapy is one of the best ways of inducing the tubercle bacillus to acquire drug resistance. But Sergei—along with about thirty other Vladimir inmates—was to be sent home this month, in all likelihood carrying infectious, drug-resistant tuberculosis with him. He was to spend the harsh Siberian winter cooped up in a tiny wooden house with his wife and children. The one thing that might protect his family was that they might already be infected with latent tuberculosis. Quiescent infection with *Mycobacterium tuberculosis* likely confers some immunity to the drug-resistant strains now pouring out of Russia's vast prison network. In Siberia, the incidence of tuberculosis has trebled in the decade since Sergei was arrested.[3]

Handing the X-rays back to the doctor, I smiled encouragingly at Sergei and wished him luck. He made a small, polite bow and said nothing, as he was once again coughing. But he managed a smile as he tried to suppress his paroxysm; the other prisoners also murmured their farewells. After the doctor and I left the crowded cell, and we were more or less alone, my questions began in earnest. Although she had heard them all before, she listened patiently.

With what drugs were Sergei and the other patient-prisoners being treated? I asked. Are you having trouble with drug supply? Do the prisoners take their medications? Is each dose directly observed? Is there adequate food? My uniformed colleague nodded politely. Food was scarce, she allowed, but we're managing to scrape by. Some of the guards, although themselves grossly underpaid, shared their own food with the prisoners (the sharing, and selling, of vodka is already much commented upon). Sergei was receiving isoniazid, rifampin, and ethambutol—three of the strongest (the so-called first-line) drugs; his previous regimen had included streptomycin. The dosages were correct, and the staff indeed observed him taking the pills. Yet each month, his doctor explained, microscopic examination of Sergei's sputum continued to reveal signs of persistent tuberculosis.

My final question, and perhaps the first one my colleague found pertinent, concerned microbial resistance to drugs. Most tuberculosis patients who fail treatment do so because they're not taking their medications regularly. In the Russian Federation, this can be a result of the commonplace drug stockouts or the patients' failure to take their drugs. But with directly observed therapy, failure to respond to powerful drugs is usually a sign that the tubercle bacillus has become resistant to them. An infecting strain that is resistant to at least isoniazid and rifampin—the two most powerful first-line drugs—is termed "multidrug-resistant tuberculosis" (MDRTB).

When patients have MDRTB, they require longer periods of treatment—about two years of a multidrug regimen. This compares with the six to nine months of treatment needed for disease caused by drug-susceptible strains. Several of the less powerful second-line drugs, which are required to treat MDRTB, are also more toxic, with side effects such as nausea, abdominal pain, and even psychosis; as a result, it's harder to manage patients who are receiving them. Five first-line drugs are available for treating tuberculosis; at most, eight second-line drugs also have proven effective, if less so than isoniazid and rifampin, against *M. tuberculosis*. But strains of MDRTB exist that are resistant to all the first-line and most of the second-line drugs. (The Partners In Health team had treated patients in Peru who were sick with strains that were resistant to ten and even twelve drugs. Most such patients require adjuvant surgery for any hope of cure.)

Did Sergei's doctor think drug resistance might be a problem among the more than nine hundred patients in her care? "Oh, yes," she replied. "Many are resistant to the drugs. There are, as you might say, superbugs loose in our jails and prisons. We know how to manage the cases, even the drug-resistant ones. But we don't have the resources." The annual medication budget for the entire Vladimir colony was the equivalent of about two thousand dollars, less than a fifth of what it had been a decade earlier, when drugs were virtually free and plentiful—and there were, by all accounts, fewer cases and far less drug resistance. Thus, the colony could now afford only an irregular supply of certain first-line drugs and no second-line drugs. The facility was also chronically short of syringes, masks, X-ray film, and other supplies.[4]

Conditions in Russia's TB colonies are nothing short of dismal. Having visited far worse prisons in Latin America, I'm quick to note that jails and prisons in Russia are far cleaner than, for example, the squalid *cachots* of Haiti. The Russian prison medical facilities were somehow both dingy and clean. The prison personnel, at least the medical corps, struck me as professional and conscientious. They were, by and large, well liked by the prisoners.[5] Indeed, they compared favorably to many of their international interlocutors. But the overall effect of a modern Russian TB colony is one of gloom, shabbiness, and desuetude, amid a stark lack of necessary supplies. The prisons were either too hot or too cold, airless in winter, and always short of light. Morale was poor, but not as poor as I had expected. Throughout the Russian Federation, prison medical staff continued to show up for work, whether paid or not.

Some of these doctors and nurses have themselves fallen ill with MDRTB. It's believed that, if left untreated, each smear-positive pulmonary tuberculosis patient can, in turn, infect a dozen or more new contacts every year.[6] The transmission rate is surely even higher within an overcrowded penitentiary system. Authorities estimate that one in every ten (or approximately 110,000) Russian prisoners has active tuberculosis. Bad as that is, prisoners have two further strikes against them. First, even the drug-susceptible strains of the illness are being transformed into superbugs through inadequate treatment regimens. Second, prisoners who have acquired MDRTB will then infect others with drug-resistant strains. As I write this, about a quarter of the prisoners with active tuberculosis probably have MDRTB.[7] If Sergei has MDRTB and is receiving a regimen based on first-line drugs, he will not be cured—but his germs may acquire more drug resistance even as he follows his well-intentioned and well-trained doctor's orders.

What of prisons elsewhere in the former Soviet Union? In the past few years, I have examined detainees in Latvia, Azerbaijan, and Kazakhstan. In each of these places, my fears were confirmed: tuberculosis is out of control throughout the region's jails and prisons. Just as it was in the time of Dostoyevsky and Chekhov, tuberculosis is again the leading cause of death of young prisoners. According to the International Committee of the Red Cross, it accounts for up to 80 percent of deaths in many prisons.[8] Worse, highly resistant strains are already entrenched there. An epidemiological catastrophe has come to pass inside Russia's prisons and in many others throughout the former Soviet Union: ineffective treatment regimens have produced drug-resistant disease, and since only the susceptible strains are being treated effectively, the proportion of drug-resistant cases continues to grow.

International expert opinion has tended to blame poor treatment outcomes on the hapless TB services, both prison and civilian, or on a lin-
gering "Soviet culture," rather than on the social and economic conditions that are at the heart of both the epidemic of imprisonment and the
epidemic of tuberculosis.[9] Worse still, many international experts continue to insist that the prescription for Russia's runaway TB epidemic
must include only the wise use of first-line drugs—this at a time when
fully half of all patients with active disease are sick with strains resistant
to isoniazid or streptomycin.[10]

No epidemic of drug-resistant disease on this scale has ever before
been documented. It's unquestionably true that prisons were an important factor in New York's MDRTB epidemic of the early 1990s. The
New York State Department of Health reported that this outbreak consisted of 1,279 cases from 1991 to 1994, with no figures available for
1990.[11] According to a report issued by city health authorities, fully 80
percent of all MDRTB cases could be traced back to prisons and homeless shelters.[12] By some estimates, the New York epidemic cost more
than $1 billion to bring under control. But compare that with what is
unfolding in Russia. There I've visited prison colony after prison
colony—more than fifty such facilities exist—and in each one, hundreds
of detainees with drug-resistant tuberculosis languish untreated. The
Russian MDRTB epidemic is already so widespread that no single country, and certainly not one in the midst of economic turmoil, could ever
hope to assume complete financial and technical responsibility for its
control.

The natural history of tuberculosis teaches us that the disease is most
effectively propagated by crowding people into small spaces and then
denying them access to adequate nutrition. Prisons within the Russian
Federation are thus as effective a means of fanning a TB epidemic as
might be imagined. But it need not be so. According to human rights
groups, including Penal Reform International, Russia's federal penitentiary system (GUIN) is more open to reform than in the past. Mistreatment of detainees continues, however, and ill-functioning court and judicial systems hamper attempts at reform. Amnesty International reports
that in 1995 Yuri Kalinin, then head of GUIN, now Deputy Minister of
Justice, acknowledged the poor state of pre-trial detention centers. Conditions there, he said, "can be classified as torture under international
standards; that is, deprivation of sleep, air, and space."[13]

When the head of what was recently known as the "gulag" acknowledges publicly that prison conditions are tantamount to torture, human

rights groups needn't focus on forcing such confessions. That is, if the jailers are quick to admit that prison conditions are deplorable, what role, really, remains for sustained public pressure to have the Ministry of Justice officials unveil the truth—a truth now obvious to all? The next step, obviously, is to push for the social and economic rights of those incarcerated. Here pragmatic solidarity—on an international scale—will do more for the prisoners than, say, letters or demonstrations. Curing the prisoners before their release is the best way to respect their rights and also the best way to prevent further transmission to prison staff and to the civilian population.

AN INNOVATIVE STRATEGY FOR TREATING MDRTB

In Sergei's home region, Kemerovo Oblast, almost a tenth of the populace is in detention or on probation. In September 1998, Governor Aman Tuleyev told a group of visiting tuberculosis experts that prisons there are filled with a new type of detainee: young, poor, and convicted not of crimes against the state but of crimes against property. In Russia as a whole, nearly 1 million people out of a population of more than 150 million are in prison.[14] Only the United States, with close to 2 million prisoners out of a population of 272 million, rivals that ratio. Whatever the efficacy of imprisonment as a deterrent to nonviolent crime in a country caught in the grip of economic crisis, one thing is certain: better habitats for epidemics of airborne disease could hardly be found than those provided by Russia's overcrowded prisons.

Concerned about the serious tuberculosis problem, GUIN officials opened the prisons in 1996 to foreign nongovernmental medical organizations. The Public Health Research Institute (PHRI) was at the forefront of these groups. PHRI had helped bring New York City's MDRTB epidemic to heel, and Alex Goldfarb, a Russian-born microbiologist on the PHRI staff, convinced financier and philanthropist George Soros to fund TB control efforts in Russia. I was called in as a consultant to that project in 1998, after it became clear that up to half of all prisoners were failing to respond to internationally recommended treatment regimens.

Partners In Health has a particular and hard-won expertise in the treatment of MDRTB. In 1992 a Catholic priest who was a cofounder of Partners In Health went to a sprawling slum in Lima, Peru, as a relief worker. Three years later he fell ill. It started insidiously, he told us, with fevers, night sweats, and chronic diarrhea. He lost weight and developed

a cough. We urged him to return home to Boston. There he was diagnosed with tuberculosis and put on a regimen of first-line drugs. Two
weeks later he was dead. At about the time of his funeral, we found out
why: a culture of the TB strain that had infected him showed resistance
to all four of the drugs he had received. He had died of MDRTB.

We at Partners In Health were faced with more than our own grief.
We had an obligation to the residents of the shantytown where he had
worked, for we were certain that there would be cases similar to his
among them. Sure enough, when we began looking in the slums of Lima,
we found hundreds of patients who had failed first-line drug therapy. In
a few families, every adult was sick with—or had already died from—re-
fractory tuberculosis. When we performed drug-susceptibility tests of my-
cobacteria obtained from the survivors, we discovered that more than 90
percent of them were afflicted with resistant strains of the organism.[15]

Having diagnosed resistance to first-line drugs, we embarked on a
treatment regimen using second-line drugs, including cycloserine and
capreomycin. Similar treatments had been tried before elsewhere, but
chiefly in older patients whose tuberculosis was complicated by other
concurrent disease, such as emphysema, or in younger patients co-
infected with HIV. Ours was the first such treatment program—at least
in an impoverished setting—for younger patients with otherwise un-
complicated medical histories. Public health officials in Peru and the
United States, as well as from the World Health Organization, cautioned
that we could not expect good results. And the less powerful second-line
drugs, which require a long course of treatment, would be prohibitively
costly, they said. They warned that second-line drugs were up to one hundred times more expensive than first-line drugs. In China, according to
the World Bank, it is possible to purchase an entire course of therapy
based on first-line drugs for well under a hundred dollars.[16] The cost of
a much longer regimen of second-line drugs, on the other hand, can run
to tens of thousands of dollars.

But the crucial point for us was that second-line drugs could cure where
first-line drugs had failed. We pressed on. Private donors in the United
States (with Partners In Health trustee Tom White providing the lion's
share) helped us finance the acquisition of the expensive second-line drugs,
and soon we had more than fifty patients in treatment. (Thanks to generous funding, we are now poised to "scale up" this project to cover the
entire country of Peru.) Most of the first fifty had excellent responses to
therapy, even though they were precisely the patients termed "untreatable" by local and international authorities. Most had already failed sev-

eral previous therapies based on first-line drugs and were locally referred to as *crónicos*. But at the close of eighteen to twenty-four months of treatment, over 80 percent of these patients showed no signs of persistent disease. This is why doctors from as far afield as Russia wanted to know more about our treatment program, and it is also why I have been visiting TB detention centers there, including, in September 1998, Colony 33 in Sergei's home region of Kemerovo Oblast.

THE CONSEQUENCES OF NOT TREATING MDRTB

Colony 33 houses more than thirteen hundred prisoners diagnosed with tuberculosis. Three years ago, as it became increasingly clear that tuberculosis was epidemic within Russia's penitentiary system, GUIN joined with the Belgian branch of the relief organization Médecins Sans Frontières (Doctors Without Borders) in a treatment program. There was a sense of excitement as they collaborated to treat their first group of patients with a standardized, directly observed regimen based on first-line drugs.

But something went wrong in Colony 33. Many prisoners remained smear-positive—that is, with tubercle bacilli still in their sputum—after months of therapy. At the end of a six- to eight-month treatment regimen, less than half of the first cohort of prisoners were declared cured—and some of these "cures" later developed signs of recrudescent disease. Many hypotheses were advanced to explain this failure, but only one panned out: the prisoners who failed therapy were sick with MDRTB. Nevertheless, second-line drugs have yet to be provided as part of donor-supported treatment to the MDRTB patients of Colony 33. Doctors there told me that death rates were still high and that—every week, it seemed—a couple of young men would begin coughing up blood and die. Others were wasting away slowly.

The Russian and European physicians based in Colony 33 were unsure how to proceed. Most of the Europeans had not had significant previous experience treating tuberculosis; the Russians were more familiar with the disease, but their treatment strategies were under attack by influential advisers based in a number of expert bodies. Discrepant suggestions began to pour in. Many experts argued that Siberian prisoners with MDRTB were simply "untreatable." The logic used in making this claim was sometimes clinical, sometimes economic. To this point, the latter set of arguments had held sway: treatment of MDRTB in "resource-poor" settings—and Colony 33 was manifestly short of resources—was "not cost-effective."

The great irony, in 1998, was that some patients—all those with MDRTB—were receiving a wholly ineffective treatment on the grounds of cost-effectiveness. How did this come to pass inside the prisons of the former Soviet Union? The spectacle of prisoners receiving directly observed therapy with the wrong drugs is related to rigid adherence to a strategy called DOTS—an acronym for "directly observed therapy, short-course." DOTS is a good therapy for pan-susceptible TB, but its success depends on the efficacy of the antibiotics used. In the setting of obvious "therapeutic chaos" and the collapse of the Soviet-era TB infrastructure, international advisers hewed to the line that DOTS was the only way to treat TB.

Even if one agrees (as I do) that DOTS should be the cornerstone of tuberculosis control around the world, what about Sergei and the thousands of others who are already sick with strains resistant to these first-line drugs? One unintended result of not treating MDRTB is that patients with persistently positive smears are denied access, month after month, to the tests and drugs they need. They then spread the mutant organisms to others. Genetic fingerprinting was already demonstrating epidemic spread within the prison system.[17] How could the epidemic be stopped without second-line drugs?

One answer was euphemistically called "cohorting"—isolating patients with MDRTB within a barbed wire compound. This strategy was being practiced in Colony 33. But even without resorting to human rights arguments, one could readily see the flaw in this plan: when the prisoners behind barbed wire had served their sentences—if they survived their sentences—they were released.

The only defensible way to stop transmission is to treat the patients correctly, which in this case meant the use of second-line drugs. Those influential in shaping international health policy, including experts from the World Bank, resisted the use of the second-line drugs in nations receiving "aid."[18] (The Russian Federation had of course recently fallen into this club.) Sometimes the reasons for their reluctance cited the necessity of having a robust tuberculosis control program in order to prevent resistance from emerging in the first place; more often, the high cost of the drugs was mentioned.

Discussions of prevention were obviously tardy. It was too late to prevent an epidemic of MDRTB. Some, mostly nonclinicians, argued that the patients were untreatable. The work of Partners In Health in Haiti and Peru, however, had shown that MDRTB can be treated successfully in settings of overwhelming poverty. All that was left, then, was the recurrent mantra that the drugs were too expensive to be cost-effective. But this mantra was repeated without honest investigation of *why* the drugs, long off patent, were so expensive. Thus has the notion of cost-effectiveness become one of the chief means by which we manage (and perpetuate) modern inequality.

The GUIN physicians, although familiar with short rations, were uncomfortable with the logic of cost-effectiveness. Furthermore, although they were in the supplicant position, many did not agree that the patients were untreatable. They knew about the second-line drugs, some of which had been widely used in the Soviet era, and also about adjuvant surgery for MDRTB. On paper, patients who failed standardized short-course chemotherapy and were deemed to have MDRTB were declared untreatable and transferred to an "isolation unit" surrounded by barbed wire. But many were in fact receiving, as a desperate measure, alternative treatment regimens, some of which included second-line drugs. These nonstandardized, last-resort efforts did not, however, receive the financial support of the project's European partners. Among physicians and nurses, to say nothing of patient-prisoners, a palpable tension reigned in Colony 33.

Clearly, it will take massive amounts of aid and political will to replicate the successful Peruvian strategy in the overwhelmed TB colonies of Russia, where politicians have reduced the already inadequate prison funding. As a result, exasperated GUIN officials have talked about giving amnesty to one hundred thousand prisoners, a substantial number of whom are likely to have active tuberculosis. Lawmakers have blocked that move for now. What will become of these young men with tuberculosis? Some will surely die in prison; GUIN officials maintain that those who are still alive when their sentences are up will be released on schedule. Like Sergei, they will carry prison-acquired strains of tuberculosis back home with them. Most of these will be drug-resistant strains.

THE RIGHT TO EFFECTIVE THERAPY

Three months after my visit to Colony 33, I returned to Russia for a conference on human rights and penal reform. At a Moscow gathering of GUIN officials and international advocates of prison reform, both sides agreed that the size of the prison population must be reduced, that detainees must be brought to trial with much greater dispatch, and that punishments other than detention must be attempted. But there was acrimony, too. A prominent jurist from Poland took the prison officials to task "for allowing ten thousand prisoners to starve to death in the preceding year." The GUIN officials looked more confused than defensive. That can't be true, they whispered to each other. *That* many? From hunger? I sat quietly, a few rows back, too travel-weary to suggest that whatever the accuracy of the figure, it was not hunger alone but also epidemic tuberculosis that was killing many of the country's young convicts. And it was killing some of their guards and other prison staff as well.

Sitting in the human rights conference, among like-minded people, I felt mostly exasperation. Doesn't it matter that we get the story right? Dying from starvation and torture is surely not the same thing as dying from drug-resistant tuberculosis. Isn't it important that critics, both local and imported, understand the complex series of events and processes that have conspired to make tuberculosis once again the leading cause of deaths within Russia's prisons?

The human rights gathering in Moscow made it clear to me that competing ideologies were fogging the view of what was causing so much suffering and death within the penitentiary system. The advocates of penal reform and the human rights community, accustomed to shouting at an unresponsive bureaucracy, had failed to note important facts about disease and death within the Russian jails and prisons. If starvation were the only problem, then food alone would go a long way toward relieving it. And when Médecins Sans Frontières began supplementing the food supply in Colony 33, the death rate dropped dramatically. But the cure rate did not rise much. Food cures starvation, not tuberculosis. If the problem were merely garden-variety tuberculosis, then DOTS alone would stop TB within the Russian penitentiary system. But short-course chemotherapy is not much more effective against MDRTB than is food. Moreover, the problem was not a matter of denied political rights that could be restored through a sudden political act: the evil did not all lie with the erstwhile gulag. Much of it could be traced to the pricing mechanisms and social policies current in the "free world." Thus all sides had gotten it wrong, and they were also failing to note that GUIN officials were asking for assistance, which they had never done before. Moreover, these officials made it easy for me to visit their prisons—far easier than it had been to deal with the corresponding prison administrations in Haiti or the United States.

With the international human rights and prison reform communities crying for amnesties, and GUIN only too happy to agree, what will happen next? To what care will these young men with drug-resistant tuberculosis be released? Prospects outside the prison gates are no less unsettling. Public health departments within Russia and in many parts of the former Soviet Union show a markedly diminished capacity to treat tuberculosis among civilians. The Soviet medical system had been able to keep the disease in check. During the Soviet era, drugs were centrally produced and distributed, and screening was frequent and nearly universal. Patients were strictly managed, often with mandatory stays in sanatoriums. Rates of tuberculosis in Russia dropped throughout the twentieth century, lagging behind Western Europe but clearly on the same downward arc. But all this has changed, in the civilian sector as well as within the penitentiary system. Between 1990 and 1996, rates increased almost threefold, by some estimates. Even according to the most conservative estimates of the World Health Organization, the rates at least doubled, with 111,075 new cases reported in 1996 alone. Estimates classify one in five new cases as drug-resistant. Since 1996, incidence has continued to increase at a steady rate; the number of new cases reported is more than 130,000.[19]

The threat represented by those figures is all too real. And there's no closing the gates on the airborne foe. A single plane ride is enough to transport tuberculosis from one country to another. Of course, transmission of this sort, though dramatic and well-documented, is rare. Far more common is the incessant bombardment of prisoners by the bacilli coming from the lungs of their untreated, or incorrectly treated, jailmates. No less common is the hidden-away suffering of a family that will never board a plane to any destination. But since proximity to the nonpoor is, dreadfully enough, the chief source of hope for those now without treatment, I will spell it out: an epidemic of these proportions cannot be contained by national boundaries any more than it can be contained by prison bars.

One of the most celebrated events of the late twentieth century was "the fall of the Berlin Wall." While East Germans celebrated the crumbling of this unlovely structure, a lot more crumbling was about to ensue. The steady dismantling of the Soviet-era health infrastructure occurred at the same time that the social safety net was ripped apart.[20] As job security disappeared, petty criminality rose. Arresting the impoverished is one of the oldest tricks in the book—what the sociologist Loïc Wacquant calls "the police-and-prison management of poverty."[21] And if Sergei struck me as looking more like an accountant than a felon, it's perhaps because there's little in his nature, but much in his surroundings, that led him to crime. Honest assessments, though late in coming, reveal the true dimensions of the Russian tragedy:

Even before its independence in December 1991 Russia had inherited the corrupt state apparatus, but without the restraining rule of the Communist party. The Russian Federation was in no shape to replace party rule with the rule of law. The corrupt piratization (*piratizatsiya*) of state assets and extensive further criminalization of government and the economy left Russia in the grip of venal, and often deadly, countercommunities. Disunited democrats and a weak, impoverished civil society were hardly a countervailing match for that.

The mismatch between corruption and democratization opened the way to massive violations of economic and social rights. The Soviet-era priority of economic and social rights has been blotted out by social calamity.[22]

Sergei's lungs have been destroyed by the tubercle bacillus. But this is only the distal event in a long and complicated story. The story stands to gain many more chapters, because the fall of the Wall has meant a rapid rise in travel to and from the former Soviet Union. In the Baltic region, where visitors moving between St. Petersburg and the major seaboard cities of Scandinavia number in the millions, how can there not be a rise in drug-resistant tuberculosis? How can there not be such a rise in dozens of countries, if the disease is treated effectively on one side of the sea but not the other?[23] If the number of travelers to and from Russia and Europe has risen exponentially over the past decade, how can the exponential rise of tuberculosis within Russia's porous prisons not have epidemiological impact wherever microbial traffic is facilitated by human movement? If the standard of care in New York City includes rapid identification and effective, specific treatment of drug-resistant tuberculosis, why should we expect medical officers within Russia's Ministry of Justice to be willing to implement an inferior standard of care for the likes of Sergei?

It is shameful that the world's international health and prison reform experts are calling for less than the highest quality of care for the incarcerated. Yet shame, it seems, rarely moves experts. Perhaps that is why, in the corridors of power, drug-resistant tuberculosis and other "emerging infectious diseases" have now been declared "national security issues."[24] When those responsible for protecting U.S. interests at home and abroad learn that treating prisoners who have multidrug-resistant tuberculosis with first-line drugs will not cure them, they will probably do the math—they're good at math—and will learn that most young men with pulmonary tuberculosis can live a long time. They will learn, too, that large-scale amnesties are being planned for tens of thousands of prisoners with tuberculosis. And if they have reasonable intelligence, they will learn that the cheerleaders of modern capitalism have pushed for a massive reduction in health care expenditures within the former Soviet Union. Although these cheerleaders and their technical consultants term this reduction "health care reform," it ensures that people who acquired drug-resistant tuberculosis in prison will find little help in the civilian sector. And, like all humans, these people will move—in and out of prison and in and out of Russia.

Thus prisoners like Sergei, who by now no doubt has made his way back to western Siberia, are epidemiologically important. But the case for prompt and effective therapy for all forms of active tuberculosis, everywhere, must also be made on human rights grounds. I was surprised to discover that some within the global community of prison reform experts have questioned aggressive advocacy on behalf of prisoners sick with drug-resistant tuberculosis. If effective therapy for MDRTB is not available within the civilian sector, goes this line of reasoning, then it cannot be made available to prisoners. Heaven forfend that we would risk having higher health care standards within prisons and jails.

Managing inequality almost never includes higher standards of care for those whose agency has been constrained, whether by poverty or by prison bars. In Chapter 7, I argue that precisely such a strategy should be used within prisons. Careful research shows that many of these young men, arrested for crimes against property, enter jail uninfected by *M. tuberculosis*. Well before they ever come to trial, however, many become sick with tuberculosis; some die of this disease before being convicted of any crime. Visits to these prisons and jails have taught me that the incarcerated know very well the risk they run. But *they* cannot run from the risk.

Surely it is an irony of the global era that the stewards of power will take international health experts to task for failing to, in their lingo, "contain a threat" such as this one. If the guardians of Fortress America prove to be the most ardent champions of effective therapy for Russian prisoners with tuberculosis, it will be because we in the human rights and international health communities have failed, and failed miserably, to move resources to the places where they are most needed. Sub-Saharan Africa stands as the greatest rebuke to our inaction on these scores, but Russian prisoners with an airborne disease have become yet another reminder of the "unsustainability" of any approach based on differential valuation of human life.

—January 1999

POSTSCRIPT: DECEMBER 23, 2000

I heard the bells on Christmas Day
Their old, familiar carols play,
And wild and sweet
The words repeat
Of peace on earth, good-will to men!

And in despair I bowed my head;
"There is no peace on earth," I said;
"For hate is strong
And mocks the song
Of peace on earth, good-will to men!"

Henry Wadsworth Longfellow,
Christmas Bells

Siberia is in many ways a nice place to visit in the winter. The thick drifts of clean snow are breathtaking; fine local vodka and beer run freely to slake thirst and lessen the chill of the dark afternoons. Preparations for Christmas are underway. Even inside the Tomsk penitentiary, where we are visiting medical colleagues, prisoners compete to see who can make the most beautiful ice sculpture. A pair of comical bears, one of them with a wrapped present, greets all those who enter the dilapidated complex, after the electric doors buzz and clang shut behind them.

As temperatures drop to 30 below zero, prison windows are closed as tightly as the doors. It is warm inside, but deadly: the air in the cells is thick and teeming with the organism that causes tuberculosis. In less than a decade, rates of tuberculosis in western Siberia have more than trebled, with case notifications reaching 117 per 100,000 people who live here in the oblast of Tomsk. Rates are forty to fifty times higher within its prisons. And this prison, like the others described in this book, is swollen to bursting as petty crime has risen sharply in the wake of social and economic upheaval.

As elsewhere, the Tomsk prisons and jails have served as breeding grounds for difficult-to-treat strains of drug-resistant tuberculosis. In a 1998 survey of 212 prisoners with active, pulmonary tuberculosis, three quarters had drug-resistant tuberculosis. Among prisoners with a history of previous antituberculous therapy—and this was the majority—most had resistance to more than one first-line drug.[25] The mean age of the Tomsk patients was twenty-seven years old. Here as elsewhere, the disease is again the leading cause of death of prisoners.

The mutant microbes are not long deterred by prison bars. Inside the nearby Tomsk civilian sanatorium, one-third of all patients suffer from MDRTB. According to the director, no fewer than half of the past year's deaths in the hospital resulted from MDRTB. Many of these patients have been in prison; some are prison staff. But some patients appear to have become infected in hospitals and other institutions. Still others are homeless coughers or alcoholics.

Prisons, hospitals, homeless shelters, addiction, and drug-resistant tuberculosis—this cycle should sound familiar. The epidemiology of MDRTB in Tomsk recalls the tuberculosis crisis discovered a decade ago in the prisons of New York City, where hundreds of millions of dollars were expended to improve tuberculosis treatment and control. Few would argue that these dollars were poorly spent.

But precisely this argument—that tuberculosis control is too costly, especially if it involves treating prisoners with MDRTB—continues to hamper efforts to check the most serious epidemic of tuberculosis ever to hit an industrialized country. Tomsk Oblast alone, with its million or so souls, probably has more MDRTB patients than New York did at the height of the U.S. outbreak. But the tuberculosis services in Tomsk have a budget that amounts to less than 5 percent of that of New York's tuberculosis bureau.

Impossible not to note that many of Russia's rubles have ended up in dollar accounts in New York, Switzerland, and the Caribbean. Perhaps this cash flow helps explain why aggressive tuberculosis control—which necessarily includes treatment of all the afflicted—is "cost-effective" in New York but not in Siberia. In fact, the logic of cost-effectiveness was invoked to justify extraordinary expenditures in New York:

> The costs of the resurgence of tuberculosis have been phenomenal. From 1979 through 1994, there were more than 20,000 excess cases of the disease in New York City.... Each case cost more than $20,000 in 1990 dollars, for a total exceeding $400 million. In addition, as many as one third of patients with tuberculosis were rehospitalized because of inadequate follow-up.... There were additional expenditures for renovation of Rikers Island...[and for] the renovation of hospitals.... Care will be required for those who become ill in the years and decades to come. These costs easily exceed $1 billion and may reach several times that amount. Thus, *despite their cost,* efforts to control tuberculosis in the United States are likely to be highly cost effective.[26]

What is to be done? Most international health experts have argued that Russia needs to pare back its large, unwieldy tuberculosis control system, which relied on in-patient services and individualized treatment regimens. Patients should be treated at home, say the international experts; all Russian patients should be treated with standardized doses of the same drugs—what is termed "short-course chemotherapy." But the Russians counter that many of their patients have complex social problems (it's hard to treat people at home if they have no home, for instance, and alcoholics cannot always adhere to out-patient therapy). Their "case mix" is too complex, they say, for a one-size-fits-all approach to tuberculosis treatment and control.

MDRTB certainly proves their point. If someone is sick with MDRTB, giving that patient short-course chemotherapy is tantamount to doing nothing—worse than nothing, given the toxicity of the drugs. As for cutting back expenditures in the midst of a burgeoning epidemic, we can only note that it is unwise suddenly to start conserving water when your house is on fire.

That these complexities are only now acknowledged, more than a decade into the epidemic, is a shame—and, for some patients, an irreparable one. But some groups are trying to repair this damage. Here in Tomsk, a novel effort is bringing together all parties—the Russians and their international interlocutors; doctors and nurses and patients; prison and civilian authorities; public and private donors—in order to make sure that every patient receives high-quality care. For several years, a British nongovernmental agency and PHRI have worked with Tomsk's civilian and prison authorities to respond to resurgent tuberculosis effectively and in a coordinated manner. What was missing was the ability to treat patients who had MDRTB. That meant second-line drugs, specialized laboratory capacity, and some technical assistance. To us, that meant pragmatic solidarity.

A few months ago, after careful evaluation of local capacity to use the drugs correctly, Partners In Health purchased some of the second-line medications required by the prisoner-patients. And this week, civilians with MDRTB will finally have access to the drugs that might save their lives; scores of prisoners are already being treated or slated for treatment. Adequate resources to rebuild the tuberculosis infrastructure, which includes increased laboratory capacity, are finally being brought to bear on this problem. But the project will be difficult to implement and sustain.[27] Many of these patients will die, even though they are at last receiving the therapy they need. This is because it's late in the game for most of the afflicted, who have already failed treatment with short-course chemotherapy. Most have failed multiple rounds of inadequate treatment, and their disease worsens with each passing day. And the epidemic grows.

Critics argue that the comprehensive approach costs too much, especially if it cannot promise universal cure. Admittedly, the costs are high, if nowhere near as high as rumor has it. But the worst of the expense lies with the medications, and there is no reason for their high and fluctuating prices: the drugs have been off patent for decades, and we know that the same companies sell the same drug at wildly different prices in different countries.[28] Drug prices should not constitute the chief barrier to effective therapy for all patients, regardless of infecting strain. With less complaining, and more coordination, international public health authorities could have brought these prices down rapidly, as we have learned by our efforts to do so.[29]

Critics further argue against treatment for MDRTB patients in order to conserve resources for more readily treated patients. But this zero-sum approach does not ask why funds are so short, does not even acknowledge the vast sums of money shipped out of Russia—gained, no doubt, from the sale of public property—as part of the equation. Critics of universal treatment do not always remember that all tuberculosis patients in New York, including those with MDRTB, were treated. This special effort did not draw money away from garden-variety tuberculosis control. Quite the contrary: MDRTB has almost disappeared from New York, but funding remains robust. The specter of "killer TB strains loose in the subway" (as the headlines went) was enough to generate support for a more adequate tuberculosis service.

Opponents of universal tuberculosis treatment, reasoning from misguided notions of cost-effectiveness, fail to acknowledge that MDRTB is not exclusively a disease of poor people in distant places. The disease is infectious and airborne. Treating only one group of patients looks inexpensive in the short run, but it will prove disastrous for all in the long run. For those already sick with the disease, including many of the young men now making ice sculptures in the prison courtyard, there will be no long run.

PART II

ONE PHYSICIAN'S PERSPECTIVE ON HUMAN RIGHTS

A discourse on human rights must begin with the right to life that is the right precisely of the poor.

Jon Sobrino, *Spirituality of Liberation*

Article 25:

Everyone has the right to a standard of living adequate for the health and well-being of himself and of his family, including food, clothing, housing and medical care and necessary social services, and the right to security in the event of unemployment, sickness, disability, widowhood, old age or other lack of livelihood in circumstances beyond his control.

Article 27:

Everyone has the right freely to participate in the cultural life of the community, to enjoy the arts and to share in scientific advancement and its benefits.

Everyone has the right to the protection of the moral and material interests resulting from any scientific, literary or artistic production of which he is the author.

Universal Declaration of Human Rights

ON ANALYTIC PERSPECTIVE

In recent years an anthropology of suffering has
emerged as a new kind of theodicy, a cultural inquiry
into the ways that people attempt to explain the presence of pain, affliction, and evil in the world. At times
of crisis, in moments of intense suffering, people everywhere demand an answer to the primal existential
question: "Why me, oh God? Why me, of all people?
Why now?" The quest for meaning may be posed to
vindicate an indifferent God, to quell one's self doubt,
or to restore faith in an orderly and righteous world.

Nancy Scheper-Hughes,
"Sacred Wounds: Writing with the Body"

A FRIEND OF MINE, an anthropologist, suggested that I explain why I felt
this book was divided into two parts. The first half of *Pathologies of
Power* is called "Bearing Witness" because it relies on eyewitness accounts
and on my own interviews (whether as physician or anthropologist). The
second half of the book consists of a series of essays about the analytic
perspective that informs my critique of human rights as conventionally
defined. "Analytic perspective" may be too grand a term, and by quali-
fying it as "one physician's perspective on human rights" I mean to be
humble in two ways. The first is fairly conventional, and I mention it only
in passing: this critique comes from a particular vantage point, that of a
physician-anthropologist in service to the poor. Many would prefer to
hear an analysis of human rights by human rights experts, most of whom
are trained in law and jurisprudence rather than in my two disciplines.

The second strand of humility is less commonly encountered in scholarly writing, so I will outline it here. Those who consider themselves
stringent about matters such as "theory" and "analysis" may well find
these essays insufficient. Theirs, however, are not the critiques to which
I seek to respond in these pages. Rather, I am humbled by the suffering
of the destitute sick and also by human rights abuses as conventionally
defined. These also affect primarily the poor.

Given that such an "analytic perspective" is as much a stance as an analysis, and given that the stance is one of humility before the suffering of the poor, where does one turn for inspiration? As Chapter 1 noted, liberation theology has been one of my intellectual resources. Liberation theology, curiously enough, is the branch of theology most likely to turn to social theory, history, political economy. This would seem like a very indirect way for an anthropologist to delve into the social sciences. But liberation theology adds something not found in any discipline, including Marxist analyses. It adds this constant interrogation: *how is this relevant to the suffering of the poor and to the relief of that suffering?* Thus, unlike most forms of social analysis, liberation theology seeks to yoke all of its reflection to the service of the poor.

This helps to explain, perhaps, why I put medicine first in the title of Part II. Scholarship, including anthropology, is not always readily yoked to the service of the poor. Medicine, I have discovered, is. At its best, medicine is a service much more than a science, and the latest battery of biomedical discoveries, in which I rejoice, has not convinced me otherwise. Medicine becomes pragmatic solidarity when it is delivered with dignity to the destitute sick. Elsewhere I have argued that physicians need social theory (including anthropology) in order to resocialize their understanding of who becomes sick and why, and of who has access to health care and why. We also need to resocialize our understanding of human rights abuses. As I've tried to show, these abuses are no more random in distribution than is, say, typhoid or AIDS.

In short, this "one physician's perspective on human rights" may be summed up as follows: just as the poor are more likely to fall sick and then be denied access to care, so too are they more likely to be the victims of human rights abuses, no matter how these are defined. By including social and economic rights in the struggle for human rights, we help to protect those most likely to suffer the insults of structural violence. It is my belief that the liberation theologians, in advocating preferential treatment for the poor, offer those concerned with human rights a moral compass for future action. A preferential option for the poor, and all perspectives rooted in it, also offers a way out of the impasse in which many of us caregivers now find ourselves: selling our wares and services only to those who can afford them, rather than making sure that they reach those who need them most. Allowing "market forces" to sculpt the outlines of modern medicine will mean that these unwelcome trends will continue until we are forced to conclude that even the practice of medicine can constitute a human rights abuse.

CHAPTER 5

HEALTH, HEALING, AND SOCIAL JUSTICE

INSIGHTS FROM
LIBERATION THEOLOGY

If I define my neighbor as the one I must go out to look for, on the highways and byways, in the factories and slums, on the farms and in the mines—then my world changes. This is what is happening with the "option for the poor," for in the gospel it is the poor person who is the neighbor par excellence....

But the poor person does not exist as an inescapable fact of destiny. His or her existence is not politically neutral, and it is not ethically innocent. The poor are a by-product of the system in which we live and for which we are responsible. They are marginalized by our social and cultural world. They are the oppressed, exploited proletariat, robbed of the fruit of their labor and despoiled of their humanity. Hence the poverty of the poor is not a call to generous relief action, but a demand that we go and build a different social order.

Gustavo Gutiérrez, The Power of the Poor in History

Not everything that the poor are and do is gospel. But a great deal of it is.

Jon Sobrino, Spirituality of Liberation

MAKING A PREFERENTIAL OPTION FOR THE POOR

For decades now, proponents of liberation theology have argued that people of faith must make a "preferential option for the poor." As discussed by Brazil's Leonardo Boff, a leading contributor to the movement, "the Church's option is a preferential option *for the poor, against their poverty*." The poor, Boff adds, "are those who suffer injustice. Their poverty is produced by mechanisms of impoverishment and exploitation. Their poverty is therefore an evil and an injustice."[1] To those concerned with health, a preferential option for the poor offers both a challenge and an insight. It challenges doctors and other health providers to make an option—a choice—for the poor, to work on their behalf.

The insight is, in a sense, an epidemiological one: most often, diseases themselves make a preferential option for the poor. Every careful survey, across boundaries of time and space, shows us that the poor are sicker than the nonpoor. They're at increased risk of dying prematurely, whether from increased exposure to pathogens (including pathogenic situations) or from decreased access to services—or, as is most often the case, from both of these "risk factors" working together.[2] Given this indisputable association, medicine has a clear—if not always observed—mandate to devote itself to populations struggling against poverty.

It's also clear that many health professionals feel paralyzed by the magnitude of the challenge. Where on earth does one start? We have received endless, detailed prescriptions from experts, many of them manifestly dismissive of initiatives coming from afflicted communities themselves. But those who formulate health policy in Geneva, Washington, New York, or Paris do not really labor to transform the social conditions of the wretched of the earth. Instead, the actions of technocrats—and what physician is not a technocrat?—are most often tantamount to managing social inequality, to keeping the problem under control. The limitations of such tinkering are sharp, as Peruvian theologian Gustavo Gutiérrez warns:

> Latin American misery and injustice go too deep to be responsive to palliatives. Hence we speak of social revolution, not reform; of liberation, not development; of socialism, not modernization of the prevailing system. "Realists" call these statements romantic and utopian. And they should, for the reality of these statements is of a kind quite unfamiliar to them.[3]

Liberation theology, in contrast to officialdom, argues that genuine change will be most often rooted in small communities of poor people; and it advances a simple methodology—*observe, judge, act*.[4] Throughout Latin America, such base-community movements have worked to take stock of their situations and devise strategies for change.[5] The approach is straightforward. Although it has been termed "simplistic" by technocrats and experts, this methodology has proven useful for promoting health in settings as diverse as Brazil, Guatemala, El Salvador, rural Mexico, and urban Peru. Insights from liberation theology have proven useful in rural Haiti too, perhaps the sickest region of the hemisphere and the one I know best. With all due respect for health policy expertise, then, this chapter explores the implications—so far, almost completely overlooked—of liberation theology for medicine and health policy.[6]

Observe, judge, act. The "observe" part of the formula implies analysis. There has been no shortage of analysis from the self-appointed apostles of international health policy, who insist that their latest recipes become the cornerstones of health policy in all of Latin America's nations.[7] Within ministries of health, one quickly learns not to question these fads, since failure to acknowledge the primacy of the regnant health ideology can stop many projects from ever getting off the ground. But other, less conventional sources of analysis are relevant to our understanding of health and illness. It's surprising that many Catholic bishops of Latin America, for centuries allied with the elites of their countries, have in more recent decades chosen to favor tough-minded social analysis of their societies. Many would argue that liberation theology's key documents were hammered out at the bishops' conventions in Medellín in 1968 and in Puebla in 1978. In both instances, progressive bishops, working with like-minded theologians, denounced the political and economic forces that immiserate so many Latin Americans. Regarding causality, the bishops did not mince words:

> Let us recall once again that the present moment in the history of our peoples is characterized in the social order, and from an objective point of view, by a situation of underdevelopment. Certain phenomena point an accusing finger at it: marginalized existence, alienation, and poverty. In the last analysis it is conditioned by structures of economic, political, and cultural dependence on the great industrialized metropolises, the latter enjoying a monopoly on technology and science (neocolonialism).[8]

What began timidly in the preparation for the Medellín meeting in 1968 was by 1978 a strong current. "The Puebla document," remarks Boff, "moves immediately to the structural analysis of these forces and denounces the systems, structures, and mechanisms that 'create a situation where the rich get richer at the expense of the poor, who get even poorer.' "[9] In both of these meetings, the bishops were at pains to argue that "this reality calls for personal conversion and profound structural changes that will meet the legitimate aspirations of the people for authentic social justice."[10]

As Chapter 1 noted, liberation theology has always been about the struggle for social and economic rights. The injunction to "observe" leads to descriptions of the conditions of the Latin American poor, and also to claims regarding the origins of these conditions. These causal claims have obvious implications for a rethinking of human rights, as Gutiérrez explains:

> A structural analysis better suited to Latin American reality has led certain Christians to speak of the "rights of the poor" and to interpret the defense of human rights under this new formality. The adjustment is not merely a matter of words. This alternative language represents a critical approach to the laissez-faire, liberal doctrine to the effect that our society enjoys an equality that in fact does not exist. This new formulation likewise seeks constantly to remind us of what is really at stake in the defense of human rights: the misery and spoliation of the poorest of the poor, the conflictive character of Latin American life and society, and the biblical roots of the defense of the poor.[11]

Liberation theologians are among the few who have dared to underline, from the left, the deficiencies of the liberal human rights movement. The most glaring of these deficiencies emerges from intimate acquaintance with the suffering of the poor in countries that are signatory to all modern human rights agreements. When children living in poverty die of measles, gastroenteritis, and malnutrition, and yet no party is judged guilty of a human rights violation, liberation theology finds fault with the entire notion of human rights as defined within liberal democracies. Thus, even before judgment is rendered, the "observe" part of the formula reveals atrocious conditions as atrocious.

The "judge" part of the equation is nonetheless important even if it is, in a sense, pre-judged. We look at the lives of the poor and are sure, just as they are, that *something is terribly wrong*. They are targets of structural violence. (Some of the bishops termed this "structural sin.")[12] This is, granted, an a priori judgment—but it is seldom incorrect, for analysis of social suffering invariably reveals its social origins. It is not primarily cataclysms of nature that wreak havoc in the lives of the Latin American poor:

> All these aspects which make up the overall picture of the state of humanity in the late twentieth century have one common name: oppression. They all, including the hunger suffered by millions of human beings, result from the oppression of some human beings by others. The impotence of international bodies in the face of generally recognized problems, their inability to effect solutions, stems from the self-interest of those who stand to benefit from their oppression of other human beings. In each major problem there is broad recognition of both the moral intolerableness and the political non-viability of the existing situation, coupled with a lack of capacity to respond.

> If the problem is (or the problems are) a conflict of interests, then the energy
> to find the solution can come only from the oppressed themselves.[13]

Rendering judgment based on careful observation can be a powerful experience. The Brazilian sociologist Paulo Freire coined the term *conscientization,* or "consciousness raising," to explain the process of coming to understand how social structures cause injustice.[14] This "involves discovering that evil not only is present in the hearts of powerful individuals who muck things up for the rest of us but is embedded in the very structures of society, so that those structures, and not just individuals who work within them, must be changed if the world is to change."[15] Liberation theology uses the primary tools of social analysis to reveal the mechanisms by which social structures cause social misery. Such analysis, unlike many fraudulently dispassionate academic treatises, is meant to challenge the observer to judge. It requires a very different approach than that most often used by, say, global health bureaucrats. It requires an approach that implicates the observer, as Jon Sobrino notes:

> The reality posed by the poor, then, is no rhetorical question. Precisely as
> sin, this reality tends to conceal itself, to be relativized, to pass itself off as
> something secondary and provisional in the larger picture of human
> achievements. It is a reality that calls men and women not only to recognize
> and acknowledge it, but to take a primary, basic position regarding it.
> Outwardly, this reality demands that it be stated for what it is, and de-
> nounced.... But inwardly, this same reality is a question for human beings
> as themselves participants in the sin of humankind.... the poor of the
> world are not the causal products of human history. No, poverty results
> from the actions of other human beings.[16]

How is all of this relevant to medicine? It is more realistic, surely, to ask how this could be considered irrelevant to medicine. In the wealthy countries of the Northern hemisphere, the relatively poor often travel far and wait long for health care inferior to that available to the wealthy. In the Third World, where conservative estimates suggest that one billion souls live in dire poverty, the plight of the poor is even worse. How do they cope? They don't, often enough. The poor there have short life expectancies, often dying of preventable or treatable diseases or from accidents. Few have access to modern medical care. In fact, most of the Third World poor receive no effective biomedical care at all. For some people, there is no such thing as a measles vaccine. For many, tuberculosis is as lethal as AIDS. Childbirth involves mortal risk. In an age of explosive development in the realm of medical technology, it is unnerving to find that the discoveries of Salk, Sabin, and even Pasteur remain irrelevant to much of humanity.

Many physicians are uncomfortable acknowledging these harsh facts of life and death. To do so, one must admit that the majority of premature deaths are, as the Haitians would say, "stupid deaths." They are completely preventable with the tools already available to the fortunate few. By the criteria of liberation theology, these deaths are a great injustice and a stain on the conscience of modern medicine and science. Why, then, are these premature deaths not the primary object of discussion and debate within our professional circles? Again, liberation theology helps to answer this question. First, acknowledging the scandalous conditions of those living in poverty often requires a rejection of comforting relativism. Sobrino is addressing fellow theologians, but what he writes is of relevance to physicians, too:

> In order to recognize the truth of creation today, one must take another tack in this first, basic moment, a moment of honesty. The data, the statistics, may seem cold. They may seem to have precious little to do with theology. But we must take account of them. This is where we have to start. "Humanity" today is the victim of poverty and institutionalized violence. Often enough this means death, slow or sudden.[17]

A second reason that premature deaths are not the primary topic of our professional discussion is that the viewpoints of poor people will inevitably be suppressed or neglected as long as elites control most means of communication. Thus the steps of observation and judgment are usually difficult, because vested interests, including those controlling "development" and even international health policy, have an obvious stake in shaping observations about causality and in attenuating harsh judgments of harsh conditions. (This is, of course, another reason that people living in poverty are cited in this book as experts on structural violence and human rights.)

Finally, the liberation theologians and the communities from which they draw their inspiration agree that it is necessary to *act* on these reflections. The "act" part of the formula implies much more than reporting one's findings. The goal of this judging is not producing more publications or securing tenure in a university: "in order to *understand* the world, Latin American Christians are taking seriously the insights of social scientists, sociologists, and economists, in order to learn how to *change* the world."[18] Sobrino puts it this way: "There is no doubt that the only correct way to love the poor will be to struggle for their liberation. This liberation will consist, first and foremost, in their liberation at the most elementary level—that of their simple, physical life, which is what is at stake in the present situation."[19] I could confirm his assessment with my own experiences in Haiti and elsewhere, including the streets of some of the cities of the hemisphere's most affluent country. What's at stake, for many of the poor, is physical survival.

The results of following this "simple" methodology can be quiet and yet effective, as in the small-scale project described in the next section. But careful reflection on the inhuman conditions endured by so many in this time of great affluence can of course also lead to more explosive actions. Retrospective analysis of these explosions—the one described in Chapter 3 of this volume, for example—often reveals them to be last-ditch efforts to escape untenable situations. That is, the explosions follow innumerable peaceful attempts to attenuate structural violence and the lies that help sustain it. The Zapatistas, who refer often to early death from treatable illnesses, explain it this way in an early communiqué:

> Some ask why we decided to begin now, if we were prepared before. The answer is that before this we tried other peaceful and legal roads to change, but without success. During these last ten years more than 150,000 of our indigenous brothers and sisters have died from curable diseases. The federal, state, and municipal governments' economic and social plans do not even consider any real solution to our problems, and consist of giving us handouts at election times. But these crumbs of charity solve our problems for no more than a moment, and then, death returns to our houses. That is why we think no, no more, enough of this dying useless deaths, it would be better to fight for change. If we die now, we will not die with shame, but with the dignity of our ancestors. Another 150,000 of us are ready to die if that is what is needed to waken our people from their deceit-induced stupor.[20]

APPLYING PRINCIPLES OF LIBERATION THEOLOGY TO MEDICINE

To act as a physician in the service of poor or otherwise oppressed people is to prevent, whenever possible, the diseases that afflict them—but also to treat and, if possible, to cure. So where's the innovation in that? How would a health intervention inspired by liberation theology be different from one with more conventional underpinnings? Over the past two decades, Partners In Health has joined local community health activists to provide basic primary care and preventive services to poor communities in Mexico, Peru, the United States, and, especially, Haiti—offering what we have termed "pragmatic solidarity." Pragmatic solidarity is different from but nourished by solidarity per se, the desire to make common cause with those in need. Solidarity is a precious thing: people enduring great hardship often remark that they are grateful for the prayers and good wishes of fellow human beings. But when sentiment is accompanied by the goods and services that might diminish unjust hardship, surely it is enriched. To those in great need, solidarity without the pragmatic component can seem like so much abstract piety.

Lest all this talk of structural violence and explosive responses to it seem vague and far-removed from the everyday obligations of medicine, allow me to give examples from my own clinical experience. How does liberation theology inform medical practice in, say, rural Haiti? Take tuberculosis, along with HIV the leading infectious cause of preventable adult deaths in the world. How might one observe, judge, and act in pragmatic solidarity with those most likely to acquire tuberculosis or already suffering from it?

The "observation" part of the formula is key, for it involves careful review of a large body of literature that seeks to explain the distribution of the disease within populations, to explore its clinical characteristics, and to evaluate tuberculosis treatment regimens. This sort of review is standard in all responsible health planning, but liberation theology would push analysis in two directions: first, to seek the root causes of the problem; second, *to elicit the experiences and views of poor people* and to incorporate these views into all observations, judgments, and actions.

Ironically enough, some who understand, quite correctly, that the underlying causes of tuberculosis are poverty and social inequality make a terrible error by failing to honor the experience and views of the poor in designing strategies to respond to the disease. What happens if, after analysis reveals poverty as the root cause of tuberculosis, tuberculosis control strategies ignore the sick and focus solely on eradicating poverty? Elsewhere, I have called this the "Luddite trap," since this ostensibly progressive view would have us ignore both current distress and the tools of modern medicine that might relieve it, thereby committing a new and grave injustice.[21] The destitute sick ardently desire the eradication of poverty, but their tuberculosis can be readily cured by drugs such as isoniazid and rifampin. The prescription for poverty is not so clear.

Careful review of the biomedical and epidemiological literature on tuberculosis does permit certain conclusions. One of the clearest is that the incidence of the disease is not at all random. Certainly, tuberculosis has claimed victims among the great (Frederic Chopin, Fyodor Dostoyevsky, George Orwell, Eleanor Roosevelt), but historically it is a disease that has ravaged the economically disadvantaged.[22] This is especially true in recent decades: with the development of effective therapy in the mid-twentieth century came high cure rates—over 95 percent—for those with access to the right drugs for the right amount of time. Thus tuberculosis *deaths* now—which each year number in the millions—occur almost exclusively among the poor, whether they reside in the inner cities of the United States or in the poor countries of the Southern hemisphere.[23]

The latest twists to the story—the resurgence of tuberculosis in the United States, the advent of HIV-related tuberculosis, and the development of strains of tuberculosis resistant to the first-line therapies developed in recent decades—serve to reinforce the thesis that *Mycobacterium tuberculosis,* the causative organism, makes its own preferential option for the poor.[24]

What "judgment" might be offered on these epidemiological and clinical facts? Many would find it scandalous that one of the world's leading causes of preventable adult deaths is a disease that, with the possible exception of emerging resistant strains, is more than 95 percent curable, with inexpensive therapies developed decades ago. Those inspired by liberation theology would certainly express distaste for a disease so partial to poor and debilitated hosts and would judge unacceptable the lack of therapy for those most likely to become ill with tuberculosis: poverty puts people at risk of tuberculosis and then bars them from access to effective treatment. An option-for-the-poor approach to tuberculosis would make the disease a top priority for research and development of new drugs and vaccines and at the same time would make programs to detect and cure all cases a global priority.

Contrast this reading to the received wisdom—and the current agenda—concerning tuberculosis. Authorities rarely blame the recrudescence of tuberculosis on the inequalities that structure our society. Instead, we hear mostly about biological factors (the advent of HIV, the mutations that lead to drug resistance) or about cultural and psychological barriers that result in "noncompliance." Through these two sets of explanatory mechanisms, one can expediently attribute high rates of treatment failure either to the organism or to uncooperative patients.

There are costs to seeing the problem in this way. If we see the resurgence or persistence of tuberculosis as an exclusively biological phe-

nomenon, then we will shunt available resources to basic biological research, which, though needed, is not the primary solution, since almost
all tuberculosis deaths result from lack of access to existing effective therapy. If we see the problem primarily as one of patient noncompliance,
then we must necessarily ground our strategies in plans to change the
patients rather than to change the weak tuberculosis control programs
that fail to detect and cure the majority of cases. In either event, weak
analysis produces the sort of dithering that characterizes current global
tuberculosis policy, which must accept as its primary rebuke the shameful death toll that continues unabated.

How about the "act" part of the formula advocated by liberation theology? In a sense, it's simple: heal the sick. Prompt diagnosis and cure
of tuberculosis are also the means to prevent new infections, so prevention and treatment are intimately linked. Most studies of tuberculosis in
Haiti reveal that the vast majority of patients do not complete treatment—which explains why, until very recently, tuberculosis remained
the leading cause of adult death in rural regions of Haiti. (It has now
been surpassed by HIV.) But it does not need to be so. In the country's
Central Plateau, Partners In Health worked with our sister organization,
Zanmi Lasante, to devise a tuberculosis treatment effort that borrows a
number of ideas—and also some passion—from liberation theology.

Although the Zanmi Lasante staff had, from the outset, identified and
referred patients with pulmonary tuberculosis to its clinic, it gradually
became clear that detection of new cases did not always lead to cure,
even though all tuberculosis care, including medication, was free of
charge. In December 1988, following the deaths from tuberculosis of
three HIV-negative patients, all adults in their forties, the staff met to reconsider the care these individuals had received. How had the staff failed
to prevent these deaths? How could we better observe, judge, and act as
a community making common cause with the destitute sick?

Initially, we responded to these questions in differing ways. In fact,
the early discussions were heated, with a fairly sharp divide between
community health workers, who shared the social conditions of the patients, and the doctors and nurses, who did not. Some community health
workers believed that tuberculosis patients with poor outcomes were the
most economically impoverished and thus the sickest; others hypothesized that patients lost interest in chemotherapy after ridding themselves
of the symptoms that had caused them to seek medical advice. Feeling
better, they returned as quickly as possible to the herculean task of providing for their families. Still others, including the physicians and nurses,

attributed poor compliance to widespread beliefs that tuberculosis was a disorder inflicted through sorcery, beliefs that led patients to abandon biomedical therapy. A desire to focus blame on the patients' ignorance or misunderstanding was palpable, even though the physicians and nurses sought to cure the disease as ardently as anyone else involved in the program.

The caregivers' ideas about the causes of poor outcomes tended to coalesce in two directions: a *cognitivist-personalistic* pole that emphasized individual patient agency (curiously, "cultural" explanations fit best under this rubric, since beliefs about sorcery allegedly led patients to abandon therapy), and a *structural* pole that emphasized the patients' poverty. And this poverty, though generic to outsiders like the physicians from Port-au-Prince, had a vivid history to those from the region. Most of our tuberculosis patients were landless peasants living in the most dire poverty. They had lost their land a generation before when the Péligre dam, part of an internationally funded development project, flooded their fertile valley.[25]

More meetings followed. Over the next several months, we devised a plan to improve services to patients with tuberculosis—and to test these discrepant hypotheses. Briefly, the new program set goals of detecting cases, supplying adequate chemotherapy, and providing close follow-up. Although they also continued contact screening and vaccination for infants, the staff of Zanmi Lasante was then most concerned with caring for smear-positive and coughing patients—believed to be the most important source of community exposure. The new program was aggressive and community-based, relying heavily on community health workers for close follow-up. It also responded to patients' appeals for nutritional assistance. The patients argued, often with some vehemence and always with eloquence, that to give medicines without food was tantamount to *lave men, siye atè* (washing one's hands and then wiping them dry in the dirt).

Those diagnosed with tuberculosis who participated in the new treatment program were to receive daily visits from their village health worker during the first month following diagnosis. They would also receive financial aid of thirty dollars per month for the first three months; would be eligible for nutritional supplements; would receive regular reminders from their village health worker to attend the clinic; and would receive a five-dollar honorarium to defray "travel expenses" (for example, renting a donkey) for attending the clinic. If a patient did not attend, someone from the clinic—often a physician or an auxiliary nurse—would make a visit to the no-show's house. A series of forms, including a detailed initial interview schedule and home visit reports, regularized these arrangements and replaced the relatively limited forms used for other clinic patients.

Between February 1989 and September 1990, fifty patients were enrolled in the program. During the same period, the clinical staff diagnosed pulmonary tuberculosis in 213 patients from outside our catchment area. The first fifty of these patients to be diagnosed formed the comparison group that would be used to judge the efficacy of the new intervention. They were a "control group" only in the sense that they did not benefit from the community-based services and financial aid; all tuberculosis patients continued to receive free care.

The difference in the outcomes of the two groups was little short of startling. By June 1991, forty-six of the patients receiving the "enhanced package" were free of all symptoms, and none of those with symptoms met radiologic or clinical diagnostic criteria for persistent tuberculosis. Therefore, the medical staff concluded that none had active pulmonary tuberculosis, giving the participants a cure rate of 100 percent. We could not locate all fifty of the patients from outside the catchment area, but for the forty patients examined more than one year after diagnosis, the cure rate was barely half that of the first group, based on clinical, laboratory, and radiographic evaluation. It should be noted that this dismal cure rate was nonetheless higher than that reported in most studies of tuberculosis outcomes in Haiti.[26]

Could this striking difference in outcome be attributed to patients' ideas and beliefs about tuberculosis? Previous ethnographic research had revealed extremely complex and changing ways of understanding and speaking about tuberculosis among rural Haitians.[27] Because most physicians and nurses (and a few community health workers) had hypothesized that patients who "believed in sorcery" as a cause of tuberculosis would have higher rates of noncompliance with their medical regimens, we took some pains to address this issue with each patient. As the resident medical anthropologist, I conducted long—often very long—and open-ended interviews with all patients in both groups, trying to delineate the dominant explanatory models that shaped their views of the disease. I learned that few from either group would deny the possibility of sorcery as an etiologic factor in their own illness, but I could discern no relationship between avowal of such beliefs and compliance with a biomedical regimen. That is, the outcomes were related to the quality of the program rather than the quality of the patients' ideas about the disease.

Suffice it to say, this was not the outcome envisioned by many of my colleagues in anthropology.

Although anthropologists are expected to underline the importance of *culture* in determining the efficacy of efforts to combat disease, in Haiti we learned that many of the most important variables—initial exposure to infection, reactivation of quiescent tuberculosis, transmission to household members, access to diagnosis and therapy, length of convalescence, development of drug resistance, degree of lung destruction, and, most of all, mortality—are all strongly influenced by *economic* factors. We concluded that removing structural barriers to "compliance," when coupled with financial aid, dramatically improved outcomes in poor Haitians with tuberculosis. This conclusion proved that the community health workers, and not the doctors, had been correct.

This insight forever altered approaches to tuberculosis within our program. It cut straight to the heart of the compliance question. Certainly, patients may be noncompliant, but how relevant is the notion of compliance in rural Haiti? Doctors may instruct their patients to eat well. But the patients will "refuse" if they have no food. They may be told to sleep in an open room and away from others, and here again they will be "noncompliant" if they do not expand and remodel their miserable huts. They may be instructed to go to a hospital. But if hospital care must be paid for in cash, as is the case throughout Haiti, and the patients have no cash, they will be deemed "grossly negligent." In a study published in collaboration with the Zanmi Lasante team, we concluded that "the hoary truth that poverty and tuberculosis are greater than the sum of their parts is once again supported by data, this time coming from rural Haiti and reminding us that such deadly synergism, formerly linked chiefly to crowded cities, is in fact most closely associated with deep poverty."[28]

Similar scenarios could be offered for diseases ranging from typhoid to AIDS. In each case, poor people are at higher risk of contracting the disease and are also less likely to have access to care. And in each case, analysis of the problem can lead researchers to focus on the patients' shortcomings (for example, failure to drink pure water, failure to use condoms, ignorance about public health and hygiene) or, instead, to focus on the conditions that structure people's risk (for example, lack of access to potable water, lack of economic opportunities for women, unfair distribution of the world's resources). In many current discussions of these plagues of the poor, one can discern a cognitivist-personalistic pole and a structural pole. Although focus on the former is the current fashion, one of the chief benefits of the latter mode of analysis is that it encourages physicians (and others concerned to pro-tect or promote health) to make common cause with people who are both poor and sick.

Tuberculosis aside, what follows next from a perspective on medicine that is based in liberation theology? Does recourse to these ideas demand loy-alty to any specific ideology? For me, applying an option for the poor has never implied advancing a particular strategy for a national economy. It does not imply preferring one form of development, or social system, over another—although some economic systems are patently more pathogenic than others and should be denounced as such by physicians. Recourse to the central ideas of liberation theology does not necessarily imply sub-scription to a specific body of religious beliefs; Partners In Health and its sister organizations in Haiti and Peru are completely ecumenical.[29] At the same time, the flabby moral relativism of our times would have us believe that we may now choose from a broad menu of approaches to delivering effective health care services to the poor. This is simply not true. Whether you are sitting in a clinic in rural Haiti, and thus a witness to stupid deaths from infection, or sitting in an emergency room in a U.S. city, and thus the provider of first resort for forty million uninsured, you must ac-knowledge that the commodification of medicine invariably punishes the vulnerable.

A truly committed quest for high-quality care for the destitute sick starts from the perspective that health is a fundamental human right. In contrast, commodified medicine invariably begins with the notion that health is a desirable outcome to be attained through the purchase of the right goods and services. Socialized medicine in industrialized countries is no doubt a step up from a situation in which market forces determine who has access to care. But a perspective based in liberation theology highlights the fundamental weakness of this and other strategies of the affluent: if the governments of Scandinavian countries and that of France, for example, then spend a great deal of effort barring noncitizens from access to health care services, they will find few critics within their bor-ders. (Indeed, the social democracies share a mania for border control.) But we will critique them, and bitterly, because access to the fruits of sci-ence and medicine should not be determined by passports, but rather by need. The "health care for all" movement in the United States will never be morally robust until it truly means "all."

Liberation theology's first lesson for medicine is similar to that usually confronting healers: There is something terribly wrong. Things are not the way they should be. But the problem, in this view, is with the world, even though it may be manifest in the patient. Truth—and liberation theology, in contrast to much postmodern attitudinizing, believes in historical accuracy—is to be found in the perspective of those who suffer unjust privation.[30] Cornel West argues that "the condition of truth is to allow the suffering to speak. It doesn't mean that those who suffer have a monopoly on truth, but it means that the condition of truth to emerge must be in tune with those who are undergoing social misery— socially induced forms of suffering."[31]

The second lesson is that medicine has much to learn by reflecting on the lives and struggles of poor or otherwise oppressed people. How is suffering, including that caused by sickness, best explained? How is it to be addressed? These questions are, of course, as old as humankind. We've had millennia in which to address—societally, in an organized fashion—the suffering that surrounds us. In looking at approaches to such problems, one can easily discern three main trends: *charity, development,* and *social justice.*

Each of these might have much to recommend it, but it is my belief that the first two approaches are deeply flawed. Those who believe that charity is the answer to the world's problems often have a tendency— sometimes striking, sometimes subtle, and surely lurking in all of us— to regard those needing charity as intrinsically inferior. This is different from regarding the poor as powerless or impoverished because of historical processes and events (slavery, say, or unjust economic policies propped up by powerful parties). There is an enormous difference between seeing people as the victims of innate shortcomings and seeing them as the victims of structural violence. Indeed, it is likely that the struggle for rights is undermined whenever the history of unequal chances, and of oppression, is erased or distorted.

The approach of charity further presupposes that there will always be those who have and those who have not. This may or may not be true, but, again, there are costs to viewing the problem in this light. In *Pedagogy of the Oppressed,* Paulo Freire writes: "In order to have the continued opportunity to express their 'generosity,' the oppressors must perpetuate injustice as well. An unjust social order is the permanent fount of this 'generosity,' which is nourished by death, despair, and poverty." Freire's conclusion follows naturally enough: "True generosity consists precisely in fighting to destroy the causes which nourish false charity."[32] Given the twentieth century's marked tendency toward increasing economic inequity in the face of economic growth, the future holds plenty of false charity. All the recent chatter about "personal responsibility" from "compassionate conservatives" erases history in a manner embarrassingly expedient for themselves. In a study of food aid in the United States, Janet Poppendieck links a rise in "kindness" to a decline in justice:

> The resurgence of charity is at once a *symptom* and a *cause* of our society's failure to face up to and deal with the erosion of equality. It is a symptom in that it stems, in part at least, from an abandonment of our hopes for the elimination of poverty; it signifies a retreat from the goals as well as the means that characterized the Great Society. It is symptomatic of a pervasive despair about actually solving problems that has turned us toward ways of managing them: damage control, rather than prevention. More significantly, and more controversially, the proliferation of charity *contributes* to our society's failure to grapple in meaningful ways with poverty.[33]

It is possible, however, to overstate the case against charity—it is, after all, one of the four cardinal virtues, in many traditions. Sometimes holier-than-thou progressives dismiss charity when it is precisely the virtue demanded. In medicine, charity underpins the often laudable goal of addressing the needs of "underserved populations." To the extent that medicine responds to, rather than creates, underserved populations, charity will always have its place in medicine.

Unfortunately, a preferential option for the poor is all too often absent from charity medicine. First, charity medicine should avoid, at all costs, the temptation to ignore or hide the causes of excess suffering among the poor. Meredeth Turshen gives a jarring example from apartheid South Africa:

> South African paediatricians may have developed an expertise in the understanding and treatment of malnutrition and its complications, but medical expertise does not change the system that gives rise to malnutrition nor the environment to which treated children return, an environment in which half of the children die before their fifth birthday. Malnutrition, in this context, is a direct result of the government's policies, which perpetuate the apartheid system and promote the poor health conditions and human rights violations.[34]

Second, charity medicine too frequently consists of second-hand, castoff services—leftover medicine—doled out in piecemeal fashion. How can we tell the difference between the proper place of charity in medicine and the doling out of leftovers? Many of us have been involved in these sorts of good works and have often heard a motto such as this: "the homeless poor are every bit as deserving of good medical care as the rest of us." The notion of a preferential option for the poor challenges us by reframing the motto: the homeless poor are *more* deserving of good medical care than the rest of us.[35] Whenever medicine seeks to reserve its finest services for the destitute sick, you can be sure that it is option-for-the-poor medicine.

What about development approaches?[36] Often, this perspective seems to regard progress and development as almost natural processes. The technocrats who design development projects—including a certain Péligre dam, which three decades ago displaced the population we seek to serve in central Haiti—plead for patience. In due time, the technocrats tell the poor, if they speak to them at all, you too will share our standard of living. (After a generation, the reassurance may be changed to "if not you, your children.") And certainly, looking around us, we see everywhere the tangible benefits of scientific development. So who but a Luddite would object to development as touted by the technocrats?

According to liberation theology, progress for the poor is not likely to ensue from development approaches, which are based on a "liberal" view of poverty. Liberal views place the problem with the poor themselves: these people are backward and reject the technological fruits of modernity. With assistance from others, they too will, after a while, reach a higher level of development. Thus does the victim-blaming noted in the earlier discussion of tuberculosis recur in discussions of underdevelopment.

For many liberation theologians, developmentalism or reformism cannot be rehabilitated. George Pixley and Clodovis Boff use these terms to describe what they consider an "erroneous" view of poverty, in contrast to the "dialectical" explanation, in which the growth of poverty is dependent on the growth of wealth. Poverty today, they note, "is mainly the result of a contradictory development, in which the rich become steadily richer, and the poor become steadily poorer." Such a poverty is "internal to the system and a natural product of it."[37] Developmentalism not only erases the historical creation of poverty but also implies that development is necessarily a linear process: progress will inevitably occur if the right steps are followed. Yet any critical assessment of the impact of such approaches must acknowledge their failure to help the poor, as Leonardo and Clodovis Boff argue:

> "Reformism" seeks to improve the situation of the poor, but always within existing social relationships and the basic structuring of society, which rules out greater participation by all and diminution in the privileges enjoyed by the ruling classes. Reformism can lead to great feats of development in the poorer nations, but this development is nearly always at the expense of the oppressed poor and very rarely in their favor. For example, in 1964 the Brazilian economy ranked 46th in the world; in 1984 it ranked 8th. The last twenty years have seen undeniable technological and industrial progress, but at the same time there has been a considerable worsening of social conditions for the poor, with exploitation, destitution, and hunger on a scale previously unknown in Brazilian history. This has been the price paid by the poor for this type of elitist, exploitative, and exclusivist development.[38]

In his introduction to *A Theology of Liberation,* Gustavo Gutiérrez concurs: we assert our humanity, he argues, in "the struggle to construct a just and fraternal society, where persons can live with dignity and be the agents of their own destiny. It is my opinion that the term *development* does not well express these profound aspirations."[39] Gutiérrez continues by noting that the term "liberation" expresses the hopes of the poor much more succinctly. Philip Berryman puts it even more sharply: " 'Liberation' entails a break with the present order in which Latin American countries could establish sufficient autonomy to reshape their economies to serve the needs of that poor majority. The term 'liberation' is understood in contradistinction to 'development.' "[40]

In examining medicine, one sees the impact of "developmental" thinking not only in the planned obsolescence of medical technology, essential to the process of commodification, but also in influential analytic constructs such as the "health transition model."[41] In this view, societies as they develop are making their way toward that great transition, when deaths will no longer be caused by infections such as tuberculosis but will occur much later and be caused by heart disease and cancer. But this model masks interclass differences *within* a particular country. For the poor, wherever they live, there is, often enough, no health transition. In other words, wealthy citizens of "underdeveloped" nations (those countries that have not yet experienced their health transition) do not die young from infectious diseases; they die later and from the same diseases that claim similar populations in wealthy countries. In parts of Harlem, in contrast, death rates in certain age groups are as high as those in Bangladesh; in both places, the leading causes of death in young adults are infections and violence.[42]

The powerful, including heads of state and influential policymakers, are of course impatient with such observations and respond, if they deign to respond, with sharp reminders that the overall trends are the results that count. But if we focus exclusively on aggregate data, why not declare public health in Latin America a resounding success? After all, life expectancies have climbed; infant and maternal mortality have dropped. But if you work in the service of the poor, what's happening to that particular class, whether in Harlem or in Haiti, always counts a great deal. In fact, it counts most. And from this vantage point—the one demanded by liberation theology—neither medicine nor development looks nearly so successful. In fact, the outcome gap between rich and poor has continued to grow.

In summary, then, the charity and development models, though perhaps useful at times, are found wanting in rigorous and soul-searching examination. That leaves the social justice model. In my experience, people who work for social justice, regardless of their own station in life, tend to see the world as deeply flawed. They see the conditions of the poor not only as unacceptable but as the result of structural violence that is human-made. As Robert McAfee Brown, paraphrasing the Uruguayan Jesuit Juan Segundo, observes, "unless we agree that the world should not be the way it is . . . there is no point of contact, because the world that is satisfying to us is the same world that is utterly devastating to them."[43] Often, if these individuals are privileged people like me, they understand that they have been implicated, whether directly or indirectly, in the creation or maintenance of this structural violence. They then feel indignation, but also humility and penitence. Where I work, this is easy: I see the Péligre dam almost every week.

This posture—of penitence and indignation—is critical to effective social justice work. Alas, it is all too often absent or, worse, transformed from posture into posturing. And unless the posture is linked to much more pragmatic interventions, it usually fizzles out.

Fortunately, embracing these concepts and this posture do have very concrete implications. Making an option for the poor inevitably implies working for social justice, working with poor people as they struggle to change their situations. In a world riven by inequity, medicine could be viewed as social justice work. In fact, doctors are far more fortunate than most modern professionals: we still have a sliver of hope for meaningful, dignified service to the oppressed. Few other disciplines can make this claim with any honesty. We have a lot to offer right now. In Haiti and Peru and Chiapas, we have found that it is often less a question of "development" and more one of redistribution of goods and services, of simply sharing the fruits of science and technology. The majority of our efforts in the transfer of technology—medications, laboratory supplies, computers, and training—are conceived in just this way. They end up being innovative for other reasons: it is almost unheard of to insist that the destitute sick receive high-quality care as a right.

Treating poor Peruvians who suffer from multidrug-resistant tuberculosis according to the highest standard of care, rather than according to whatever happens to be deemed "cost-effective," is not only social justice work but also, ironically enough, innovative. Introducing antiretroviral medications, and the health systems necessary to use them wisely, to AIDS-afflicted rural Haiti is, again, viewed as pie-in-the-sky by international health specialists but as only fitting by liberation theology. For example, operating rooms (and cesarean sections) must be part of any "minimum package" of health services wherever the majority of maternal deaths are caused by cephalopelvic disproportion. This is obvious from the perspective of social justice but controversial in international health circles. And the list goes on.

A preferential option for the poor also implies a mode of analyzing health systems. In examining tuberculosis in Haiti, for example, our analysis must be *historically deep*—not merely deep enough to recall an event such as that which deprived most of my patients of their land, but deep enough to remember that modern-day Haitians are the descendants of a people enslaved in order to provide our ancestors with cheap sugar, coffee, and cotton.

Our analysis must be *geographically broad*. In this increasingly interconnected world ("the world that is satisfying to us is the same world that is utterly devastating to them"), we must understand that what happens to poor people is never divorced from the actions of the powerful. Certainly, people who define themselves as poor may control their own destinies to some extent. But control of lives is related to control of land, systems of production, and the formal political and legal structures in which lives are enmeshed. With time, both wealth and control have become increasingly concentrated in the hands of a few. The opposite trend is desired by those working for social justice.

For those who work in Latin America, the role of the United States looms large. Father James Guadalupe Carney, a Jesuit priest, put his life on the line in order to serve the poor of Honduras. As far as we can tell, he was killed by U.S.-trained Honduran security forces in 1983.[44] In an introduction to his posthumously published autobiography, his sister and brother-in-law asked starkly: "Do we North Americans eat well because the poor in the third world do not eat at all? Are we North Americans powerful, because we help keep the poor in the third world weak? Are we North Americans free, because we help keep the poor in the third world oppressed?"[45]

Granted, it is difficult enough to "think globally and act locally." But perhaps what we are really called to do, in efforts to make common cause with the poor, is to think locally *and* globally and to act in response to both levels of analysis. If we fail in this task, we may never be able to contend with the structures that create and maintain poverty, structures that make people sick. Although physicians and nurses, even those who serve the poor, have not followed liberation theology, its insights have never been more relevant to our vocation. As international health experts come under the sway of the bankers and their curiously bounded utilitarianism, we can expect more and more of our services to be declared "cost-ineffective" and more of our patients to be erased. In declaring health and health care to be a human right, we join forces with those who have long labored to protect the rights and dignity of the poor.

CHAPTER 6

LISTENING FOR
PROPHETIC VOICES

A CRITIQUE OF
MARKET-BASED MEDICINE

As of 1999, more than 43 million people in the United States
did not hold any form of public or private health insurance,
while health-care expenditures totaled more than one trillion
dollars annually, equivalent to about 14 percent of the gross
domestic product. Many people with insurance coverage still
experienced major barriers to access, due to copayments or
other deductible provisions. Most strikingly, every proposal
for a national health program in the United States, intended
to address the problems of inadequate access and high costs,
failed. As the United States enters the new millennium, it
remains the only economically developed country without a
national health program that ensures universal access to
care.... The structures of oppression and the social origins of
illness...have emerged as even greater problems as corporate
penetration of health care has increased.

Howard Waitzkin, *The Second Sickness*

But tell me, this physician of whom you were just speaking, is
he a moneymaker, an earner of fees or a healer of the sick?

Plato, *The Republic*

The Old Testament prophets cannot have had a very easy time of it, and
not because their primary work was as clairvoyants or seers. Prophetic
voices were more often raised in protest against the social conditions endured by widows, orphans, and the poor majority. These voices were
raised in opposition to structural violence—the poverty and inequality
that meant opulent excess for a few and misery for most. Many prophets
were regarded by their literate contemporaries as certifiably mad; few
were heeded.

In some ways, the prophets failed, for the inequities they deplored still endure. A growing and globalizing market economy has not, as promised, lifted all boats.[1] Instead, increasing wealth has meant entrenched excess and squalor. We read in the newspapers of famine and strife, but also of the stunning sales of luxury items. The Roaring Nineties were notable for waiting lists for $4,000 handbags and $44,500 watches; $75,000 cars sold like hotcakes. The new millennium dawned not with Armageddon but rather with the spectacular success of free-market capitalism, so long as "success" is measured in terms of gross national product, the number of billionaires, or the volume of the stock exchange. Although recent events—including the attacks of September 11, 2001, and the very public unraveling of a giant "energy" company that in fact did little in the way of generating energy—have dampened the fervor of the preceding decade, it is clear that rich countries remain rich, and most rich people remain very, very rich. The much-discussed collapse of the stock market has not come to pass; it is not even clear that markets have contracted in any significant, enduring way. As both wealth and poverty continue to rise, many of the most affluent have managed to escape with their capital gains intact. "America," observes Christopher Jencks in a recent review, "does less than almost any other rich democracy to limit economic inequality."[2]

Indeed, a less heartening picture emerges when economic and other forms of social inequality are scrutinized, for they are growing at an even more rapid pace. Inequality is very much the sign of our times.[3] By almost every measure, social inequalities—both within affluent societies and across borders—have risen sharply over the past two or three decades.[4] The social pathologies associated with rising inequality give pause to even the cheerleaders of neoliberal economics. More thoughtful students of inequality are persuaded that there are many reasons to limit it. "My bottom line," concludes Jencks after decades of studying the topic, "is that the social consequences of economic inequality are sometimes negative, sometimes neutral, but seldom—as far as I can discover—positive."[5]

It's clear that modern biomedicine, like the global economy, is booming. Never before have the fruits of basic science been so readily translated into life-promoting technologies. Headlines abound with news of sequencing the entire human genome, of effective organ transplants, of new drug development. Every affliction, even many of the indignities of normal aging, must have its response, as the therapeutic armamentarium grows and the desire for health makes the pharmaceutical industry the most profitable of all major industries.[6] But inequalities of access and outcome increasingly dominate the health care arena, too. Every victory is marred by a troubling counter-story: protests of indigenous people against the Human Genome Project; grisly stories of organs stolen or coerced from the poor for transplant to the bodies of those who can pay; great enthusiasm, on the part of drug companies, for the development of new drugs to treat baldness or impotence while antituberculous medicines are termed "orphan drugs" and thus deemed not worthy (based on profitability) of much attention from the drug companies.[7]

Medicine-as-commerce is at the heart of each of these stories, just as it is at the heart of some of the good trends and most of the bad ones. It is clear enough that biotech and pharmaceutical firms can work miracles. But it is also true that they lean heavily on public funding and end up making a great deal of private profit. Even more troublesome are the rapidly growing investor-owned health plans. They go under many names, including health-maintenance organizations. Although some of these are not-for-profit, many have in common a basic strategy: selling "product" to "consumers" rather than providing care to patients.[8]

In an essay critiquing the shift toward the commodification of health care, Edmund Pellegrino argues that health care cannot be considered a commodity, one like food or clothes, that fits into its appointed place in the American free-market system. The highly championed view of market forces as the ideal mechanism driving the distribution of goods and services in a democratic society cannot be extended to the medical profession. The ends and purposes of medicine are unique, since they are linked to issues of individual trust and common good: "healing [is] a special kind of human activity governed by an ethic that serves those ends and not the self-interests of physicians, insurance plans, or investors."[9]

What happens when health becomes a commodity and doctors conduct "commercial transactions" with patients, in a climate where managed-care corporations are the "providers"? Pellegrino cautions that business ethics do not translate well to medicine:

> Inequalities in distribution of services and treatments are not the concerns of free markets. Denial[s] of care for patients who could not pay were not unknown in the past. But they were not legitimated as they are in a free market system where patients are expected to suffer the consequences of a poor choice in health care plans.... In this view, inequities are unfortunate but not unjust. Some simply are losers in the natural and social lottery. The market ethos does not *per se* foreclose altruism, but neither does it impose a moral duty to help.[10]

Theoretically, if the market ethos rules health care, "physicians would be justified in refusing care" on the grounds that "patients are responsible for their own health."[11]

In the United States, investor-owned health plans have rapidly transformed the way we confront illness. Despite much talk of "cost-effectiveness" or "reform," the primary feature of this transformation has been the consolidation of a major industry with the same goal as other industries: to turn a profit.[12] Emboldened by obscenely large salaries and stock options, the captains of this emerging industry are unselfconscious, almost shameless, about their plans for American medicine. One commentary, in advancing a "code of ethics for the medical-industrial complex," puts it boldly enough: "Make a profit: economies involving scarcity are bad for everyone.... Therefore, be good to people and make money."[13] Furthermore, the health care system should "help people buy what they want....Therefore, people should be allowed to purchase health care packages that provide limited or less than optimal care. As a matter of justice, they should also be allowed to receive only the health care services that their coverage allows."[14] Writing in the *New England Journal of Medicine,* one of the cheerleaders for this new, soulless trend stated flatly: "there is no longer a role for non-profit health plans in the new health care environment."[15]

Neither is there a role for the "fungible" patients, as one acidic commentary notes:

> There is no room in a free market for the non-player, the person who can't "buy in"—the poor, the uninsured, the uninsurable. The special needs of the chronically ill, the disabled, infirm, aged, and the emotionally distressed are no longer valid claims to special attention. Rather, they are the occasion for higher premiums, more deductibles, or exclusion from enrollment. There is no economic justification for the extra time required to explain, counsel, comfort, and educate these patients and their families since these cost more than they return in revenue.[16]

The "new health care environment" has, of course, deep cultural resonance with the affluent, inegalitarian society from which it springs. Supporters of medicine for profit do not hesitate to class their endeavor as part of the American Way: "Freedom of choice is valued more highly than equality of outcome, and...our commitments to beneficence are limited, as reflected by the absence of a constitutional right to receive welfare services. These we take to be the broad moral assumptions of American health care policy."[17]

Can we still hear, in this "new health care environment," today's prophetic voices? Unless we make our world a place free of structural violence, we cannot completely obliterate these voices. We can only ignore them, and we seem to be doing a rather good job on this score. But the experiences of those who are sick and poor—and, often enough, sick because they're poor—remind us that inequalities of access and outcome constitute the chief drama of modern medicine. In an increasingly interconnected world, inequalities are both local and global, as examples from my own practice illustrate. These stories also ask us to decide whether or not we believe that health care is a basic human right.

BRENDA AND THE EXCUSES OF OUR TIMES

Brenda, a native of Boston, had advanced AIDS when she first came to my clinic. She doesn't know how she acquired HIV—increasingly, people don't[18]—but she guessed it was through the father of her first child, since he'd used heroin. Brenda herself had never done so. Twenty-eight years old when I met her, she was already almost blind from CMV retinitis. She weighed eighty-nine pounds and had great difficulty taking care of her children, even with help. After learning of her diagnosis, she had set herself the goal of seeing her oldest child graduate from high school. In subsequent years, she downgraded her aspirations. Since Andrew was seven in 1995, the year she lost her vision, she hoped to see him graduate from junior high school.

In 1997, however, Brenda allowed her hopes to rise. She'd heard about the powerful new combination of drugs that seemed to revive even the near-dead, and she herself knew a woman with AIDS who, on these drugs, went from bedridden to buoyant—at least, that was Brenda's impression—in a matter of months.

At last, thought Brenda, who in taking other antiretroviral drugs had suffered through side effects ranging from pancreatitis to unremitting nausea, only to learn that these medications had little demonstrable effect on the progression of her disease. *At last.*

But there was a glitch. In the course of her previous (ineffective) therapies, she had been labeled "noncompliant." This, in any case, was the opinion of some of those who had cared for her. This label made it difficult for her to be accepted into the clinical trials that are so often the only affordable source of these drugs. The *New York Times* reported in 1997 that doctors in New York City were rationing protease inhibitors and other new antiretrovirals, saving them for those they deemed likely to comply.[19]

Although there's no doubt that physicians do this with the best of intentions, such strategies are seriously flawed. First, research has shown that physicians are poor predictors of which patients will comply with prescribed regimens.[20] Second, those least likely to comply are usually those least able to comply. Among my patients, at least, structural violence and its products—including racism, addiction, lack of insurance, lack of employment, lack of stable housing, domestic violence—constrain their ability to comply with complex drug regimens. For example, many patients living with HIV also care for children. They have no access to day care and can't afford babysitters or other help. In the everyday hurly-burly, which involves getting kids ready for school, their own health concerns fade to insignificance. During many visits to patients' houses, I have recognized as genuine their surprise when I ask them whether they've taken their morning medications. They apologetically head for the medicine cabinet, if they have one, and for a glass of water. Willful noncompliance is, often enough, what we term a "diagnosis of exclusion."

Third, rationing effective therapies can actually serve to deepen the gaps between the rich and the poor. If marginally effective treatments for HIV disease are not available to the poor, then their health suffers only marginally. But if highly effective therapies—such as the more active "cocktails" of antiretroviral drugs—are unavailable to those living in poverty, then class-based inequalities of outcome worsen with time.[21] Through such mechanisms, our failure to ensure that people like Brenda receive such medications is tantamount to what the Latin American bishops cited in Chapter 5 termed "structural sin."[22]

The excuses of our times can be ingenious; failure to provide access to treatment becomes reframed as failure to adhere to prescribed drug regimens. Under the headline "Precious Pills," the *Wall Street Journal* ran a front-page story about protease inhibitors and responses to them.[23] A subheading read, "Gotta Clean Up Your Act," a reference to one New York caregiver's admonition to his patients who were seeking access to the (then new) drugs. This "perceived" noncompliance of the poor (but not of other classes of patients) is reframed, in turn, as a public health issue. Not only are "precious pills" wasted on such patients, but *their* noncompliance is seen as leading to new drug-resistant strains of HIV. Thus does denial of access to treatment ingenuously become transformed into a rational public health strategy, as poor patients are warned to "clean up their acts"—for their own good and for the public good. But what, exactly, do we tell our patients, many of whom, like Brenda, are as likely to lack "day planners" as they are day care? If I could acknowledge that their lives have been damaged by the poverty they face every day, by racism, and, often enough, by gender inequality, if only I could say this in an appropriate way, I would. If I could tell them that they deserve the best medical care we can deliver, I'd tell them that, too. There are many things I'd like to tell them, but somehow I cannot bring myself to recommend that they "clean up their acts."[24]

Perhaps it's time that we clean up our own. When some colleagues and I published a volume called *Women, Poverty, and AIDS,* we berated fellow physicians and academics for our collective failure to appreciate how gender inequality and poverty were putting millions of women at risk for HIV infection. Although we've received many supportive letters in response to the book, these tended to come from community activists and providers. Some of the scholars who wrote to us were resentful that we had critiqued their work as not mindful enough of the plight of poor women. (The irritation and defensiveness of fellow academics and policymakers have in fact been a staple in all our work on behalf of the destitute sick.) But the entire point of the volume was to analyze massive failure. The failure of public health measures to prevent AIDS from becoming, in a single generation, the leading cause of death for young women living in poverty. The failure of researchers to bring into relief the mechanisms by which poverty and gender inequality create situations of risk for poor women. The failure of physicians to insist that HIV care be available to poor women. The failure to care enough about a catastrophe that, increasingly, primarily affects the poor. Indeed, by what measure is the AIDS pandemic among women not a failure?

Because she lives in such an affluent country, and hard by one of its most famous teaching hospitals, Brenda eventually got her medications. And she's doing much better. Although her visual impairment is irreversible, she gained twenty pounds during the course of 1998. She once again hopes to see her children graduate from high school. During one clinic visit, she termed her improvement "miraculous." Although she has since had many ups and downs, Brenda is still responding to combination therapy.

For the millions of HIV-infected women "hidden away," as it were, in Haiti and sub-Saharan Africa, no such miracle has occurred. Because we have allowed market forces to determine who has access to these newer drugs, we have a situation in which those most likely to benefit do not yet appear on the radar of those charged with developing strategies to contain the epidemic in these regions. As Chapter 8 discusses, the destitute sick have not even been acknowledged as an ethical problem for modern medicine, much less an emergency: "There are at least 34 million HIV-infected people in the world, at least 30 million of them poor. Poor not just by American standards, but by world standards: living on less than $2 a day. AIDS specialists rarely say this bluntly, but the majority of those 30 million people have simply been written off, because the first priority for the first few billion dollars is prevention, not treatment."[25]

SANOÎT AND THE DISPOSABLE MILLIONS

I spend more than half my time seeing patients in the Clinique Bon Sauveur in Cange, Haiti. The facility, which I have described elsewhere, serves largely the landless poor and the peasants of the Central Plateau's arid highlands.[26] As mentioned in Chapter 2, this clinic is the most crowded one in central Haiti. The reason is simple: it's the only facility available to the poorest of the poor. Medicines are not sold at the Clinique Bon Sauveur, since selling medications means that those who cannot pay do not receive therapy at all: we are the provider of last resort. Instead, doctors, rather than a patient's social standing, decide who needs what medications.

On most mornings, the clinic courtyard is thronged with hundreds waiting to see a doctor or a nurse. Even several years ago, when Sanoît's mother brought him there, we were seeing tens of thousands of patients each year. Our patients certainly needed to be patient, since they could count on spending an entire day waiting to be seen, especially if their physicians or nurses felt that they needed laboratory studies or X-rays. Sanoît showed up in the clinic looking like a little stick figure. He was already nine years old, but he weighed only thirty-five pounds. He was coughing and had a fever, and we thought he had pneumonia. We prescribed antibiotics and suggested that he be brought back to the clinic in a couple of weeks for follow-up.

Two weeks to the day, Sanoît's mother brought him back. He was worse, a mere skeleton. This time, we took a chest X-ray and diagnosed pulmonary tuberculosis. In retrospect, the diagnosis should have been made more promptly, as his mother had been a tuberculosis patient some years earlier. But tuberculosis is difficult to detect in children, and examination of his sputum on that earlier day had not suggested the diagnosis. Besides, he and his family lived in a shack less than an hour north of the clinic. They would come back, we reasoned, if he happened to become sicker. We should have guessed, perhaps, that they might not return until the day of their appointment. Regardless of what went wrong, Sanoît was even more gravely ill on the day he was at last diagnosed, and he knew it.

"Am I going to die?" he asked quietly, as if curious.

"No, you're not going to die."

Sanoît, I recall, looked doubtful. I know little about child psychology, but this kid, I believe, had seen enough deaths to conclude that he was not going to survive tuberculosis. Tuberculosis had almost killed his mother; it had taken the lives of many he knew.

Of course, Sanoît did not die. He received, in addition to his antituberculous medications, a tiny amount of financial and nutritional aid. His mother, a quiet woman who had had nine other children, looked as relieved by the meager social assistance as by the diagnosis and free treatment. Sanoît began gaining weight immediately. Within a month, most of his symptoms were gone; nine months later, he was declared cured. We still see him now and again, but not because he is ill or has sequelae of his disease: he is now a small but healthy teenager.

In short, Sanoît recovered beautifully. The same cannot be said for the other disposable people. Fifty years after the introduction of combination therapy that is almost 100 percent effective, tuberculosis remains (along with AIDS) the world's leading infectious cause of readily preventable adult deaths. If the World Health Organization is correct, tuberculosis killed between two and three million people in 1997—more than died that year from complications of HIV infection, and perhaps more than have died in any one year since 1900.[27] And this happens in almost complete silence, in large part because tuberculosis victims are usually poor. Lee Reichman has underlined this point by observing that, if tuberculosis were ever taken seriously, discussions about it "would have to be moved to the local football stadium to accommodate all interested parties."[28]

Although calls for patients to clean up their acts also ring out in the tuberculosis literature, it is again clear that those least likely to "comply" with treatment recommendations are precisely those least able to comply. Thus are the poor—people like Sanoît and his mother—put at risk of tuberculosis, at risk of having no access to treatment, and at risk of being blamed for their own misfortune and for infecting others.

OLGA AND THE IRONIES OF POST-PERESTROIKA RUSSIA

Olga was pale and thin, and she coughed throughout our two interviews. Her spectacles were far too large for her face; she reminded me of the U.S. novelist Joyce Carol Oates. I noticed that the tips of Olga's fingers were deformed by "clubbing," a sign of chronic lung disease seen most often in older people who have smoked for decades or who have lung tumors. Olga has never smoked; her lung pathology is tuberculosis.

Olga, thirty-two years old in 1998, was a native of Tomsk Oblast. Her family had once been farmers, tilling the rich black soil north of the city. Although her father had worked for two decades in a nuclear power plant, they still had the family farm, which had never really been "sovietized." In recent years, they had come to rely on its harvests, something that for Olga belonged to the distant past of her grandparents.

She had been living in Tomsk, a university city with about half a million inhabitants, since the mid-eighties, having come there to work in a research laboratory. She had started at the bottom, washing glassware, and was also responsible for ordering reagents for a biogenetics laboratory affiliated not with one of Siberia's famous "closed cities" but rather with the university. Olga had been taking classes there and was an avid reader of English literature ("in translation," she added quickly). She also helped to organize an annual film festival and had been seeing a medical student. They had planned to marry.

"That," she said with a small smile, "was before everything went to pieces." Shortly after perestroika, even before the formal dissolution of the USSR, government funding for research began to dwindle. Then it "simply disappeared." She and the other employees lost their jobs "softly, without fanfare." They were not fired; they simply went unpaid. "The lab is still open," she noted. "But only the professors come in, and they don't come in the winter, since there's so little heat." Throughout the city, it was much the same. Olga lived in a charmingly dilapidated wooden house—Tomsk is famous for them—along with several other people who used to work in either the university or one of the top-secret laboratories a bit further up the broad Tom River. Only one of her six housemates still has a job.

Olga's employers assured her that her job was secure if the laboratory ever received its funding. But after a few months without a paycheck, Olga was forced to rely on her family for money and food. "It was discouraging, since my father is a pensioner, and I was the one to send them money."

She fell ill in 1993. "Bronchitis, I was told." But her boyfriend, although still in his pre-clinical years, was quick to suggest tuberculosis. She was treated with antibiotics for several months, to no effect. In October of that year, she was diagnosed with left-upper lobe collapse as a result of tuberculosis. This was a shock to her, as the disease was regarded as uncommon in both her parents' families and in the university community where she worked. "I thought, just then, that things could not get worse."

They did. Olga's first treatment, which was provided by the city's tuberculosis service, was interrupted several times by drug stockouts. "Other patients had it worse, because many of them had nowhere to live and not a lot to eat." She responded to the treatment, only to relapse in the summer of 1995. "Even then, they thought I had drug-resistant tuberculosis, but by this time [a European nongovernmental organization] had started restructuring the tuberculosis service, and there were many things that they would not pay for." Among the services discouraged by the Europeans were drug-susceptibility testing, fluorography, surgery of any sort, and treatment with any drugs other than those deemed first-line. There was even debate as to whether patients termed "chronic," such as Olga, would qualify for services funded by the relief organizations that were becoming increasingly visible in Siberia.

Olga became sicker still. She lost a great deal of weight and in the autumn of 1995 had several episodes of hemoptysis, one of which landed her in the hospital for a week. By the new year, she said, "I was pretty depressed, even though I had stopped coughing up blood." Her boyfriend left for further training in Novosibirsk; she heard little from him after that. "Not that I blame him," she said. "I was not a lot of fun to be around. And I'm a danger to others."

By the time we met, Olga already knew that she was sick with drug-resistant tuberculosis. She likely had multidrug-resistant tuberculosis—that is, she was already sick with a strain resistant to both isoniazid and rifampin—but this had not yet been confirmed. What is known is that, fully three years earlier, the strain devouring her lungs was already resistant to isoniazid, ethambutol, and streptomycin. (Olga had copies of all these results, which came from a Russian clinical laboratory, and also reports of her chest films.) These lab data are relevant because, at the time we last spoke, she was being treated with a regimen consisting of precisely those medications plus rifampin. The great irony: she was receiving, at best, "cryptic monotherapy"—rifampin was the only drug to which her infecting strain might still be susceptible—even though her treatment had been designed by the very international experts who had accused the Russians of using monotherapy.

I asked her whether she thought this treatment, her third, would cure her. "No," she replied, "but it's the only thing they have. They say the other medicines are too expensive. I know the name of some of the ones I need, and my brother tried to get them for me in Moscow. They were there, but they were too expensive, since you need to take several of them for a long time." Olga did not blame the people caring for her, but she felt sure that she would have received better treatment if she'd fallen ill a decade earlier.

Olga also worried that she didn't have much time left. "I see two options. I want to get better. No one will marry me now, and I won't be able to teach, but I'm not ready to give up....I want the second-line drugs. Either [the nongovernmental organization] will come through on its promise of helping patients with drug-resistant tuberculosis or I will go with the professor."

Olga was referring to a well-known tuberculosis specialist, a professor at the medical school and the director of the tuberculosis sanatorium. He had evaluated Olga and recommended surgery and a long stay in his facility. The Europeans had counseled against it, referring as they often did to "antiquated Soviet approaches" to tuberculosis treatment. But they did not offer an alternative to yet another round of treatment with the same drugs that had already proven ineffective, and Olga had already decided that she would not undergo that. She'd had hearing loss even before starting her current regimen, which still contained the offending agent.

I later spoke with the professor about Olga's plight. He remembered her immediately, even though he had seen hundreds of patients with drug-resistant tuberculosis. "Of course, she needs both surgery and a multidrug regimen. We know the drugs she needs, the second-line drugs. But our budget has been severely cut, and we have to play along with the new rules being set here." I had the strong sense that he wanted to say more, but he was also indebted to the foreign nongovernmental organizations that had decreed that patients like Olga were in effect not eligible for treatment. He was more anxious than bitter, I thought.

Neither is Olga bitter. "Things were a lot better here ten, fifteen years ago," she said with a sigh. "There's no one here that would disagree. We all had jobs back then....Everything our parents fought for has gone down the drain, and now all of these laboratories and research centers have been closed. We don't have money any more, and that's why these organizations are here. We have to be grateful, I guess, for what we've got."

Why doesn't Russia "have money any more"? Why have the research institutes, laboratories, "closed cities," and classrooms shut down? Flying out of Tomsk on Tomsk Air, in a slightly dilapidated Tupolev jet, one wonders what happened, say, to the Russian aircraft industry. Fifteen years ago, the Tomsk airport was a much busier place, with forty-seven departures a day. Now Tomsk is just another shrinking Russian city, its airport as empty as its hospitals and laboratories.

Some justify opposition to the aggressive treatment of MDRTB in developing countries as public health *realpolitik,* but careful systemic analysis casts doubt on such notions. Although our failure to effectively confront tuberculosis is obvious, the hypothesis that we lack sufficient means to cure all tuberculosis cases, everywhere and regardless of susceptibility patterns, is not supported by data. There is plenty of money—even in many poor countries. The degree of accumulated wealth in the world today is altogether unprecedented, but this accumulation has occurred in tandem with growing inequality.

Simply following the money trail reveals both the range of available capital and also the degree to which resource flows are transnational. Russia's economic contraction has been profound and is tightly tied to the market-based economies led by the Western cheerleaders of perestroika. After the collapse of the former Soviet Union, at the goading of Western economic advisers, the Russian Federation sold off the majority of its assets at bargain prices. By April 2000, estimates of capital flight out of Russia since 1993, the year Olga's illness began, topped $130 billion. Less than a decade after its liberation from communism, Russia was rated the world's most indebted country. As this book goes to press, there are signs of economic recovery for the Russian Federation. But this will likely come too late for Olga and others like her.

In the global era, we often engage in fraudulent analyses of what bounds our "communities" and where they fit in larger social webs. If I were one of the Masters of the Universe, I'd try and get folks like us to adopt a motto such as "think globally, act locally." In terms of analysis, those who direct modern commerce are far ahead of us. They understand the artificiality of borders and the gains to be made from differentials in price and supply; they exploit the whole world. Meanwhile, the forces of healing, which deal in the priceless and universal value of health, are trammeled by parochialisms of place and creed.

Olga is still sick with a drug-resistant strain of tuberculosis. As noted in the postscript to Chapter 4, our own group, Partners In Health, is determined to see her treated with the drugs to which her infecting strain is susceptible. Our efforts on her behalf may ultimately fail, but they will not have failed to call into question the cynical calculus by which some lives are considered valuable and others expendable.

HEALTH CARE "REFORMS" VERSUS PROGRESS WITH JUSTICE

Of all the forms of inequality, injustice in health is the
most shocking and the most inhumane.

> Attributed to Dr. Martin Luther King Jr.

How do these stories fit into the local moral worlds of our clinics and hospitals? How do they interrogate our convictions regarding health care as a human right? All three vignettes point to the fact that with all of our technological power, our magnetic resonance scans, and our protease inhibitors, we allow not only the continuation but the *entrenchment* of inequalities. The justification for this sad state of affairs is usually economic: we're told that we live in a time of "shrinking health resources." But is this really so? Look at profits in the managed-care companies. In the mid-1990s, the *Wall Street Journal* described these companies as "money machines so awash in cash that they don't know what to do with it all."[29] A *New York Times* headline noted, "Penny Pinching HMOs Showed Their Generosity in Executive Paychecks."[30] The CEO of one managed-care company received a salary of $370,604 and stock options worth more than $15 million; other, more dramatic examples could be offered.[31]

This trend has continued unabated, as a recent Families USA report points out: "With costs of health care coverage soaring, one aspect of health plan company expenses has kept pace: compensation packages for top executives."[32] In looking at salaries, bonuses, and other benefits for ten multistate for-profit health plans, the report found that in 2000, the twenty-five highest-paid executives in these companies made a total of $201.1 million in annual compensation—not counting unexercised stock options, which were valued at $1.1 billion.[33] One detractor of managed care, Leon Eisenberg of Harvard Medical School, asks, "Where do health care profits come from? . . . Is it from efficiency? . . . Does a significant portion of health care profits come from care that is not given?"[34] One has to wonder what, in addition to growing inequality, is being managed in this arena of for-profit health care.

Again, perhaps it is we physicians who need to clean up our acts. Increasingly, the inequalities that we're told to countenance are inimical to good medicine.[35] Even stop-gap measures, such as the federal program designed to make AIDS and tuberculosis therapies available to the poor, are under heavy fire by politicians who guess, with a confidence bordering on arrogance, that they and theirs are never likely to need such drugs.

In the face of unprecedented bounty and untold penury, where are the prophetic voices in medicine? Instead of forthright demands for access to care, we have foggy-minded critiques of technology. Take a look at "medical ethics," a staple of medical school curricula. What is defined, these days, as an ethical issue? End-of-life decisions, medicolegal questions of brain death and organ transplantation, and medical disclosure issues dominate the published literature. In the hospital, the quandary ethics of the individual constitute most of the discussion of medical ethics. The question "When is a life worth preserving?" is asked largely of lives one click of the switch away from extinction, lives wholly at the mercy of the technology that works to preserve some. The countless people whose life course is shortened by unequal access to health care are not topics of discussion. To hear dead silence in the realm of medical ethics, you have to look at access for poor people, especially those who, like Brenda and Sanoît and Olga, can be hidden away. Absent from the grand debates about whether or not health care is a right, bioethics now finds itself in the position of scrambling to interpret clinical failures, as for-profit medical care has wreaked havoc even in a setting of great affluence. Larry Churchill puts it this way:

> Perhaps it is not too immodest to claim that bioethicists have had some influence...replacing medical paternalism with patient self-determination and serving as a constructive force in the establishment of more rights and protections for research subjects. Advocacy for a fair system of health care, however, has failed miserably, at least so far. But more disconcerting than this failure is the shift in bioethical energy over the past five years toward repairing the moral lapses and gaps in managed care, which are primarily a problem for harried physicians and insured-but-anxious middle-class citizens.[36]

How do you make a clear distinction between life and death, between death and prolonged coma, between two technologies with near-even chances of failure? These are subtle decisions and have weighty consequences. I would be the last to trivialize them. But their formulation assumes a great many givens—a wealth of clinical alternatives, a battery of life-support mechanisms, access to potentially unlimited care. These are the quandaries of the fortunate. But in working for the health of the poor, we are faced with a different set of moral issues. Will this patient get any treatment at all? Will her survival be considered less precious than a fourteen-dollar savings in basic medicines? These are not typically quandaries that the well-instructed medical ethicist can resolve by deciding when or where to flip a switch.[37]

Some involved in ethics would have you believe that technological advances are in and of themselves bad. I believe the Luddites are dead wrong. We *all* should have access to the fruits of modern technology, especially those who most need it. As health care "reforms" move forward, this technology is, increasingly, at the disposal only of those who can pay for it. We thus find ourselves at a crossroads: health care can be considered a commodity to be sold, or it can be considered a basic social right. It cannot comfortably be considered both of these at the same time. This, I believe, is the great drama of medicine at the start of this century. And this is the choice before all people of faith and good will in these dangerous times.

REDISCOVERING SOCIAL JUSTICE

What is medicine about? Is it about maximizing the incomes of physicians or health care organizations? Do patients and their suffering exist in some fundamental sense for the benefit of the physician, the hospital, or the stockholder? Or do physicians and the entire medical enterprise of which they are a part exist for the benefit of patients and the relief of human suffering?

Richard Gunderman, "Medicine and the Pursuit of Wealth," 1998

There is no more place in this country than in any other for self-congratulation on the quality of the medical care that has been developed until the utmost has been achieved in making it available to all levels of society, in all places and at all times.

Dr. Joseph Garland, former editor of the *New England Journal of Medicine*, 1952

It stands to reason that, as beneficiaries of growing inequality, we don't like to be reminded of misery and squalor and failure. Our popular culture provides us with no shortage of anesthesia. I can refer to "our" popular culture because, increasingly, the beneficiaries of inequality share a transnational culture in which elements of both work and leisure are regimented by tastes cultivated in affluent societies. This is not to argue that local cultures are unimportant; nor would I argue that resistance to dominant cultures is insignificant. But many posit a soul-numbing equation between conspicuous consumption and modern existence, a formula said to lead millions to intellectual and moral oblivion. There are, of course, more subtle means of manufacturing consent: modes of explaining the world, including social inequalities and the violence they engender, are also undergoing a form of globalization, as are rights discourses.[38]

And yet the voices, the faces, the suffering of the sick and the poor are all around us. Can we see and hear them? Well-defended against troubling incursions of doubt, we the privileged are precisely the people most at risk of remaining oblivious, since this kind of suffering is not central to our own personal experience.

Can we tune in to the prophetic voices in our midst? One of my former medical students, Anthony Mitchell, is also a preacher. He shared with me one of his sermons. Delivered in December 1998 at the Greater Piney Grove Baptist Church in Atlanta, Georgia, the homily is called "Who Has the Last Word?"

> We live in a time where Herod is in control....If you stand up and do as John the Baptist did, say a few simple words—such as *That is not right; this is not how it should be done; this is not how we should treat one another; this is not how we should live*—you are risking death. Sometimes we forget that the Christian life is a risky life, a life that might cost you your own life. This is the context of the text, and also the context of the miracle....This is the Gospel. This is where it is preached, in dangerous times.

These are indeed dangerous times. In the name of "cost-effectiveness," we cut back health benefits to the poor, who are more likely to be sick than the nonpoor. We miss our chance to heal. In the setting, we're told, of "scarce resources," we imperil the health care safety net. In the name of expedience, we miss our chance to be humane and compassionate.[39]

Herod remains in control, but this is also the context of the miracle: it is in precisely such contexts that we have the privilege of reasserting our humanity. Against a tide of utilitarian opinion and worse, we are offered the chance to insist, *This is not how it should be done.* Indeed, this is always what healers were called upon to say, but now the stakes are even higher. The world is a very different place now than when the prophets roamed the land. Medical technology has changed. We have great laboratories, diagnostic capabilities, and effective medications for a host of diseases.

Certainly, distributing these developments equitably would be expensive. Certainly, excess costs must be curbed. But how can we glibly use terms like "cost-effective" when we see how they are perverted in contemporary parlance? You want to help the poor? Then your projects must be "self-sustaining" or "cost-effective." You want to erase the poor? Hey, knock yourself out. The sky's the limit.

Similar chicanery is used with a host of other terms, ranging from "appropriate technology" to "community." Through analytic legerdemain—the world is composed of discretely bounded nation-states, some rich, some poor, and each with its unique destiny—we're asked to swallow what is, ultimately, a story of growing inequality.

Is this the best we can do? Attempting to provide a "basic minimum package" for the poor is something that should be done apologetically, not proudly. Even the World Health Organization, which has invested heavily in promoting cost-effectiveness as a means of assessing health care services, recognizes the sharp limitations of this method in improving the health of the poor and thus addressing inequalities of outcome:

> Cost-effectiveness by itself is relevant for achieving the best overall health, but not necessarily for the second health goal, that of reducing inequality. Populations with worse than average health may respond less well to an intervention, or cost more to reach or to treat, so that a concern for distribution implies a willingness to sacrifice some overall health gains for other criteria.[40]

The "other criteria" in question are equity criteria, but the language of social justice is increasingly absent from public health parlance. Perhaps we need a new lexicon for this "new health care environment," or perhaps we need to rediscover an old one.[41] A compelling lexicon of social medicine must be linked to a return to social justice, to a struggle against the tide of opinion. If we fail to resist the current trends, we risk sapping biomedicine of its vast power and ourselves of our humanity. If we lived in a utopia, simply practicing medicine would be enough. But no matter how you slice it, we live in a dystopia. Increasingly, in this "new environment," inequalities of access and outcome characterize medicine. These inequalities could be the focus of our collective action as morally engaged members of the healing professions, broadly conceived. For we have before us an awesome responsibility—to prevent social inequalities from being embodied as bad health outcomes. We have the technology. The future of medicine depends on continuing to invest heavily in basic and applied research and trusting in scientific method. But our success in this arena forces another even more important choice.

Throughout human history, the sick have relied on healers of one stripe or another. Throughout human history, there have been talented healers and there have been charlatans. But never before has medicine tapped the full promise of science and technology. These were twentieth-century developments, and we are now faced with a twenty-first-century decision: where will healers stand in the struggle for health care as a human right? This question is posed acutely by the suffering of the destitute sick. But even in the most affluent countries, there is, in the global era, no hiding from the question—or from the imperative to respond.

CHAPTER 7

CRUEL AND UNUSUAL
DRUG-RESISTANT TUBERCULOSIS
AS PUNISHMENT

> Incarceration is a prosperous industry, and one with a glow-
> ing future—as is true of all the others linked to the great
> hiding away of the American poor.
>
> Loïc Wacquant, *Les Prisons de la Misère*

> All the men were used to their fetters, they all regarded them
> as an accomplished fact with which it was useless to argue. It
> is unlikely that anyone ever gave the matter an instant's
> thought, since during all those years it never even once oc-
> curred to the doctors to petition the authorities for the re-
> moval of the fetters from a convict who was seriously ill,
> especially in cases of tuberculosis....It may be objected by
> someone that a convict is a villain and so unworthy of bless-
> ings, but can it be right to aggravate the punishment of those
> whom the wrath of God has smitten in this way?
>
> Fyodor Dostoyevsky, *The House of the Dead*

TUBERCULOSIS AND PRISONS

It's easy to find, in the long and grim history of punishment, inventive
ways of making prisoners suffer. The crudest of these are usually known
as penal torture, a practice roundly condemned by all governments—
and practiced, still, by many. This chapter does not focus on whether the
term "torture" aptly describes capital punishment, hard labor, flogging,
or isolation, although I'm fairly certain that we can and must make fine-
grained distinctions when we can. Nor does it address, as Chapter 4 does,
the experience of tuberculosis within prisons. Rather, this chapter discusses *tuberculosis as punishment.*

Tuberculosis has a long history of association with prisons. In the
pre-chemotherapeutic era, "consumption" was in many settings the
major cause of prison mortality. In the mid-nineteenth century, for example, TB caused an estimated 80 percent of all U.S. prison deaths. In
Boston, Philadelphia, and New York, in any case, about 10 percent of

all prisoners died from the disease.[1] In our own post-antibiotic era, prisoners continue to endure TB risks well in excess of those faced by individuals not in prison. In most countries, TB prison rates five to ten times the national average are not uncommon, and outbreaks can lead rapidly to TB rates more than one hundred times the national average.[2]

This is not to say that there's nothing new under the sun. On the contrary, it's easy to discern novel developments. We are living in an era in which new myths and mystifications about both TB and prisoners abound. We are living in a global economy with its own rapidly changing "geoculture," a transnational social phenomenon that interacts in novel ways with local cultures, themselves rapidly mutating.[3] Alterations in telecommunications and a proliferation of regulations and laws are linked to all manner of human rights discourses, themselves linked both to emerging geoculture and to more established cultural traditions. The degree of transnational travel and trade is unprecedented.

Society and human behavior have changed. *Mycobacterium tuberculosis,* the organism that causes TB, has changed too. Multidrug-resistant tuberculosis (MDRTB) is a relatively recent development, one that has emerged only in the past two or three decades as a frightening concomitant of drug development. Unfortunately, the TB bacillus has mutated more quickly than our own ability to respond with new and effective drugs. And MDRTB is difficult to treat and carries a high case-fatality rate when not treated. It is also stubbornly entrenched in many of the prisons of the former Soviet Union.

This chapter examines TB—and, particularly, MDRTB—in prisons during an era in which neither bars nor national boundaries confine the disease. Let us remember that MDRTB treatment is available for the fortunate few; others, including most prisoners, are summarily informed that their affliction is incurable. Accordingly, I write both as a clinician specializing in the treatment of tuberculosis and as an anthropologist trying to comprehend the myths and mystifications that hamper effective interventions.

KEY CONCEPTS

To examine the problem at hand critically, it's necessary to define or explain certain terms and concepts. For example, patients who relapse after TB therapy do not necessarily have MDRTB; indeed, most of them do not. The term "MDRTB" implies resistance to at least isoniazid (INH) and rifampin (RIF), the two most powerful antituberculous drugs. When a patient who is infected with a TB strain resistant to INH and RIF is treated with a regimen based on these two first-line agents, he or she is unlikely to be cured. Although this might seem obvious, many experts have advocated one-size-fits-all empiric regimens based on first-line drugs—even in the middle of MDRTB outbreaks. This call to downplay the complexity of local epidemics is linked most often to the push for "directly observed therapy, short-course" (DOTS). DOTS has proven to be a very effective strategy for controlling tuberculosis and also for preventing the emergence of MDRTB strains. But the two drugs on which the DOTS strategy is based are the very two to which all MDRTB patients are, by definition, resistant. Thus recommendations that *all* patients with active tuberculosis receive DOTS should not be made with any confidence in the middle of an epidemic of MDRTB. Such recommendations are made, often enough, because the second-line drugs that might cure patients with MDRTB are held to be too expensive for use in precisely those countries or settings in which they are most needed. Second-line drugs are not deemed "cost-effective," in the confused and morally flabby jargon of our day.

INH/RIF-based regimens not only fail to cure patients with MDRTB, they may also lead to iatrogenic worsening of an individual patient's patterns of resistance. That is, the infecting strain is exposed to brief courses of drugs that do not kill the microbe but that can induce further resistance, rendering even carefully designed subsequent regimens less effective. My colleagues and I have called this the "amplifier effect" of short-course chemotherapy.[4]

Of course, there are other ways to amplify the problem. TB is an airborne pathogen. It is coughed into the air in what are known as "droplet nuclei," and these may be inhaled by anyone who shares air with an infectious person. The number of droplet nuclei coughed into the air and the rate of ventilation (air changes per unit of time) are key determinants of risk of infection. Complex mathematical formulas describe transmission dynamics, but suffice it to say that overcrowded prisons with poor ventilation are particularly effective amplification systems for the spread of TB whenever prompt diagnosis and effective therapy are unavailable. Adding HIV to the equation increases the likelihood that new infections will progress to active and contagious TB, further amplifying outbreaks and driving up mortality.

Prisons have gates, but they are highly permeable institutions, with a great deal of interaction with surrounding communities (the "outside world"). This occurs not only through guards and other employees but also because detention is often brief. In the United States, for example, there are about fourteen million arrests each year.[5] Thus what goes on inside prisons and jails is of great relevance to the public's health, as we'll see in examining data from the United States and Russia. It is for all of these reasons that certain correctional facilities have been felicitously termed "infectious prisons."[6]

Another bit of terminology bears consideration. "Acquired MDRTB" occurs when patients do not or cannot adhere to therapy, and intermittent selective pressures allow drug-resistant mutants to become the dominant infecting strain. "Primary MDRTB" occurs when others are infected and fall ill with MDR strains. When poorly conceived regimens further amplify preexisting resistance, primary MDRTB may be misdiagnosed as acquired MDRTB. The difference is critical in prisons.

A review of the literature reveals many discrepant claims about the nature of the prison-tuberculosis association.[7] For example, whereas one survey argues that prisons are "particularly difficult environments" in which to treat TB and that prisoner education is "often hopeless," another review concludes more hopefully that, "with on-site services and confined patients, [correctional institutions] are all suited for public health interventions, health professional education and epidemiologic study."[8] And although the literature seems to show that TB treatment outcomes among prisoners are often poor, there's little agreement as to why. Few studies have examined the contribution of endemic drug resistance to poor clinical outcomes in prisons.[9] Some commentators argue that poor treatment outcomes are the result of the structural constraints of working within underfunded prison systems; others seem to blame the prisoners, often by focusing on alleged psychological or even "cultural" traits. Still others refer to the fragility of the patient-doctor relationship when the latter works for the system that is punishing the former. Because generalizations are hazardous, allow me to turn to the issue of tuberculosis in the prisons of two countries, the United States and Russia.

TAKING A CLOSER LOOK: THE UNITED STATES AND RUSSIA

The United States and Russia hold world records in many prison statistics, taking the prize, most notably, for the highest per capita rates of imprisonment in the world. The United States continues to be the uncontested world leader in detention, although the new Russia almost edged ahead. Of every 100,000 U.S. citizens, 690 are incarcerated, the majority for nonviolent offenses;[10] the rate for Russians, in turn, is 676 per

100,000. For the sake of comparison, note that in many European countries the rate ranges from 60 to 130 per 100,000.[11]

What do we know about epidemics of MDRTB in U.S. prisons? To
begin, it is clear that several of what are termed "nosocomial outbreaks"
began not in hospitals but in prisons. In the largest U.S. outbreak, which
began in New York City in 1989, fully 80 percent of all index cases could
be traced to jails and prisons.[12] The U.S. Centers for Disease Control
(CDC) had sounded the alarm before the New York MDRTB epidemic,
noting the steady and dramatic rise in TB incidence within prisons. In
the New York state correctional system, for example, average annual TB
incidence increased from 15.4 per 100,000 inmates in 1976–78 to 105.5
per 100,000 in 1986.[13] Much of the rise was associated with HIV, but
intramural TB transmission—that is, transmission within the institution—was clearly affecting HIV-negative inmates, wardens, visitors, and
surrounding communities: at least eleven prison outbreaks were recorded
between 1985 and 1989.[14]

These warnings went largely unheeded, as did new guidelines to prevent intramural transmission.[15] By 1991, the Rikers Island jail, which
had experienced a threefold increase in census during the 1980s, had
one of the highest TB case rates in the nation: 400 to 500 cases per
100,000 population.[16] The record shows a dozen more prison epidemics, many with fatalities, between December 1990 and December
1992. By the time the dust settled, it was clear that a mutant strain of
M. tuberculosis resistant to all five first-line drugs was implicated in
most of the deaths. In the New York prison system, for example,
MDRTB was diagnosed in at least thirty-three inmates, 84 percent of
whom died of the disease; one correctional officer was fatally
afflicted.[17]

The prison epidemics were amplified, certainly, by HIV. At the time
of the outbreaks, New York inmates were already saddled with the nation's highest reported rates of HIV infection.[18] But the explosion of TB
in prisons was even more intimately tied to government policies, most
notably those of the Reagan and Bush administrations. In addition to
dismantling the country's TB infrastructure—budgets were slashed
throughout the 1970s as well—the government declared its "war on
drugs" in 1982. One of the newer ruses for managing inequality and
criminalizing poverty, it became in large part a war on drug users and
petty traffickers rather than on those who run or finance the drug trade,
and rates of drug-related arrest and imprisonment skyrocketed during
the first decade of the program.[19] In 1980, there were approximately ten

thousand new commitments for drug offenses; in 1990, more than one hundred thousand. Sentencing mirrored the inequalities of U.S. society: by 1995, some 7 percent of all African American adult males were interned.[20] As Loïc Wacquant has remarked, the state of New York counts more men of color in its prisons than in its public universities.[21] It is important to note that these trends reflect changes in policy rather than changes in behavior.

These policies have had a profound impact. By 1990, 4.3 million men and women—2.35 percent of the U.S. adult population—were in prison or jail or were on probation or parole. This explosion, a 63 percent increase over 1984, left most U.S. detention facilities filled well beyond their original capacity. Prisons without proper ventilation were soon crammed with inmates who had high baseline rates of infection with both HIV and *M. tuberculosis*. A 1993 review noted: "Expansion of physical facilities has not kept pace with the doubling of prison and jail populations in the past decade, nor did it contemplate the risk of transmission of airborne disease."[22]

Yet the connection between the "war on drugs" and drug-resistant tuberculosis was noted early on by those working in the correctional system.[23] Just as detention facilities were not designed to warehouse such large numbers of prisoners, so too was the prison medical system ill prepared to manage the resulting TB crisis. A lack of TB diagnostic capabilities was further compounded by HIV co-infection, which was associated with atypical presentations of active TB that were even more difficult to diagnose.[24] More critically, overburdened providers could not track patients' adherence to antituberculous therapy, and the resulting lack of consistency sparked increased rates of acquired resistance to first-line drugs. In the sardine-can atmosphere of prisons in the 1980s, MDRTB transmission soon led to high rates of primary MDRTB infection in a vulnerable and captive population.

HIV and prison are thus two reasons for the preponderance of males in the U.S. tuberculosis case rates: more than 70 percent of new "excess" TB cases were diagnosed among men, most of them poor African Americans and Latinos living in cities.[25] Among urban African American men, for example, rates of TB jumped *more than 1500 percent* between 1985 and 1990.[26] Many of those afflicted lived in shared spaces: prisons, jails, homeless shelters, drug-treatment programs, and public hospitals. Molecular epidemiology subsequently showed that TB outbreaks tied such institutions together in a vast chain, conveying the mutant strains rapidly across the nation.[27]

Little public outcry was heard, however, until prison wardens, health professionals, and other such "innocent" parties began to fall ill. Then, as Laurie Garrett describes, "panic broke out."[28] Articles began to appear in newspapers and other print media.[29] "This publicity caused such alarm in one upstate New York community," write the authors of one review, "that its hospitals refused to care for inmates, even in life-threatening emergencies."[30] With unions of health care workers and prison employees pressing for their own protection (more than for that of the incarcerated), the Occupational Safety and Health Administration and other regulatory bodies laid down guidelines designed to contain nosocomial and institutional transmission. Court-ordered caps on the number of inmates were issued to several of the key prisons and jails.[31] Several detention facilities were upgraded, and others were built to permit respiratory isolation. Enhanced awareness and surveillance led to earlier identification of drug-resistant cases, and improved outcomes ensued. The CDC recommended culture and drug-susceptibility testing on all isolates of *M. tuberculosis* (reversing a previous recommendation that had termed such testing "no longer cost-effective").

These tardy interventions were, in the end, effective. But what was the cost of the delay? The MDRTB outbreaks, to an important extent the result of imprudent cost-cutting and ill-advised public policy, led to a massive outlay of public monies, especially in New York City. In addition to treatment costs, the upgrading of hospitals and detention facilities cost big money: a new facility for Rikers Island, for example, cost $113 million. In a helpful review, Garrett sums it up well:

> When all the costs of the 1989–94 MDR-TB epidemic were totaled it was clear that more than $1 billion was spent to rein in the mutant mycobacteria. Saving perhaps $200 million in budget cuts during the 1980s eventually cost America an enormous sum, not only in direct funds but also in lost productivity and, of course, human lives.[32]

The MDRTB misadventures also led many professionals to reevaluate the "war on drugs," widely regarded as totally ineffectual by both the medical and jurisprudence communities. "Prisons are terrible institutions," observed Dr. Robert Cohen, whose experience as medical director of the Rikers Island facility forever changed his views on prisons and on drug policy. "The problem of drug abuse is much better approached with a medical model than with a crime-and-punishment model."[33]

Crime-and-punishment models bring us to modern Russia, where prison conditions perhaps recall Kafka more than Dostoyevsky. As Chapter 4 described, the tuberculosis-prison story is even grimmer in Russia than in the United States. Russia has recently been demoted to the status of a developing country, and it is embracing, according to many observers, "Western" (read, American) ways of managing inequality. Writing of the growing influence of U.S. penal policy in Europe, Wacquant remarks that "the influence of Washington, on both economic and penal fronts, is felt even more strongly in Latin America and—supreme irony of history—in numerous countries of the former Soviet Empire."[34] As rates of incarceration rose within Russia, so too did rates of tuberculosis, with both trends tightly linked to economic decline. In 1990, TB incidence in Moscow was 27 per 100,000 population; by 1993, it had almost doubled, to 50 per 100,000. The situation was worse in Siberia, where incidence went from 43 to 94 per 100,000 during the same period.[35]

And the degradation continues. International health officials announced at a news conference in Copenhagen on March 24, 1998, that TB incidence had risen another 50 percent in Russia between 1994 and 1996. "We have never seen such an increase before," commented Arata Kochi, director of the World Health Organization's Global TB Programme. About a quarter of a million cases were announced in 1996, and officials further warned that these infections respected no borders: from Scandinavia to Israel, new cases of drug-resistant tuberculosis were diagnosed in immigrants from the Baltic states or elsewhere in the former Soviet Union.[36] By the close of the millennium, rates had surpassed 100 per 100,000 in many parts of the Russian Federation.

Russia's increase in TB rates cannot be attributed to HIV or to ill-conceived drug policy. Nor can it be attributed to the attitudes and practices of the local TB specialists, who have had their funding cut, in many instances, by more than 90 percent. Rather, the collapse of the public health system, a part of the broader social disruption registered there, is the heart of the problem; and prisons, it transpires, are central both to the amplification of the TB problem and to the mortality trends.[37] "In the Russian Federation," notes one review, "there is evidence from tuberculosis control programmes in the community that a high proportion of patients have served time in prisons, and that having been in jail is a major risk factor for the development of multidrug resistant strains of *M. tuberculosis*." The same report cites tuberculosis death rates as high as 24 percent, with the disease causing from 50 to 80 percent of all prison deaths.[38] Prison officials do not deny the problem. As one of them remarked, "The three major problems facing our correctional system are underfunding, overcrowding, and tuberculosis. Simply being in prison is one of Russia's biggest risk factors for TB."[39]

With so many TB deaths in prison and with such a high rate of imprisonment, it is less surprising to learn that tuberculosis has become the single leading contributor to increased mortality among young Russian men. Why are these patients dying from an eminently treatable disease? Although HIV has only recently been introduced to the formula, it has already emerged as a significant problem within Russian prisons and among others at risk of tuberculosis, including injection drug users.[40] Some Russian patients die because they have no access to therapy; others die because they have access to the wrong kind of therapy. As in the U.S. outbreaks, many of these prisoners have MDRTB, but in Russia many are receiving the very medications to which their infecting strains are already resistant. Still others, it is said, are dispirited enough to give up. Poor conditions in Russian jails and prisons led to prison riots in 1992, and these were harshly repressed. During the 1990s, conditions deteriorated even further until those responsible for making the arrests (and for the military) turned Russia's vast prison system over to the Ministry of Justice, which was led by more enlightened forces. But even prison reformers could not stop the complex biosocial processes then underway: rising social inequality led to rising crime, which led in turn to rising rates of imprisonment. Rates of imprisonment doubled during the course of the decade. Prison-seated epidemics of tuberculosis were sure to follow.

Overcrowding in Russian prisons is now far greater than in U.S. facilities. In the United States, legislation was passed to ensure that each prisoner was allotted 80 square feet of space. In Russia, the space allotment was increased from 27 to 43 square feet.[41] But site visits to prisons and jails reveal an actual parameter far below 27—especially in pretrial detention centers, where more than two hundred thousand people currently languish.[42] And more and more of those detained have or develop active tuberculosis. In these conditions, even brief pre-trial detention often means intense bombardment with viable TB bacilli. The average duration of pre-trial detention is now ten months. One journalist observed that, in these crowded holding centers, "a death sentence stalks people who have not yet been convicted of a crime."[43]

Pre-trial detention, certainly, is more Kafka-esque than Dostoyevskean. The criminal justice bureaucracy, though large and complex, cannot begin to keep up with the current demand. Matrosskaya Tishina, a jail in central Moscow built for two thousand prisoners, currently holds five thousand—no small number of them with active tuberculosis. Moscow's chief of corrections reports that, within the jail, seventy detainees died in the first nine months of 1996—a majority of them from tuberculosis. And the problem has since worsened. For example, Mischa Chukanov, then twenty-two years old, was arrested in February 1997 for petty larceny— he and another young man were accused of stealing a crate of watches from a Moscow warehouse. He waited seventeen months for his case to come to trial. But shortly before his first post-arrest encounter with a judge, Mischa was diagnosed with active pulmonary tuberculosis. After almost four months of treatment, he remained smear-positive—with evidence of tubercle bacilli in his sputum—suggesting that he might never respond to conventional therapy. By his own account, he felt worse and had lost almost thirty pounds since his arrest. Tried and convicted *in absentia*, he was slated for transfer from the Matrosskaya Tishina sickbay to a TB prison colony. "It can't be worse than here," he said.[44]

What are the TB penal colonies like? Russia has about fifty of them, one of which is described in greater detail in Chapter 4. The colonies house almost seventy-one thousand prisoners—half of them under twenty-five years of age. Mischa Chukanov is to be transferred to a colony located in a town of about thirty thousand, about 100 kilometers east of Moscow, a trip of two hours through well-tended fields and thick forests of birch and fir. The colony's dreary barracks, when I saw them, were depressing and overcrowded. Prisoners with tuberculosis were allotted 4 square meters per person. But the facility was clean, the guards and correctional officials cooperative, and the prisoners did not appear malnourished.

The colony's medical director told me that of 909 prisoners, well over 800 suffered from active tuberculosis. The mean age was forty and falling, though teenagers were sent to another facility. The prison had been designed, she explained, for patients who had already received the "intensive phase" of treatment and who, smear-negative, were slated to complete therapy in the colony. In recent years, however, patients arrived with nothing more than a diagnosis. They were transferred, smear-positive, from the facility in which they'd been diagnosed. To tend to these sick prisoners, she had an ancillary staff of forty-three, most of them from the community and several of them prisoners themselves. HIV was not yet a problem, although hepatitis B and syphilis were endemic among the prisoners. "Our medical capacity," she told me, "is altogether inadequate."

Asked about TB outcomes, the medical director was very forthcoming: cure rates were low. Why? She denied that prisoners showed widespread reluctance to be treated:

On the contrary, the patients are very interested in treatment. They want to recover—especially the younger ones. A very small percentage of them refuse treatment, and usually do so because of some extenuating circumstance or misunderstanding. For example, some patients with liver disease are under the impression that they cannot tolerate the drugs. With a minimal amount of explanation, they too accept TB therapy.

Furthermore, all patients, she insisted, receive directly observed therapy. The explanation for low cure rates lay elsewhere. "We know how to manage the cases," she explained wearily, "even the drug-resistant ones. But we don't have the resources." An annual medication budget of 14,000 rubles—not much more than $2,000—meant an irregular supply of first-line drugs and no supply whatsoever of second-line drugs, even though many patients, especially those infected in prison, were known to have drug-resistant disease.[45] Although no survey of drug susceptibility had ever been conducted, the medical director estimated that fully half of all prisoners had drug-resistant TB.

Just how low are the cure rates? The colony's general plan is to treat patients with active TB and then transfer them back to regular prisons. But fewer than one hundred prisoners were transferred last year, reported the chief warden as he listened quietly to his medical director. Far more common is another scenario: the prisoners remain in the colony until they are released. The warden informed us that of thirty prisoners slated for release that month, twenty-seven were known to have active, infectious TB. "We can't really cure them," added the doctor, "so we do our best to keep them alive."

Post-release care is not under the jurisdiction of the correctional system, and there was little coordination between the Ministry of Interior and the Ministry of Health. Now that the Ministry of Justice has taken over the management of the prisons, there is reason to believe that post-release care can be improved. The historical record shows that serious effort is required if prisoners are to receive proper care once they become civilians. "[The prisoners] are released, and many have not finished therapy," continued the prison doctor. "We send them out with prescriptions rather than the medications. By law, they have a right to the medications for free. But that's on paper. In reality, we know that the medications are no longer available for free. Sometimes they are not available at all." Asked about transmission to family members, she replied, "We have no statistics, but we fear the worst. We certainly have cases in which a father comes here as a convict, and we later meet his son—also a convict and also with active TB."

Concern about this state of affairs was visible in the prisoners' faces. I already cited the case of Sergei, a thirty-two-year-old man arrested in eastern Siberia in 1988. He is now only four months away from the end of an eleven-year sentence for fraud. He was diagnosed with TB while working in the TB infirmary, a job he earned for good behavior. He was treated but relapsed later in the course of his sentence. He is now slated to return to his wife and children in Siberia, but he's still sick. "Of course I'm worried I won't be better by the time my sentence is up," he said, "and that I will give my illness to my family."

The double jeopardy faced by Russian detainees is not lost on those working on their behalf. One penal reform activist observed, "Sometimes, the prison officers and medical staff are doing the best they can, and the inmates understand that poor conditions are not the fault of the prison staff but rather of the whole criminal justice system."[46] A former dissident, also now a prisoners' rights activist, agrees, but his assessment is even more dour: "During my six years in Soviet prisons, I lived through many horrors." But "it is certain," he adds, "that conditions in normal jails were not this bad even under Stalin."[47] As Chapter 4 pointed out, the Ministry of Justice—now responsible for the penitentiary system—has deplored prison conditions quite publicly. "We do not wish to house prisoners in such awful conditions," Deputy Minister Yuri Kalinin told me in January 2000. "It makes no sense for anyone concerned with justice to see young men arrested for minor crimes condemned to die of tuberculosis."

In summary, the collapse of the Soviet Union, with its infamous gulags and "psychiatric prisons," has led to a *worsening* of TB care for prisoners, even as it has increased their risk of contracting the disease. The cost of this degradation is in some ways incalculable, and not merely in terms of human lives. The virtual disappearance of social services and a disregard for human dignity fuel a growing cynicism in Russia, weakening chances for the development of a truly open society.

WHAT SHOULD BE DONE?

There is no doubt, then, that MDRTB in prisons—a subset of the problem of tuberculosis in prisons—is a significant public health issue and also a peculiarly modern human rights challenge. How have the public health and human rights communities responded? It is not hyperbole to say that much of the commentary on the problem reveals both a lack of vision and an ignorance of MDRTB management. Some international health experts throw their hands up, as if the ongoing spread of MDRTB and the mounting death toll were reflections of a *force majeure,* beyond the scope of human intervention. Although we have evidence to the contrary, one of the most commonly heard excuses is that MDRTB is simply untreatable.[48] Since drug stockouts are a major problem, it's also argued that drugs are "unavailable" or "too expensive." But is it really a question of drug distribution, when Coca-Cola and McDonald's have introduced their products into the far reaches of Siberia without much difficulty?

Other excuses abound. We have heard them in Peru, the United States, Geneva, and Russia: the patients refuse treatment; they're noncompliant; they hide drugs in their mouths and spit them out later; they falsify lab results. Some argue that prisoners with TB are simply "too antisocial to be treated." It's also been said that "prison culture" in Russia undermines efforts to treat—another example of the conflation of structural violence and cultural difference. When international experts or those responsible for addressing tuberculosis in prisons are the ones offering these excuses, one fears that hunches and impressions and prejudices are being translated into public policy. Cohorting and permanent isolation without treatment have been proposed as "solutions," with little objection from human rights activists.[49] Indeed, international humanitarian organizations have in some instances been the primary architects of cohorting schemes in certain Russian oblasts.

What about those who propose action on behalf of prisoners with tuberculosis? Even in these circles, we're offered long lists of pitfalls. For example, Hernán Reyes and Rudi Coninx report on the Red Cross experience in six Ethiopian prisons, in which a TB program was abandoned because of a high rate of default—62 percent of the patients in an Addis Ababa prison defaulted. And, notes the report, these partially treated prisoners were unlikely to receive therapy elsewhere: "the national tuberculosis program for the general population was unable to provide treatment."[50] The situation in Russia is depicted as singularly discouraging. There, even laboratory results must be regarded with suspicion, since "wealthy prisoners" may "put pressure on laboratory technicians to find bacilli in negative sputum samples" in order to have access to antituberculous drugs that can be sold in the prison black market.[51]

Recognizing the gravity of the situation, the International Committee of the Red Cross, working with the World Health Organization, called a meeting in Baku, Azerbaijan, where an estimated seven hundred prisoners were sick with TB. Many of them, it is clear, have MDRTB. Disturbingly, 89 percent of the patients who remained smear-positive after they had received first-line drugs were found to have MDRTB. Furthermore, fully 24 percent of all consecutive patients initiating therapy were diagnosed with MDRTB. It is not clear from the report what therapy was offered to these prisoners, but the Baku Declaration issued at this meeting called on "governments, ministries of justice and interior and state security and health to work together towards providing prisoners with adequate health care and the means to cure tuberculosis, and Prison health services to implement DOTS."[52] Unfortunately, this strategy will not work well in the Baku prisons. If 24 percent of all comers already have MDRTB, and the majority have drug-resistant disease, DOTS will not afford a "means to cure tuberculosis." Empiric short-course regimens of first-line drugs are the wrong prescription for what ails a substantial fraction of these prisoners.

A robust human rights discourse must be underpinned by technically adequate recommendations. So what, then, is to be done? Alexander Paterson, British prison commissioner in the 1930s, put it well: "Men are sent to prison *as* punishment, not *for* punishment."[53] Paterson's aphorism reminds us that we're faced with an enormous challenge: to identify prisoners with tuberculosis, to remove them from conditions in which treatment is unrealistic, and to initiate effective therapy. In so doing, we will halt the ongoing spread of this disease, reducing the risk of making detention tantamount to a sentence of tuberculosis. And thus we will also respond, at last, to the mandate of protecting the public's health.

Enacting this plan of action requires a great deal of collaboration and good will, and it requires resources. Surveillance of drug resistance is critical, for it alone helps to steer the choice of empiric regimens, when and if empiric regimens are warranted. New field tools for rapid detection of resistance to INH and RIF are becoming available and should be deployed where they are most needed. Once patients with MDRTB are identified, further testing will be necessary to design treatment regimens, and technical assistance will be critical to ensure good outcomes. It is difficult to abort prison TB epidemics through effective therapy, but it is possible with the existing tools. This has been proven in the United States, a country hardly known for progressive prison policies. Only after the situation got totally out of hand were ample resources made available, but in the end they came bursting forth. Ironically, some prison health experts now deplore a lack of funding for TB *outside* U.S. prisons.[54]

Above all, we must avoid the temptation to throw our hands up, for that is the stance that has led us to the current impasse in Russia and elsewhere. In fact, some years of engagement with this problem lead me to conclude that the biggest pitfall of all may be resignation—not that of the prisoners but rather our own. It's for this reason that we cannot find, either in the published literature or in public health circles, a blueprint for action that would help us to respond effectively to the problem of drug-resistant tuberculosis in prisons. Nowhere can we find recommendations arguing that prisoners, precisely because they are wards of the state, must be protected from undue risk of infection. Nowhere can we find recommendations arguing that prisoners have the right to top-of-the-line therapy in part because they are prisoners and may have contracted their malady in prison. Instead, calls for effective therapy for MDRTB are often dismissed as "utopian," "unrealistic," "pie-in-the-sky," not "cost-effective."

Whether or not universal TB care sounds "utopian," the problem clearly will not improve without it. It also seems true that most prison officials in Russia and Central Europe would like to see this problem brought under control. Many prison physicians and nurses are competent and, indeed, compassionate advocates for prisoners sick with TB. Furthermore, many of the prisoners are afraid of TB and are more than willing to undergo rigorous treatment. Finally, the propositions now before us—continued directly observed therapy with short-course empiric regimens alone—simply will not work wherever MDRTB is already a problem.[55]

Prison medicine is most legitimate when it is humane. Medical interventions are most powerful when they are effective. Human rights arguments are most powerful if we really believe that all humans are equally valuable. When we do believe this, we are less likely to accept second-rate interventions and more likely instead to remediate the inequalities that are each day brought more clearly into view by a globalizing economy.

CONCLUSION: ON AGENCY AND CONSTRAINT

The branch that breaks
Is called rotten, but
Wasn't there snow on it?
        Bertolt Brecht,
        "On Sterility"

Allow me to conclude by returning to the concept of tuberculosis as punishment. "Contracting tuberculosis in prison," observes one report, "is most certainly not part of a prisoner's sentence."[56] But in many places, it most certainly is. As long as prison serves as amplifier, as long as effective treatment is not ensured, tuberculosis is part of the punishment—a package deal of new corporality. In his history of French penology, Michel Foucault charts a "displacement of the very object of the punitive operation" from the body of the offender to his "soul" or "psyche."[57] Does tuberculosis as punishment signal a return to a sort of laissez-faire penal torture, a reembodiment of discipline? Does the state's apparent impotence before the problem mean that no one is to blame for ongoing, fatal outbreaks of drug-resistant tuberculosis in prisons? That such outbreaks are accidents? Freakish natural events, microbial El Niños?

As long as they have existed, states have arrogated the power to punish. In all societies, government reserves the right to strip of their agency those individuals deemed miscreant; in some societies, including certain self-declared democracies, it reserves the right to kill criminals. But even prisoners on death row are regarded as having certain rights, including freedom from undue risk of disease. The U.S. Supreme Court has in recent times reminded us that "deliberate indifference to the serious medical needs of prisoners constitutes the unnecessary and wanton infliction of pain proscribed by the Eighth Amendment."[58]

For what it's worth, then, allowing prisoners to die of tuberculosis is illegal in the United States. While many of those who died in recent U.S. prison outbreaks were poor and voiceless, it did not take long for prisoners' rights groups to see that many detainees had been exposed, through poor planning and carelessness, to unnecessary risks. In 1981, in *Lareau v. Manson,* a group of pre-trial detainees and inmates brought suit against the Hartford (Connecticut) Community Correctional Center for exposing them to tuberculosis and other transmissible pathogens. A district circuit court ruled that failure to screen detainees for communicable diseases not only violates the Eighth Amendment's due process clause protecting pre-trial detainees but also constitutes "cruel and unusual punishment" for all inmates.[59] A federal circuit court subsequently upheld the ruling. In 1992, a group of inmates in Pennsylvania argued that the prison's lack of an adequate TB control strategy violated the rights guaranteed them under the Eighth and Fourteenth Amendments. A federal district court ruled in their favor, mandating the prompt implementation of an effective TB control program.[60]

A large number of similar cases have been reviewed in the literature, and many other cases are still pending.[61] The point is simply this: since history reveals our persistent inability to protect prisoners on principle, we must entrap ourselves into decency through public policy. The call for better policy is not an argument against human rights discourse. On the contrary, it is an argument to gird such discourse with the power to enforce.

Unbidden, to be sure, but undeniably, the globalizing economy brings into relief the self-serving relativism of the public health *realpolitik* that creates a double standard of therapy—prompt, effective MDRTB treatment for those with resources, and no treatment at all for prisoners and the poor with MDRTB. The unacceptability of such a double standard was foreseen by the architects of health internationalism. Signed into effect on July 22, 1946, the Constitution of the World Health Organization warned that "unequal development in different countries in the promotion of health and control of disease, especially communicable disease, is a common danger." The only good news, for those ardently opposed to such double standards, is that transnational TB epidemics will at least remind the affluent few that as long as these epidemics remain out of control, no one is really safe.

CHAPTER 8

NEW MALAISE

MEDICAL ETHICS AND SOCIAL
RIGHTS IN THE GLOBAL ERA

First, to what level of quality can medical ethics aspire, if it
ignores callous discrimination in medical practice against
large populations of the innocent poor? Second, how effective
can such theories be in addressing the critical issues of medical and clinical ethics if they are unable to contribute to the
closing of the gap of socio-medical disparity?

> Marcio Fabri dos Anjos, "Medical Ethics in the Developing
> World: A Liberation Theology Perspective"

Far be it from me to make ethics tremble. I tremble even at
the prospect that I will be found guilty of spreading the word
that the pants of the great man are split. For that I have already prepared a defense aimed at exonerating me of all
responsibility.... The result is that it will be very hard to
identify the guilty party, to find anyone who is singularly
responsible, if we are all rounded up by the police and
charged with inciting a riot against ethics.

> John Caputo, *Against Ethics*

DOUBLE STANDARDS OF MEDICAL "ETHICS" FOR THE DEVELOPING WORLD

On March 30, 2000, while working in rural Haiti, I received an e-mail
from a medical student. The subject line flashed by as the files reached
me through the wonder of satellite technology. "More Tuskegee," it read.[1]

The Tuskegee Syphilis Study was conducted in Alabama by the U.S.
Public Health Service from 1932 to 1972. The researchers recorded the
natural history of syphilis in an attempt to learn more about the disease
by following six hundred men, of whom about four hundred had
syphilis, throughout their lifetimes. All were African American, many
were sharecroppers, and most lived in poverty. Despite the 1947 dis-
covery of a cure for the disease—to this day, syphilis is treated with peni-
cillin—subjects were never offered that very inexpensive drug, even

though they had joined the study assuming that they would be treated. Nor were they informed of the study's real purpose.

Tuskegee ended in 1972 amid public outrage when the *Atlanta Constitution* and the *New York Times* ran front-page stories on the study. In a critical reassessment of Tuskegee, historian Allan Brandt notes, "The entire study had been predicated on nontreatment. Provision of effective medication would have violated the rationale of the experiment—to study the natural course of the disease until death."[2] It took the U.S. government decades to acknowledge its wrongdoing; President Clinton's public apology came in 1997.

My student's e-mail message contained a Reuters story about a paper published the day before in the *New England Journal of Medicine*. Under his terse subject heading, he forwarded the story, without commentary:

> BOSTON, March 29—A study of more than 15,000 people in Uganda that has raised ethical questions about AIDS research in poor countries concluded that the risk of spreading AIDS through heterosexual sex rose and fell with the amount of virus in the blood.
>
> The study, in Thursday's issue of the *New England Journal of Medicine*, also confirmed earlier research suggesting that circumcision guarded against the spread of H.I.V., the virus that causes AIDS.
>
> The research was controversial, not because of its conclusions, but because of its methodology. Unlike studies of H.I.V. in developed countries, the volunteers in the Uganda study were not offered treatment, nor did doctors inform the healthy spouse of an infected person that his or her partner harbored the virus.
>
> Instead, the team led by Dr. Thomas Quinn of the National Institute of Allergy and Infectious Diseases, tested the volunteers and tracked the spread of their illness.[3]

In brief, the randomized-control trial conducted between November 1994 and October 1998 examined the relationship between serum viral load, concurrent sexually transmitted diseases, and other known and putative HIV risk factors (for example, male circumcision and several sociodemographic and behavioral factors). The research team screened 15,127 individuals in a rural district of Uganda, of whom 415 were identified as HIV-positive with an initially HIV-negative partner. The researchers then tracked these serodiscordant couples for thirty months, following the viral load of the infected partner and the rate of seroconversion among the previously uninfected partners. The study concludes that "viral load is the chief predictor of the risk of heterosexual transmission of HIV-1." Such a finding "raises the possibility that reductions in viral load brought about by the use of antiretroviral drugs could potentially reduce the rate of transmission." Quinn and colleagues called for *more research* "to develop and evaluate cost-effective methods, such as effective and inexpensive antiretroviral therapy or vaccines, for reducing viral load in HIV-infected persons."[4]

Already, the Ugandan study has occasioned a good deal of comment. Some of it appeared in the same issue of the *New England Journal of Medicine:* "Tragically," noted a researcher from another U.S. university, "results such as these could be obtained only in places with a very high incidence and prevalence of the virus and few practical or affordable means of preventing transmission....The challenge now is to use these results *to develop prevention strategies* that can benefit everyone, especially those who participated in the research."[5]

Develop *prevention* strategies. This sounds eminently reasonable at first blush. But were more research and the development of prevention strategies the only real challenges emerging from this and other studies? I had just participated in a conference in rural Haiti—a conference attended mostly by women living in poverty, several of them also living with HIV—and the "challenge" as outlined in the paper or the accompanying commentary did not ring true to me. Prevention strategies had *already* failed those infected during the course of the Ugandan study; prevention strategies were hardly the "challenge" at hand for "those who participated in the research." The women at the meeting in rural Haiti had raised a very different set of challenges. As one asked, "What about those of us who already have HIV? Are we merely to wait for death?" Another participant said simply, "Treatment is important for sick people."

Commenting on the Ugandan study, others echoed my student. In the electronic magazine *Slate,* one writer asked: "The 15,000 Ugandan volunteers in the sample were not offered treatment nor were their healthy sex partners informed that the research subjects were HIV positive. Excuse please, but why isn't this like the [*New England Journal of Medicine*] supporting the Tuskegee experiments?"[6]

Let us leave aside the fact that there were 415 serodiscordant couples in the study, not 15,000, and the facts that the *Journal* published rather than conducted the research and that its editor wrote a highly critical commentary.[7] The point here is that even though we might dismiss comments from outside the research community as inaccurate or tendentious or worse, an understanding of the social field that generates such commentary reminds us that we live in a peculiar age. Although historians and economists warn against simplistic use of the term "globalization," rapid developments in communications clearly are changing the way we understand, experience, and manage social inequality.[8] Surely it is a novel development that research published one day in the *New England Journal of Medicine* can, within twenty-four hours, trigger heated responses from around the globe.

These and other developments in communications are reminders that, increasingly, epidemics of disease are transnational ones.[9] Research universities and development agencies now also have global reach, and, just as epidemics are transnational, so too, increasingly, is research. But although pathogens readily cross borders, the fruits of research are often delayed in customs. For example, it seems to be easy enough to use First World diagnostics—in the Ugandan study, sophisticated assays of viral load were available—even though antiretroviral therapy is deemed unfeasible, too difficult, or "cost-ineffective."[10] The most commonly encountered justification, though, is that antiretroviral therapy does not reflect "local standards of care." The devastation wrought by HIV in sub-Saharan Africa—AIDS is now far and away the leading cause of adult death across the continent and has already orphaned fourteen million children there—has brought the local-standard-of-care argument to the forefront of medical and public debate in the past few years.[11]

A 1997 article by Peter Lurie and Sidney Wolfe triggered what have become increasingly vocal attacks on the AIDS clinical trials being conducted in developing countries—studies involving, for example, what many argue are unethical placebo controls in AZT trials attempting to develop a cheaper drug regimen to prevent mother-child transmission of HIV. Udo Schüklenk cast this argument in a different light:

> In the real world there is no such thing as a fixed local standard of care. Rather, the local standard of care in, for example, India, is a standard of care determined by the prices set by Western pharmaceutical multinationals. The only reason why the [AZT placebo] trials took place at all is the pricing schedule set by the manufacturer of the drug. Glaxo-Wellcome therefore, more than anything else, determines what is described by bioethicists and clinical researchers as the "local standard of care."[12]

What does medical ethics have to say about such transnational research? The short answer: very little, so far. This in spite of the demands contained in the International Code of Medical Ethics, first drafted in Geneva in 1949, that physicians not only place the well-being of research subjects above the supposed benefits to science and society but also that they declare, "I will not permit considerations of religion, nationality, race, party politics or social standing to intervene between my duty and my patient."[13] But is it not precisely "social standing" and "national-ity" that place Ugandans at risk for becoming AIDS research subjects *and* for receiving substandard medical care? By substandard, I mean lower than the care that the researchers would expect for themselves in the unlikely event that they were to contract HIV.

It is not my intention here to focus overmuch on one particular study. Indeed, Quinn and colleagues are likely not guilty of violating the ethical codes established by their university and by their Ugandan counterparts, as they were quick to protest. They pointed out that four institutional re-view boards in the United States and Uganda had approved the study and that a data safety and monitoring board from the National Institutes of Health, composed of U.S. and Ugandan representatives, monitored their work. At no time was it recommended that the researchers provide anti-retrovirals to the participants.[14] What I am suggesting is that ethical codes and review boards are not always helpful, to put it politely. They often share an unacknowledged agreement that in fact all humans are not cre-ated equal and that this inequality accounts for both differential distri-bution of disease and differential standards of care.

It is no exaggeration to say that the majority of such international bio-medical research has inequality as its foundation. As Marcia Angell has argued:

> Research in the Third World looks relatively attractive as it becomes better funded and regulations at home become more restrictive. Despite the exis-tence of codes requiring that human subjects receive at least the same pro-tection abroad as at home, they are still honored partly in the breach. The fact remains that many studies are done in the Third World that simply could not be done in the countries sponsoring the work. Clinical trials have become a big business, with many of the same imperatives. To survive, it is necessary to get the work done as quickly as possible, with a minimum of obstacles. When these considerations prevail, it seems as if we have not come very far from Tuskegee after all.[15]

These "ironies of inequality" are doubtless the subject of much dis-cussion among people living in poverty—just as the absence of environ-mental or labor regulation in their home countries, opening up ambigu-ous forms of "development," also spurs commentary. Any anthropologist could offer examples. But the ironies are most pointed when ethical codes developed in affluent countries are quickly ditched as soon as affluent uni-versities undertake research in poor countries. Then come a series of ef-forts to develop alternative (read, less stringent) codes "appropriate" to settings of destitution. These revisions are termed "sensible," "reasonable," "realistic." Those who oppose such downgrades are branded as, at best, "utopian" and "naïve" or, at worst, "obstructionist" and even "irresponsible."

INSERTING SOCIAL JUSTICE INTO MEDICAL ETHICS

The problem here, explored throughout this book, is that our practice has not kept up with our rhetoric. In arguing that health care is a human right, one signs on to a lifetime of work dedicated to erasing double standards for rich and poor. Again, the question of social and economic rights is raised, first and loudly by the poor, and then timidly and reluctantly by the rest of us. It has taken years for the sharp critiques voiced by the poor to begin to work their way into our medical journals and ethical codes.

Without a social justice component, medical ethics risks becoming yet another strategy for managing inequality. Within the field, however, promising developments have occurred. Several years ago, an international working group from varied professions gathered in London (at Tavistock Square) to develop an initial draft of a code of ethics for those who work in health care. Members of this group were convinced of the need for a moral framework that all health care professions could relate to and that would encourage cooperation and mutual respect. The Tavistock Group's "shared ethical principles for everybody in health care" is an attempt to recapture the moral high ground of the position that health is a human right, while avoiding the relativism that has so far largely served the interests of the nonpoor.[16] The bad news is that the phrase "everybody in health care" refers to expanding medical ethics to include nurses and other health care *professionals* rather than to include those who bear the brunt of disease. The good news is that even though the poor are not mentioned in the document, something just as important is: the first of the ethical principles enumerated states that health care is a human right.[17]

Of course, this has all been said before—health care is certainly featured as a human right in the Universal Declaration of Human Rights—but the Tavistock document is a statement on *professional ethics* and, like most such statements, was formulated by members of the profession. What is the function of statements of professional ethics? Writing about codes of medical ethics, Sohl and Bassford offer a polite definition that would be challenged by few:

> While it is undeniable that a major motivation for desiring self-regulation is the pursuit of professional power, self-regulation carries with it an ethical

component, and involves a moral commitment on the part of the profession. To see this one need only think of any of the occupational groups currently trying to be recognized as having professional status. One of their first acts is to formulate and publicize a code of ethics for their members.[18]

Codes of medical ethics exist in profusion, and though some are less self-serving than others, most have, as their implicit or avowed focus, the protection of the professionals. In the Tavistock document, we have something more novel: a code crafted by professionals that starts by asserting that health care is a human right.

In subsequent discussions, some have pushed this assertion even further, to argue that *quality* health care is a fundamental human right. In a very real way, such a redefinition would bring all those who comfortably agree with the Tavistock principles to the brink of the abyss. They would have to look down at the squalid misery endured by much of humanity, with its Sisyphean burden of readily treatable pathology, and ask how a decent physician or nurse (or other health professional) should act *ethically*. More specifically, what would the world's destitute sick, wherever they languish, have to say about the key tenets of the statement? And one could ask still harder questions: Do the invisible poor come into view only when they become research subjects or immigrants, or is the next step the inclusion of everyone under the rubric "everybody"? The inclusion of all humans under the rubric "human"? The inclusion of social and economic rights under the rubric "human rights"?

I pose these questions with trepidation. But they are, in my view, far and away the most important questions for medical ethics. I agree with Jon Sobrino and others who believe that "the poor and impoverished of the world, in virtue of their very reality, constitute the most radical question of the truth of this world, as well as the most correct response to this question."[19] As a physician-anthropologist who serves the poor in Haiti, Boston, Peru, and Russia, I have no reason to back away from this stance in contemplating medical ethics, and every reason to cling to it ever more tightly.[20] Our work—analysis and praxis—takes place at an invigorating intersection of medicine, social theory, philosophy, and political analysis. And these disciplines help us to see why it is so important to socialize ethics. As humans, we are all vulnerable to sickness; as physicians, we care for the vulnerable. But some groups are far more vulnerable than others, as every serious epidemiological study has shown. For the poor in affluent countries, it is possible to document the impact of services that are inferior to those offered the nonpoor.[21] In many

resource-poor countries, it is often possible to document a complete absence of modern medical care.[22] As other chapters in this book show,
current trends are far from heartening.

A few decades ago, the impact of this injustice would have been
significant, but not invariably a matter of life and death. That is, people
lived and died, many of them unjustly, but even the well-to-do lived in
fear of microbes that could kill them, as Nancy Tomes reminds us in her
book about infectious diseases at the turn of the nineteenth century.[23]
And although the nonpoor always did better than the poor, pneumo-
coccal pneumonia and tuberculosis came with a high case-fatality rate,
regardless of social station.

Everything is different now, in large part because medicine is indeed
becoming the "youngest science," as Lewis Thomas has written.[24] Using
the basic sciences to develop new therapies and the scientific method to
evaluate their efficacy reminds us that the fight over equal access to
leeches is certainly no longer one worth wasting time on. If the medical
interventions in question are ineffective, or only marginally effective, lack
of access to these interventions, though unfair, is of limited importance.
But biomedicine can at last offer the sick truly revolutionary new therapies. In my own field, infectious disease, we have certainly seen a revolution. Antibiotics and vaccines can, for the fortunate few, virtually erase
the risk of mortality from polio, tetanus, measles, pneumonia, staphylo-
coccal and other bacterial infections, diarrheal disease, malaria, tuberculosis. Even HIV disease, the latest rebuke to undue optimism, has been
rendered, for those with access to therapy, a readily treatable disease.

Then comes the obvious irony. In the areas where I work, most premature deaths are caused by precisely these pathologies.[25]

THE LEADING ETHICAL QUESTION OF OUR TIMES

Into this irony comes bioethics. I have served on the ethics service of the
Boston teaching hospital with which I am affiliated, and of course take
each consult seriously. These consults are often enough about too much
medical care. That is, we are called to explore cases in which care is
painful, expensive, and prolonged well beyond the point of efficacy. This
is termed "medical futility." But being a clinician who works in both a
Harvard teaching hospital and rural Haiti, I can't help but make connections between the surfeit on one side—too much care—and the
paucity on the other. As an infectious-disease consultant, I feel that my
job in Haiti is to say, "Quickly, start the antibiotics," whereas my job in

Boston often comes down to saying, "Stop the antibiotics." In Haiti I am called to explain, to those who come begging for assistance, that effective treatments for HIV are not "cost-effective," whereas in Boston I spend much of my time begging patients with AIDS—some of them originally from Haiti—to take these same medications. In Boston I might be alone in witnessing this painful irony, if not for the transnational Haitian janitors who keep the hospital clean.[26]

What does bioethics have to say about this, the leading ethical question of our times? Almost nothing. Conventional medical ethics does a good job of erasing such obscene disparities, for at least four reasons. First, ethics draws strength from experience-distant disciplines such as philosophy, lending ethics debates a curious, at times almost silly, tenor, as Larry Churchill has noted:

> Bioethical disputes—as measured by the debates in journals and conferences in the United States—often seem to be remote from the values of ordinary people and largely irrelevant to the decisions they encounter in health care. In this sense, philosophical theorizing might be considered harmless entertainment, which if taken too seriously would look ridiculous, as several Monty Python skits have successfully demonstrated.[27]

There have been few attempts to ground medical ethics in political economy, history, anthropology, sociology, and the other contextualizing disciplines (although each of these would have no doubt lent its own native silliness).[28]

Second, medical ethics has been to a large extent a phenomenon of industrialized nations. This has facilitated the process of erasing the poor, since most of them live elsewhere. Thus, the great majority of the world's ethical dilemmas—and, to my mind, the most serious ones—are not discussed by the very discipline claiming expertise in such matters. The third reason that medical ethics and bioethics have been mum on the leading ethical dilemma of our times is that experts have dominated public discourse on these matters, drowning out the voices of those who have far more direct experience. To again cite Churchill:

> Ethics, understood as the capacity to think critically about moral values and direct our actions in terms of such values, is a generic human capacity. Except for sociopaths, it is common to all of us, and skill in ethics does not lend itself easily to encapsulation in theoretical categories, core competencies, or a professional speciality.[29]

A fourth reason, in part an unavoidable one, is that in the hospital we are asked to address the "quandary ethics" of individual patients. In the affluent countries where bioethics has blossomed, these have often been elderly patients for whom further care is deemed futile, even though the machine of "care" grinds on, leaving family and providers feeling a bit ground up themselves.

As the Tavistock statement notes, "The personal experience of illness is generally the principal concern of individual patients; therefore, the principal focus of the health care delivery system must be individual patients and their families or support groups."[30] This priority is altogether appropriate and should not be changed. What should be changed, rather, is that millions are denied the chance to become patients and to have an "individual focus" trained on them. Beyond the administrative borders erected around catchment areas or states or nations, legions die—not of too much care or inappropriate care but rather of no care at all. One gets the sense, in attending ethics rounds and reading the now-copious ethics literature, that these have-nots are an embarrassment to the ethicists, for the problems of poverty and racism and a lack of national health insurance figure only rarely in a literature dominated by endless discussions of brain death, organ transplantation, xeno-transplantation, and care at the end of life. When the end of life comes early—from death in childbirth, say, or from tuberculosis or infantile diarrhea—the scandal is immeasurably greater, but silence reigns in the medical ethics literature.

In an era of globalization and increased communication, this selective attention can become absurd. The world's poor already seem to have noticed that ethicists are capable of endlessly rehashing the perils of too much care, while each year millions die what the Haitians call "stupid deaths." The erasures are expedient for some, certainly, but the effaced are less easy to silence these days. One reason is that communications are different—and by and large better—in the global era. Another reason is the sheer burden of unnecessary suffering and premature death. A third is that the current trend is toward even further entrenchment of social inequality.

In the midst of all of this comes the second principle of the Tavistock document: "The care of individuals is at the center of health care delivery but must be viewed and practiced within the overall context of continuing work to generate the greatest possible health gains for groups and populations."[31] Here is a principle suited to our times. It contains its own checks and balances. A principle such as this would lead us to push for public health but at the same time resist the prevailing conditions—conditions in which it is possible, indeed deemed reasonable, for physicians to contemplate the results of a study con-

ducted among the destitute sick of Uganda and feel that the only challenge is "prevention." As the women participating in our conference in
Haiti observed, prevention comes too late for people who are already
sick and immiserated.

The self-appointed guardians of international health cannot *ethically*
erase the tens of millions already sick with HIV disease. Even using their
own, often punitive, analytic tools (for example, cost-effectiveness analysis), treatment of HIV should surely have its role among the destitute
sick of southern Africa. As Evan Wood and colleagues argue, even "limited use of antiretrovirals could have an immediate and substantial impact on South Africa's AIDS epidemic."[32] Their assessment projected
that the use of short-course prophylaxis would reduce perinatal transmission by 40 percent, preventing 110,000 infant HIV infections by
2005—at a cost of less than 0.001 percent of the national per-person
health expenditure. In a more costly scenario, triple-combination treatment for only 25 percent of the HIV-infected population would prevent
both 430,000 incident AIDS cases and a 3.1-year decline in life
expectancy.[33] Thus even without recourse to ethical reasoning—which
would lead us to ask not "if" but rather "how"—we find the world revealed to us as it really is: a place in which the absolute majority of medical ethics violations go unremarked by experts in this field.

The millions already dying during childbirth or from diseases such as
HIV and drug-resistant malaria and tuberculosis face other challenges
beyond prevention.[34] If "the care of individuals is at the center of health
care delivery," as the Tavistock statement argues, then concerns over equity won't simply go away. *In the global era, global health equity, more
than ever before, must be a goal of any serious ethical charter.* Questions
regarding social and economic rights are at the heart of what must become a new medical ethics.

EQUITY AS THE FUNDAMENTAL CORE OF A NEW MEDICAL ETHICS

I conclude by asking questions that stem from serious contemplation of
the first two principles of the Tavistock document.

*If access to health care is considered a human right, who is consid-
ered human enough to have that right?*

Looking back over the concept of human rights, we can see that social inequalities have always been used to deny some people status as fully

human. When the French promoted the "rights of the citizen," they certainly did not—and do not, for that matter—confer citizenship lightly.[35] Thus human rights were, from the beginning, quite distinct from the rights of the human. And even supposedly subaltern voices could not be depended upon to believe in human rights: when the *gens de couleur* Ogé and Chavannes traveled from colonial Haiti to revolutionary France, they went to press for the rights of mulattoes to own slaves.[36] And so it has continued, with the poor, women, black people, those of low caste, people with disabilities, children, or "aliens" from other nations—you can fill in the blanks, depending to some extent on time and place—denied the full complement of human rights.

Many quests for the rights of the disenfranchised have in truth been quests for power sharing, a process not to be confused with the struggle for social justice for all. In an affluent country like the United States, the call to a unifying nationalism across lines of race and gender often leads to a struggle for the advancement of one group at the expense of others. The identity politics of our times has a troubling subtext: *I've been wronged in the past, and I want what's coming to me.* Wallerstein calls ours "the era of groupism—the construction of defensive groups, each of which asserts an identity around which it builds solidarity and struggles to survive alongside and against other such groups."[37] The fundamental unfairness of existing social structures can be made more palatable if those with access to resources, including medical care, include "historically underrepresented minorities." But cosmetic alterations will placate those at the bottom for only so long.

Nor, if we are going to honor our calling, can health care be considered a human right accorded only to citizens of *certain* nations. People may be erased by geographical chance, by the fact of living beyond the boundaries of an affluent nation-state, but they are erased nonetheless. Physicians who reject nationalism may move to an area with grotesque burdens of disease and find themselves chided for failing to serve those who may be less sick but who carry the same passport as they do.[38]

Can medical ethics, necessarily grounded in the dilemmas faced by patients, develop a broader view of who gets sick and why? Of who has access to care and why?

This is a critical question, in any inegalitarian social field, for a robust code of medical ethics. But the second principle of the Tavistock document demands that this exercise in social medicine figure prominently in our practice. This is in no way a call for clinicians to abandon a patient-focused view. When the push for broadening access, or for attacking only the perceived roots of excess disease, leads to lowering standards of individual patient care, this Luddite approach should be criticized in strong terms. Rather, this question is simply a call for mindfulness—as a moral and analytic stance—about the strikingly patterned pathways to both sickness and care.[39] And yet medical ethics, in my experience, regards social ethics as somehow embarrassing and even inappropriate. Until we come to terms with this discomfort, we will be left with only half a principle.

Medical ethicists and physicians might reply that this is an exercise best left to epidemiologists and to those who study health care systems. But we should not pass this task on to other parties. First, we cannot always trust others to respect the rights of individual patients. Second, practitioners of many disciplines related to medicine have proven incapable of understanding the biosocial complexity that defines unequal health outcomes and health and human rights. Although disciplinary specialization has yielded great insights, the arguments in this book have tried to emphasize the cost of desocializing the concept of rights. Whether we consider Russian prisoners with drug-resistant tuberculosis, HIV-infected Cubans living within sanatoriums, Bostonians with AIDS living on the streets, or Haitians with AIDS detained on a U.S. military base, the story is the same: a failure to understand social process leads to analytic failures, with significant implications for policy and practice.[40]

How does the struggle for social and economic rights relate to, for example, a "Patient's Bill of Rights"?

Questions of erasure again loom large. Most charters of patients' rights seem unaware of the sick nonpatients who never get into the exclusive club of those who actually receive modern health care. In the broader social field in which the "bottom billion" have no access at all to modern medicine, the very real dilemmas of those who *do* have access to care have been the focus of most inquiry by medical ethicists. The right to health care would seem to be of little concern to modern medical ethics. By "modern," I mean the contemporary practice of medical ethics, which regards Nuremberg and Tuskegee as subjects of largely historical interest and ignores the Third World sick altogether, unless they happen to serve as research subjects. Thus, in discussions of medical ethics, global health equity has become the elephant in the room that no one mentions.

But whether we are talking about uninsured U.S. citizens, hapless African research subjects, or prisoners with drug-resistant tuberculosis, charters proclaiming health care as a right take on their full power only when we add the clause "by the way, we *really* mean everybody." This could be dismissed as pie-in-the-sky, but it seems better to avoid erasure and set goals high than to sink to a "pragmatism" that leads inevitably to "ethical dilemmas" (to use the polite language of academic circles; the victims of such pragmatism do not mince words in this manner).

A charter such as the one proposed in Tavistock would mean that we would no longer be more comfortable talking about "patient autonomy" than about the right to receive care when sick. Such a charter would have a great deal to say about medical research conducted by First World universities in settings of Third World poverty. It's naïve to pretend that there are no competing agendas here. At the same time, the first half of the second principle reminds me to be focused on the individual patient. And it does not exhort me to treat only patients of a certain nationality.

What do the destitute sick have to say about medical ethics?

The short answer: plenty. And as a physician-anthropologist, I get an earful. After close to two decades of work in Haiti and much experience in poor neighborhoods of Lima and Boston, I suspect that the destitute sick are in many senses our most harsh and loyal critics. They are loyal in the sense that, even though we have served them poorly, the poor continue to come to our clinics and hospitals; they continue to offer critiques of our errors, if we are willing to listen. That their commentary has not figured prominently in discussions of medical ethics should raise eyebrows, at the very least. Why do we have an extensive literature on why it is not "cost-effective" or "feasible" (or "sustainable" or "appropriate technology") to treat poor people who have complicated diseases? This opinion represents, in the view of some, another slick ruse to distract us from the fundamental ethical problem of our era: the persistence of readily treatable maladies and the growth of both science and economic inequality. Since the poor are those put at risk of sickness and then denied access to care, they are in many ways those most affected by codes of medical ethics. Within and across national boundaries, the destitute sick should be the primary judges of any code of medical ethics. Applying a "perfect" ethical code in one country alone is an impossibility in the global era. Again, we are led back to global health equity as a necessary component of any discussion of medical ethics.

*Should physicians be judged by a special calculus of
accountability?*

The short answer: of course. No other profession is accorded greater
and more intimate access to the lives of the sick and suffering. With this
great privilege comes responsibility. As Chapter 6 argued, this is not a
business contract. A fair amount has been written about the Nazi doctors, whose abuses of their professional authority led, in no small way,
to the founding of modern medical ethics.[41] Although their crimes were
perhaps no more heinous than those of other mid-range professionals
in the machinery of the Third Reich, we judge them more harshly. Such
murderous violations of the sacred contract between physician and patient are unlikely to find support in any quarter. Although these crimes
are at the extreme end of the spectrum, there is room at that end to locate the Tuskegee experiments as well. Yet Tuskegee still has its defenders, some more vocal than others.[42] And the participation of U.S.
physicians in state-sponsored executions does not cause medical licenses
to be revoked, since the death penalty is legal in the United States, and
the law of the land seems to take precedence over moral codes and professional ethics.[43]

   To return to questions of accountability, I would also warn that the
so-called "gray areas" of medical ethics are becoming more black and
white with time. So it is with the challenge of the destitute sick. Do physicians have any special obligations to go where the pathology lies heavi-
est? Virchow thought so.[44] As Chapter 5 made clear, the liberation theologians think so. And the Tavistock statement makes it clear that, even
within a code-generating professional body, the special obligation of the
healer to the destitute sick must be respected if medicine is to merit the
title "vocation."[45]

HUMAN RIGHTS IN MEDICAL ETHICS – FOR EVERYBODY

Perhaps the greatest challenge for medical ethics is to *resocialize the way
we see ethical dilemmas in medicine.* Restoring to such problems their
full social complexity is our best vaccine against the erasures documented
throughout this book. I don't feel uncomfortable doing an ethics consult
in the intensive care unit of a Boston teaching hospital, because I don't
believe a clinical ethics team is expected to discuss general social ethics
in such a context any more than other clinicians are expected to discuss
them during the course of a clinic visit. Of course, specific ethical and
practical concerns relating to the patient's social and economic context

often do—appropriately—crop up in clinical settings. But I do feel uncomfortable *writing* about these matters as if Haiti, Uganda, and Harlem
belonged to a different world.[46] They are part of the same world.

How often have we challenged the chicanery that leads us to forget
that we are part of the same world? In the United States, the subtext of
some ethical discussions has been, ironically enough, how best to manage our vast prosperity. And there is some truth in this; we are prosperous. I was en route from Moscow to the United States on the morning
after President Clinton's State of the Union address in January 2000. In
it, Clinton spoke proudly of our vast wealth and huge surpluses.[47] Yet I
was still smarting after a bitter struggle over whether food supplements
could be included in the budget of a project to treat tuberculosis within
a Russian penitentiary system full to bursting with gaunt and coughing
young men. The struggle was primarily with U.S. and European technical consultants to the World Bank, which was proposing a loan to the
Russian government as it seeks to respond to epidemic tuberculosis
within its prisons. The Russian specialists wanted to include food supplements as part of the loan. The non-Russian Bank consultants coun-
tered that the drugs would work fine with or without malnutrition.

Was this food fight emblematic of an ethical dilemma? Does being
human confer a right to survive?

We read in the Working Draft of the Tavistock statement: "Physicians
and other clinicians should be advocates for their patients or the populations that they serve but should refrain from manipulating the system
to obtain benefits for them to the substantial disadvantage of others."[48]
I suspect that the writers' intention was to exhort physicians to refrain
from exploiting some public-entitlement program in an affluent industrialized nation. But if Haiti and Uganda and Russia and Harlem are part
of the same world, we could argue just as easily that conducting research
in settings of great privation and excess burden of disease also runs the
risk of "manipulating the system," with the system in question being the
global web of connections that is increasingly visible to all of us. Much
of this research would never be considered ethical within the country
sponsoring the research; its approval by institutional review boards relies on the argument that the local standard of care—in the poor communities where the research subjects live and die—is no care at all. So
too can we wonder, as the *Financial Times* estimates capital flight out of
Russia at greater than $130 billion in seven years,[49] if our failure to fight
hard enough for food for prisoners with tuberculosis is merely a con-

cession to far more powerful forces who are only too happy to "manip-ulate the system" to the substantial disadvantage of the poor.

The concept of human rights may at times be brandished as an all-purpose and "universal" tonic, but it was developed to protect the vul-nerable. The true value of the human rights movement's central docu-ments is revealed only when they serve to protect the rights of those who are most likely to have their rights violated. The proper beneficiaries of the Universal Declaration of Human Rights—however inexpedient this point might be in our age of individualism and affluence and relativism—are the poor and otherwise disempowered. The true value of the Tavis-tock statement is that it attempts to restore the language of rights to the arena of health care. Since the burden of disease is borne by the poor and otherwise marginalized, we are offered a chance, once again, to con-template the lot of most of humanity and to ask, simply enough, if by "everybody" we truly mean everybody.

CHAPTER 9

RETHINKING HEALTH AND HUMAN RIGHTS

TIME FOR A PARADIGM SHIFT

As the global market economy pulverized traditional societies and moralities and drew every corner of the planet into a single economic machine, human rights emerged as the secular creed that the new global middle class needed in order to justify their domination of the new cosmopolitan order.

Kenneth Anderson, formerly of Human Rights Watch

From the perspective of a preferential option for the poor, the right to health care, housing, decent work, protection against hunger, and other economic, social, and cultural necessities are as important as civil and political rights or more so.

Leigh Binford, *The El Mozote Massacre*

Medicine and its allied health sciences have for too long been only peripherally involved in work on human rights. Fifty years ago, the door to greater involvement was opened by Article 25 of the Universal Declaration of Human Rights, which underlined social and economic rights: "Everyone has the right to a standard of living adequate for the health and well-being of himself and his family, including food, clothing, housing, and medical care and necessary social services, and the right to security in the event of unemployment, sickness, disability, widowhood, old age or other lack of livelihood in circumstances beyond his control."[1]

But the intervening decades have seen little progress in the efforts to secure social and economic rights, even though we can point with some pride to gains in civil or political rights. These distinctions are crucial, as a visit to a Russian prison makes clear.

In the cramped, crammed detention centers where hundreds of thousands of Russian detainees await due process, many fall ill with tuberculosis. Convicted prisoners who are diagnosed with tuberculosis are sent to one of more than fifty "TB colonies," several of which I've described in earlier chapters. I bring up these colonies again in order to illustrate the difference between civil rights and social and economic rights. Imagine a Siberian prison in which the cells are as cramped as cattle cars, the fetid air thick with tubercle bacilli. Imagine a cell in which most of the prisoners are coughing and all are said to have active tuberculosis. Let the mean age of the inmates be less than thirty years. Finally, imagine that many of these young men are receiving ineffective treatment for their disease—which, given drug toxicity, is worse than receiving a placebo—even though they are the beneficiaries of directly observed therapy with first-line antituberculous agents, delivered (however ambivalently) by European humanitarian organizations and their Russian colleagues.

If this seems hard to imagine, it shouldn't be; I have seen this situation in several prisons. As this book goes to press, most of these prisoners are still receiving directly observed doses of medications that cannot cure them. For many of these prisoners, the therapy is ineffective because the strains of tuberculosis that are epidemic within the prisons are resistant to the drugs being administered. Various observers, including some from international human rights organizations, aver that these prisoners have "untreatable forms" of tuberculosis, and few challenge this claim, even though treatment based on the standard of care used elsewhere in Europe and North America can in fact cure the great majority of such cases.[2] "Untreatable," in these debates, really means "expensive to treat." For this and other reasons, tuberculosis has again become the leading cause of death among Russian prisoners, even among those receiving treatment. One can find similar situations throughout the former Soviet Union.

Are human rights violated in this dismal scenario? Conventional views of human rights would lead one to focus on a single violation: prolonged pre-trial detention. As Chapter 4 noted, those arrested are routinely detained for up to a year before making a court appearance. In many documented cases, young detainees have died of prison-acquired tuberculosis before their cases ever went to trial. Such detention clearly violates not only Russian law but also several human rights charters to which the country is signatory. Russian and international human rights activists have focused on this problem, demanding that all detainees be rapidly brought to trial. But an impasse is quickly reached when the underfunded Russian courts wearily respond that they are working as fast as they can. The Ministry of Justice agrees with the human rights activists and is interested in amnesty for prisoners and alternatives to imprisonment. These measures may prove helpful, but they will not save those who are already sick.

What of other, complementary approaches, those invoking the rights of prisoners? Has agitation for shorter pre-trial detention, in the form of letters and other protests, proven adequate to solve the problem of prison tuberculosis? If laws were not being violated, but prisoners or former convicts continued to die of tuberculosis, would this suggest that the law is sufficient to protect the health of the vulnerable? The analysis this book presents suggests that the answers to both these questions is no. In fact, from the perspective of the poor—and most of these prisoners are poor—neither legal nor conventional human rights approaches have even begun to understand the nature of the problem.

Let us reconsider tuberculosis in Russian prisons as a question of social and economic rights. Such an exercise yields a far longer list of violations—but also a longer list of possible interventions. First, pre-trial detention is illegally prolonged and conditions are deplorable. The directors of the former gulag do not dispute this point. The head of the federal penitentiary system, speaking to Amnesty International, described the prisoners as living in "conditions amounting to torture."[3] Some of the more astute prison administrators remind their critics that the dismantling of the Soviet economy has led to a sharp rise in petty crime— "People now have to steal for food," in the words of one official[4]—which has swamped the prison system even as "economic restructuring," planned with the help of Western economic advisers, has gutted budgets for prison health care.[5]

Second, detainees are subjected to conditions that guarantee increased exposure to drug-resistant strains of *M. tuberculosis*. In other words, excess tuberculosis risks within prisons and jails should be seen as a violation of rights, a violation further compounded by a lack of commitment on the part of many—including some in the humanitarian assistance community—to providing truly effective treatment.

Third, the prisoners are denied not only adequate food but also medical care. Again, where does the blame lie? Interview medical staff in these prisons, and you will find them distraught about the funding cuts that have followed the restructuring and collapse of the Russian economy. In the words of one physician: "I have spent my entire medical career caring for prisoners with tuberculosis. And although we complained about shortages in the eighties, we had no idea how good we had it then. Now it's a daily struggle for food, drugs, lab supplies, even heat and electricity."[6]

Fourth, prisoners are dying of ineffectively treated multidrug-resistant tuberculosis. Article 27 of the Universal Declaration of Human Rights, which insists that everyone has a right "to share in scientific advancement and its benefits," leads us to raise questions of why representatives of wealthy donor nations—relief workers—are giving prisoners drugs to which their infecting tuberculosis strains have documented resistance. Thus the rights of prisoners are violated by the logic of cost-effectiveness, which argues that the appropriate drugs are too expensive for use in "the developing world" to which post-perestroika Russia has been demoted. All the prison rights activism in the world will come to naught if prisoners are guaranteed the right to treatment but given the wrong prescriptions. All the penal reform in the world will come to naught if prisoners with tuberculosis are granted amnesty only to find the civilian TB service demolished in the name of "health care reform." In short, conventional legal and human rights views on recrudescent tuberculosis in Russian prisons fail to recognize the true dimensions of the problem.

QUESTIONING "IMMODEST CLAIMS OF CAUSALITY"

This picture is further complicated by the competing explanations offered by various actors on the scene. Some international health experts insist that the heart of the problem lies with Russian physicians, who have failed to adopt modern approaches to tuberculosis control.[7] Others, basing their arguments on technical considerations or issues of cost-effectiveness, argue that multidrug-resistant tuberculosis (MDRTB) is untreatable in such settings. Experts from the international public health community have argued that it is not necessary to treat MDRTB—the "untreatable form" in question—in this region, contending that all patients should be treated with identical doses of the same drugs and that MDRTB will somehow disappear if such strategies are adopted.[8] Other experts, both Russian and international, claim that the fault for poor treatment outcomes lies with the prisoners, who are said to refuse treatment.[9]

How many of these claims are true? First, it seems absurd to lay the blame for a burgeoning tuberculosis epidemic on Russia's hapless tuberculosis specialists, given that economic restructuring (and not ill-advised clinical management strategies) has brought the nation's public health infrastructure to its knees. Second, cost-efficacy arguments against treating drug-resistant tuberculosis almost always fail to note that most of the drugs necessary for such treatment have been off-patent for years. As to assertions that MDRTB is untreatable, they are simply not true. Partners In Health has done work in Peru and Haiti showing that MDRTB can be cured in resource-poor settings.[10] By constituting a coalition of international groups able to lobby for lower prices for these drugs, we were able to drop prices of many second-line drugs by more than 90 percent in less than two years.[11] We also know from painful experience in New York prisons that failure to identify and treat MDRTB will lead to outbreaks of disease throughout a prison system, and thence on to the public hospitals and beyond. Claims that low-cost, short-course chemotherapy can eliminate the problem are thus dangerously incorrect.[12]

There is reason to suspect that the other assertion, that prisoners refuse treatment, is also false. How might this claim be assessed? One option would be to ask the concerned parties. During visits to Siberia, I have often asked prisoners with tuberculosis, "How many of you want to be treated?" All hands go up. "Why, then, is it so widely rumored that you refuse treatment?" "Hearsay," according to some. "Just not true," another will remark, "but we want treatment that will cure us." In prison after prison, it's the same story. That conventional therapy was failing to cure them was as obvious to the prisoners as it was to the medical technologists who, during each month of treatment, documented the presence of tubercle bacilli in the prisoners' sputum.

Clearly, the veracity of competing claims about a matter as complicated as epidemic MDRTB cannot be assessed by a show of hands. MDRTB in Russian prisons is an example of a complex human rights problem that requires the application of epidemiology, subspecialty clinical medicine, and a critical sociology of knowledge. Social science can also help to unmask the immodest claims of causality filling the explanatory void. Facile claims about the nature of excess deaths among prisoners are patterned and predictable. They serve recognizable (though hardly honorable) purposes. The analysis also calls for an international political economy of relief work—that is, a critical look at how humanitarian work is conducted in the global, inegalitarian era.[13]

But what, more specifically, does a focus on health bring to the struggle for human rights? This book has argued that a narrow legal approach to health and human rights can obscure the nature of violations, thereby enfeebling our best responses to them. Casting prison-based tuberculosis epidemics in terms of social and economic rights offers an entrée for public health and medicine, an important step in the process that could halt these epidemics. Conversely, failure to consider social and economic rights can prevent the allied health professions and the social sciences from making their fullest contribution to the struggle for human rights.

One of the central points of this book is that public health and access to medical care are social and economic rights; they are at least as critical as civil rights. An irony of this global era is that while public health has increasingly sacrificed equity for efficiency, the poor have become well-informed enough to reject separate standards of care. In our professional journals, these subaltern voices have been well-nigh blotted out. But we heard snatches of their rebuke recently with regard to access to antiretroviral therapy for HIV disease. For over a decade, those living with both poverty and HIV (they are tens of millions strong, even if they have no acronym) have been demanding access to effective therapy. In the past several years, these demands have become increasingly specific, as a group of rural Haitians living with HIV made clear in a declaration made public in August 2001. The patients traced the links between the right to treatment and other social and economic rights:

> It is we who are sick; it is therefore we who take the responsibility to declare our suffering, our misery, and our pain, as well as our hope. We hear many poignant statements about our circumstances, but feel compelled to say something clearer and more resounding than what we've heard from others.
>
> [We] are fortunate to have access to medications and health care even though we do not have money to buy them. Many of our health problems have been resolved with [antiretroviral] medications. Given how dire our situation was prior to treatment, we have benefited greatly. But while we feel fortunate to have access to these services, we feel great sadness for others who don't receive the same treatment we do.
>
> And in addition to our health problems, we have other tribulations. Although less preoccupied with our illness, we still have problems paying for housing. We have trouble finding employment. We remain concerned about sending our children to school. Each day we face the distressing reality that we cannot find the means to support them. Not being able to feed our children is the greatest challenge faced by mothers and fathers across the country of Haiti. We have learned that such calamities also occur in other countries. As we reflect on all these tragedies we must ask: is every human being not a person?
>
> Yes, all human beings are people. It is we, the afflicted, who speak now. We have come together...to discuss the great difficulties facing the sick. We've also brought some ideas of our own in our knapsacks; we would like to share them with you, the authorities, in the hope that you might do something to help resolve the health problems of the poor.
>
> When we the sick, living with AIDS, speak to the subject of "health and human rights," we are aware of two rights that ought to be indivisible and inalienable. Those who are sick should have the right to health care. We who are already infected believe in prevention too. But prevention will not save those who are already ill. All people need treatment when we are sick, but for the poor there are no clinics, no doctors, no nurses, no health care.

Furthermore, the medications now available are too expensive. For HIV treatment, for example, we read in the newspapers that treatment costs less than $600 per year [in developing countries]. Although that is what is quoted in press releases, here in a poor, small country like Haiti, it costs more than twice that much.

The right to health is the right to life. Everyone has a right to live. If we were not living in misery, but rather in decent poverty, many of us would not be in this predicament today.…

We have a message for the people who are here and for all those able to hear our plea. We are asking for your solidarity. The battle we're fighting—to find adequate care for those with AIDS, tuberculosis, and other illnesses—is the same as the combat that's long been waged by other oppressed people so that everyone can live as human beings.[14]

Whether or not we continue to ignore them, the destitute sick are increasingly clear on one point: making social and economic rights a reality is the key goal for health and human rights in the twenty-first century.

Although trained in anthropology, I, like most anthropologists, do not embrace the rigidly particularist and relativist tendencies popularly associated with the discipline.[15] That is, I believe that violations of human dignity are not to be accepted merely because they are buttressed by local ideology or longstanding tradition. But anthropology—in common with sociological and historical perspectives in general—allows us to place in broader contexts both human rights abuses and the discourses (and other responses) they generate. Furthermore, these disciplines permit us to ground our understanding of human rights violations in broader analyses of power and social inequality. Whereas a purely legal view of human rights tends to obscure the dynamics of human rights violations, the contextualizing disciplines reveal them to be pathologies of power. Social inequalities based on race or ethnicity, gender, religious creed, and—above all—social class are the motor force behind most human rights violations. In other words, violence against individuals is usually embedded in entrenched structural violence.

In exploring the relationships between structural violence and human rights, particularly in Part I of this book, I have drawn on my own experience serving the destitute sick in settings such as Haiti and Chiapas and Russia, where human rights violations are a daily concern (even if structural violence is not always seen as a human rights issue). I cite this experience not to make overmuch of my personal acquaintance with other people's suffering, but rather to ground a theoretical discussion in the reality that has shaped my views on health and human rights. Each

of these situations calls for us not only to recognize the relationship between structural violence and human rights violations but also to implement what we have termed pragmatic solidarity: the rapid deployment of our tools and resources to improve the health and well-being of
those who suffer this violence.

Rather than examining in detail the covenants and conventions that
constitute the key documents of the human rights movement, the goals
of this chapter are to raise, and to answer, some questions relevant to
health and human rights; to explore the promise of pragmatic solidarity
as a response to structural violence; and to identify promising directions
for future work in this field. These, I believe, are the most important issues raised by the preceding chapters, and the conclusions that follow
are the most important challenges before those who concern themselves
with health and human rights.

How Far Has the Human Rights Movement Come?

The field of health and human rights, most would agree, is in its infancy.
Attempting to define a new field is necessarily a treacherous enterprise.
Sometimes we appear to step on the toes of those who have long been
at work when we mean instead to stand on their shoulders. Human rights
law, which focuses on civil and political rights, is much older than human
rights medicine. And if vigor is assessed in the typical academic style—
by length of bibliography—human rights law is also the more robust
field. That legal documents and scholarship dominate the human rights
literature is not surprising, note Henry Steiner and Philip Alston, given
that the human rights movement has "struggled to assume so lawlike a
character."[16]

But even in legal terms, the international human rights movement is
essentially a modern phenomenon, beginning, some argue, with the
Nuremberg trials.[17] It is this movement that has led, most recently, to
the creation of international tribunals to judge war crimes in the Balkans
and in Rwanda.[18] Some fifty years after the Universal Declaration of
Human Rights, and fifty years after the four Geneva Conventions, what
do we have to show for these efforts? Do we have some sense of outcomes? When Aryeh Neier, former executive director of Human Rights
Watch, reviewed the history of various treaties and covenants from
Nuremberg to the Convention Against Torture and Other Cruel, Inhuman or Degrading Treatment or Punishment, he concluded, "Nations
have honored these obligations largely in the breach."[19]

Although few could argue against Neier's dour assessment, the past few years have been marked by a certain amount of human rights triumphalism. The fiftieth anniversary of the Universal Declaration has led to many celebrations but to few careful assessments of current realities. For some, including many in the liberation theology movement, human rights discourse is at times so divorced from reality that an "alternative language" is necessary if we are to speak of the "rights of the poor," as Gustavo Gutiérrez puts it. The basic problem, in his view, is that "liberal doctrines" about human rights presuppose "that our society enjoys an equality that in fact does not exist."[20] Jon Sobrino agrees that this lack of connection to reality is one of the reasons that liberal human rights discourses are sometimes regarded with suspicion by advocates of the poor:

> A major characterization of our era is the formulation and doctrine of human rights. And it is of no small merit for our age to have succeeded in conceptualizing and universalizing such rights—to have come to be able to speak of the right to life, to liberty, to dignity, and to so many other blessings accompanying these. But this accomplishment does not yet bring us down to basics. Reality is, after all, antecedent to doctrine, and to the philosophical or theological founding of doctrine. The concrete is antecedent to the universal.[21]

Even those within the legal community acknowledge that it would be difficult to correlate a steep rise in the publication of human rights documents with a statistically significant drop in the number of human rights abuses. Rosalyn Higgins says pointedly:

> No one doubts that there exists a norm prohibiting torture. No state denies the existence of such a norm; and, indeed, it is widely recognized as a customary rule of international law by national courts. But it is equally clear from, for example, the reports of Amnesty International, that the *great majority* of states systematically engage in torture. If one takes the view that noncompliance is relevant to the retention of normative quality, are we to conclude that there is not really any prohibition of torture under customary international law?[22]

Whether these laws are binding or largely hortatory constitutes a substantial debate in the legal literature, but such debates seem academic in the face of overwhelming evidence of persistent abuses.

When we expand the concept of rights to include social and economic rights, the gap between ideal and reality is even wider. Local and global inequalities mean that the fruits of medical and scientific advances are stockpiled for some and denied to others. The dimensions of this inequality are staggering, and the trends are bad. To cite just a few examples: By 1995, the total wealth of the top 358 "global billionaires" equaled the combined income of the world's 2.3 billion poorest people.[23] In 1998, Michael Jordan earned from Nike the equivalent of 60,000 years' salary for an Indonesian footwear assembly worker. Haitian factory workers, most of them women, make 28 cents per hour sewing Pocahontas pajamas, while Disney's U.S.-based chief executive officer makes $97,000 for each hour he toils.[24]

Although the pathogenic effects of such inequality per se are now recognized,[25] many governments, including that of the United States, do little to redress inequalities in health, while others are largely powerless to address such inequity.[26] The reasons for failure are many and varied, but even optimists allow that human rights charters and covenants have not brought an end to—and may not even have slowed—egregious abuses, however they are defined. States large and small—but especially large ones, since their reach is transnational—violate civil, economic, and social rights; and inequality both prompts and covers these violations.

There are, of course, exceptions; victories have been declared. But not many of them are very encouraging on close scrutiny. Haiti, the case I know best, offers a humbling example. In that country, the struggle for social and economic rights—food, medical care, education, housing, decent jobs—has been dealt crippling blows. Such basic entitlements, the centerpiece of the popular movement that in 1990 brought the country's first democratically elected president to power, were buried under an avalanche of human rights violations after the military coup of 1991. And although human rights groups were among those credited with helping to restore constitutional rule in Haiti, this was accomplished, to a large extent, by sacrificing the struggle for social and economic rights.[27] In recent years, it has sometimes seemed as if the movement to bring to justice those responsible for the murder and mayhem that have made Haiti such a difficult place to live has simply run out of steam. Despite a few notable exceptions—such as the sentencing of military officials responsible for the 1994 civilian massacre at Raboteau—both the legal and socioeconomic campaigns are slowed almost to a standstill.[28] Although wildly discrepant theories are advanced to explain how this struggle has been stymied, it is important to underscore the ongoing sabotage by the most powerful. Most of the most powerful, as noted in Chapter 2, are not to be found within the borders of Haiti.

Or take Argentina, a far less dependent and immiserated country by all accounts. The gruesome details of the "dirty war" are familiar to many.[29] Seeking what Neier has chillingly termed "a better mousetrap of repression," the Argentine military government began "disappearing" (as Latin Americans said in the special syntax crafted for the occasion) people it identified as leftists.[30] Many people know, now, about the death flights that took place every Wednesday for two years. Thousands of citizens the government deemed subversive, many of them students and most of them having barely survived torture, were flown from a military installation out over the Atlantic, stripped, and shoved out of the plane. A better mousetrap, indeed.

What happened next in Argentina is well documented, although it is a classic instance of the half-empty, half-full glass. Those who say the glass is half-full note that an elected civilian government subsequently tried and convicted high-ranking military figures, including the generals who shared, in the fashion of runners in a relay, the presidential office. Those who say the glass is half-empty note that the prompt pardoning and release of the criminals meant that, once again, no one has been held accountable for thousands of murders.[31] Similar stories abound in Guatemala, El Salvador, the state of Chiapas in Mexico, and elsewhere in Latin America, as I have tried to show in these pages.[32]

These painful experiences are, of course, no reason to declare legal proceedings ineffective. On the contrary, they remind us that some of what was previously hidden away is now out in the open. Disclosure is often the first step in the struggle against impunity, and human rights organizations—almost all of them nongovernmental—have at times forced unwilling governments to acknowledge what really happened. These efforts should serve as a rallying cry for those who now look to constitute international criminal tribunals.

Still, the results to date suggest that we would be unwise to place all our hopes on an approach that emphasizes legal battles. Complementary strategies and new openings are critically needed. The health and human rights "angle" can provide new opportunities and new strategies at the same time that it lends strength and purpose to a movement sorely in need of buttressing. Pragmatic solidarity with those who seem to have suffered human rights abuses—or with those most likely to suffer—is one such strategy, as discussed later in this chapter.

Can One Merely Study Human Rights Abuses?

A few years ago, the French sociologist Pierre Bourdieu and his colleagues pulled together a compendium of testimonies from those the French term "the excluded" in order to bring into relief *la misère du monde*. Bourdieu and colleagues qualify their claims for the role of scholarship in addressing this misery: "To subject to scrutiny the mechanisms which render life painful, even untenable, is not to neutralize them; to bring to light contradictions is not to resolve them."[33] It is precisely such humility that is needed, and rarely exhibited, in academic commentary on human rights. This lack of humility is even more glaringly absent within officialdom, including its human rights appendages. Indeed, Michael Ignatieff has underlined, in *Human Rights as Politics and Idolatry*, both the lack of humility and the hypocrisy that far too often pervade the statements and actions of a "human rights community" tied closely to power:

> As the West intervenes ever more frequently but ever more inconsistently in the affairs of other societies, the legitimacy of its rights standards is put into question. Human rights is increasingly seen as the language of a moral imperialism just as ruthless and just as self-deceived as the colonial hubris of yesteryear....
>
> From being the insurgent creed of activists during the Cold War, human rights has become "mainstreamed" into the policy framework of states, multilateral lending institutions like the World Bank, and the United Nations itself. The foreign policy rhetoric of most Western liberal states now repeats the mantra that national interests must be balanced by due respect for values, chief of which is human rights. But human rights is not just an additional item in the policy priorities of states. If taken seriously, human rights values put interests into question, interests such as sustaining a large export sector in a nation's defense industry, for example. It becomes incoherent for states like Britain and the United States to condemn Indonesia or Turkey for their human rights performance while providing their military with vehicles or weapons that can be used for the repression of civilian dissent. When values do not actually constrain interests, an "ethical foreign policy"—the self-proclaimed goal of Britain's Labour government—becomes a contradiction in terms.[34]

Exposing such constrictions calls for critical scholarship. Yet it is difficult merely to study human rights abuses. We know with certainty that rights are being abused at this moment. That we can study, rather than endure, these abuses is a reminder that we too are implicated in and benefit from the increasingly global structures that determine, to an important extent, the nature and distribution of assaults on dignity.

Ivory-tower engagement with health and human rights can reduce us to seminar-room warriors. At worst, we stand revealed as the hypocrites that our critics in many parts of the world have not hesitated to call us. Anthropologists have long been familiar with these critiques; specialists in international health, including AIDS researchers, have recently had a crash course.[35] It is possible, usually, to drown out the voices of those demanding that we stop studying them, even when they go to great lengths to make sure we get the message. But social scientists with more acute hearing have documented a rich trove of graffiti, songs, demonstrations, tracts, and broadsides on the subject. A hit record album in Haiti called *International Organizations* has a title cut that includes the following lines: "International organizations are not on our side. They're there to help the thieves rob and devour.... International health stays on the sidelines of our struggle."[36]

In the context of longstanding international support for sundry Haitian dictatorships, one could readily see the gripe with international organizations in general. But *international health?* The international community's extraordinary largesse to the Duvalier regime has certainly been well documented.[37] Subsequent patterns of giving, addressed as they were to the various Duvalierist military juntas, did nothing to improve the reputation of U.S. foreign aid or the international organizations; such "aid" helped to arm murderous bands and line the pockets of their leaders. Haitians saw international health "aid" either as originating from within institutions such as the U.S. Agency for International Development (USAID) or as part of the same bureaucracy that shored up dictators. Now that there is at long last a democratically elected government, however, the U.S. government has decided to pass its aid (and influence) through nongovernmental channels. The Bush administration has exercised its authority to veto already approved aid loans from the Inter-American Development Bank. Although few outside Haiti seem to be paying attention—notably, human rights organizations have had nothing to say about the hypocrisy and disregard for rights apparent in such decisions—there is widespread awareness within Haiti of what it means to be so generous to dictators and military juntas and to subsequently block a series of loans for clean water, education, and health care. Such critiques are not specific to Haiti, although Haitians have pronounced them with exceptional frankness and richness of detail. Their accusations have been echoed and amplified throughout what some are beginning to call the global geoculture.[38] A full decade before the recent debates over AIDS research in poor countries, it was possible to collect a bookful of such commentary.[39]

It is in this context of globalization, growing inequality, and pervasive transnational media influence (which both exposes and exacerbates such inequality) that the new field of health and human rights emerges. Context is particularly salient when we think about social and economic rights, as Steiner and Alston point out: "An examination of the concept of the right to development and its implications in the 1990s cannot avoid consideration of the effects of the globalization of the economy and the consequences of the near-universal embrace of the market economy."[40] This context defines our research agenda and directs our praxis. We are leaving behind the terra firma of double-blinded, placebo-controlled studies, of cost-effectiveness, and of sustainability. Indeed, many of these concepts end up looking more like strategies for managing, rather than challenging, inequality.

What, then, should be the role of the First World university, of researchers and health care professionals? What should be the role of students and others lucky enough to be among the "winners" in the global era? We can agree, perhaps, that these centers are fine places from which to conduct research, to document, and to teach. A university does not have the same entanglements or constraints as an international institution such as the United Nations or an organization such as Amnesty International or Physicians for Human Rights. Universities could, in theory, provide a unique and privileged space for conducting research and engaging in critical assessment.

In human rights work, however, research and critical assessment are insufficient. No more adequate, for all their virtues, are denunciation and exhortation, whether in the form of press conferences or reports or harangues directed at students. To confront, as an observer, ongoing abuses of human rights is to be faced with a moral dilemma: does one's action help the sufferers or does it not? As Chapter 8 argued, the increasingly baroque codes of research ethics generated by institutional review boards will not help us out of this dilemma, nor will medical ethics, so often restricted to the quandary ethics of the individual. But certain models of engagement are relevant. If the university-based human rights worker is in a peculiar position, it is not entirely unlike that of the clinician researcher. Both study suffering; both are bound to relieve it; neither is in possession of a tried-and-true remedy. Both the human rights specialist and the clinician researcher have blind spots, too.

To push the analogy further, one could argue that both lines of work carry obligations regarding the standard of care. What if we are in possession of tried-and-true remedies? Returning again to the treatment of AIDS and drug-resistant tuberculosis, we already have a great deal of knowledge regarding how best to manage both diseases. Once a reasonably effective intervention has been identified, it—and not a placebo—is considered the standard against which a new remedy must be tested. In the global era, is it wise to set, as *policy goals,* double standards for the rich world and the poor world, when we know that these are not different worlds but in fact the same one? Are the acrid complaints of the vulnerable necessary to remind us that they invariably see the world as one world, riven by terrible inequality and injustice? A placebo is a placebo is a placebo.

As an even sterner rebuke to the self-described pragmatism of those pushing for relaxed ethical practices in settings of great poverty, we once again hear the voice from liberation theology. This voice does not call for equally good treatment of the poor; it demands *preferential treatment* for the poor. And to look at many of its central documents, one would swear that the human rights movement was once headed in the same direction: fighting to protect the rights of the vulnerable, over and above the rights of the powerful. Of course, pushing for higher standards for the victims is always a utopian enterprise. Many factors might limit feasibility, but that didn't stop the authors of the Universal Declaration from setting high goals. That we have failed to meet them does not imply that the next step is to lower our sights, although this has been the default logic in many instances. Rather, the next step is to try new approaches and to hedge our bets with indisputably effective interventions.

How do we best hedge our bets? As I've argued throughout this book, providing pragmatic services to the afflicted is one obvious form of intervention. In other words, we cannot exclude social and economic rights from the campaign for health and human rights. But the spirit in which these services are delivered makes all the difference. Service delivery can be just that—or it can be pragmatic solidarity, linked to the broader goals of equality and justice for the poor. Again, my own experience in Haiti, which began in 1983, made this clear. The Duvalier dictatorship was then in power, seemingly immovable. Its chief source of external financial aid was the United States and various international institutions, many of them ostensibly charitable in nature. The local director of the USAID at the time had often expressed the view that if Haiti was underdeveloped, one could find the causes in Haitian culture.[41] The World Bank and the International Monetary Fund seemed to be part of the same giant blur of international aid organizations that Haitians associated, accurately enough, with U.S. foreign policy.

Popular cynicism regarding these transnational institutions was at its peak when my colleagues and I began working in Haiti, and that is why we chose to work through nascent community-based organizations and for a group of rural peasants who had been dispossessed of their land by a hydroelectric dam. Although we conducted research and published it, research did not figure on the wish list of the people we were trying to serve. Services were what they asked for, and as people who had been displaced by political and economic violence, they regarded these services as a rightful remedy for what they had suffered. In other words, the Haitian poor themselves believed that social and economic rights were central to the struggle for human rights. As the struggle against the dictatorship gathered strength in the mid-1980s, the language was explicitly couched in broad human rights terms. *Pa gen lapè nan tèt si pa gen lapè nan vant* (there can be no peace of mind if there is no peace in the belly). Health and education figured high on the list of demands as the Haitian popular movement began to swell.

The same has been true of the struggle in Chiapas. The Zapatista rebellion was launched on the day the North American Free Trade Agreement was signed, and the initial statement of the rebellion's leaders put their demands in terms of social and economic rights:

> We have been denied the most elemental education so that others can use us as cannon fodder and pillage the wealth of our country. They don't care that we have nothing, absolutely nothing, not even a roof over our heads, no land, no work, no health care, no food, and no education. Nor are we able freely and democratically to elect our political representatives, nor is there independence from foreigners, nor is there peace or justice for ourselves and our children.[42]

In settings such as these, we are afforded a rare clarity about choices that are in fact choices for all of us, everywhere. There's little doubt that discernment is a daily struggle. We must decide how health professionals (from providers to researchers) might best make common cause with the destitute sick, whose rights are violated daily. Helping governments shore up failing public health systems may or may not be wise. Pragmatic solidarity on behalf of Russian prisoners with tuberculosis, for example, includes working with their jailers. But sometimes we are warned against consorting with governments. In Haiti in the 1980s, it made all the difference that we formed our own nongovernmental organization far from the reach of the governments of both Haiti and the United States. In 1991, after Haiti's first-ever democratic elections brought to power the leader of the country's popular movement, we immediately began to work with the Ministry of Health. But seven months later, a military coup brought an abrupt end to that collaboration, a divorce that was to last for three long years. In Chiapas, the situation was even more dramatic. As recounted in Chapter 3, many poor communities simply refuse to use government health services. In village after village, we heard the same story. In some "autonomous zones," the Mexican army has entered these villages and destroyed local health records and what meager independent infrastructure had been developed.[43] To quote one health worker: "The government uses health services against us. They persecute us if they think we are on the side of the rebels." Our own investigations have been amply confirmed by others, including Physicians for Human Rights:

> At best, [Mexican] Government health and other services are subordinate to Government counterinsurgency efforts. At worst, these services are themselves components of repression, manipulated to reward supporters and to penalize and demoralize dissenters. In either case, Government health services in the zone are discriminatory, exacerbate political divisions, and fail utterly to address the real health needs of the population.[44]

It's not acceptable for those of us fortunate enough to have ties to universities and other "resource-rich" institutions to throw up our hands and bemoan the place-to-place complexity. Underlying this complexity is a series of very simple first principles regarding human rights, as the liberation theologians remind us. Our commitments, our loyalties, must be *primarily* to the poor and vulnerable. As a reminder of how unique this commitment is, remember that the international agencies affiliated with the United Nations, including the World Health Organization, are called to work with governments. Think, once again, of Chiapas. An individual member of any one of these international institutions may have loyalties to the Zapatistas, but no choice in his or her agency's primary interlocutor: this will be the Mexican government. That membership in a university (or hospital or local church) permits us more flexibility in making allegiances is a gift that we should not squander by mindlessly mimicking the choices of the parastatal international organizations. Close allegiance with suffering communities reminds us that it is not possible to merely study human rights abuses. But part of pragmatic solidarity is bringing to light the real story.

What Is the Difference, in Human Rights Work, between Analysis and Strategy?

If we accept the need to think both theoretically and instrumentally, we find there is a difference, in human rights work, between analysis and strategy. Failure to recognize this difference has often hobbled interventions designed to prevent or allay human rights violations. In this arena, analysis means bringing out the truth, no matter how clumsy or embarrassing or inexpedient. It means documenting, as Neier recently put it, "Who did what to whom, and when?"[45] Strategy asks a different question: What is to be done?

What is to be done? It's the oldest question around. Sometimes it's posed in a way calculated to discourage discussion, the subtext being that misery and unfairness are so ubiquitous that only hopeless romantics would discern opportunities for effective intervention. But even more often the question is asked by people of good will. I know, for example, that students often seek opportunities to play a part in diminishing structural violence or its symptoms. Too often, their contributions are diluted when they become ensnarled in institutions—foundations, aid agencies, government-affiliated groups, universities, political parties, even organized labor—that put sharp limits on activism. On the other side of the ledger are the purists, who recognize the fundamentally conservative nature of such institutions and see themselves as too good, really, to rub shoulders with those who are engaged in providing services.

How can we build an agenda for action that moves beyond good analysis? If solidarity is among the most noble of human sentiments, then surely its more tangible forms are better still. Adding the material dimension to the equation—pragmatic solidarity—responds to the needs expressed by the people and communities who are living, and often dying, on the edge. When we move beyond sentiments to action, we of course incur risks, and these deter many. But it is possible, clearly, to link lofty ideals to sound analysis.

This linkage does not always occur in human rights work, in part because of a reluctance to examine the political economy of suffering and brutality.

For example, high-minded charters are utopian strategies that may become laws to be flouted or obeyed; they are not analysis. The notion that everyone shares the risk of having his or her rights violated is reminiscent of catchy public health slogans such as "AIDS is for everyone." These slogans may be useful for social marketing, but they are redolent of the most soft-headed thinking. The distribution of AIDS is strikingly localized and nonrandom; so is that of human rights abuses. Both HIV transmission and human rights abuses are social processes and are embedded, most often, in the inegalitarian social structures I have called structural violence. Whether one examines these steep grades of inequality as an epidemiologist or as a social scientist, one comes to discern the context of risk by restoring the history and political economy of these precarious situations. There is considerable overlap between "groups at risk": if you are likely to be tortured or otherwise abused, you are also likely to be in the AIDS risk group composed of the poor and the defenseless.

Human rights can and should be declared universal, but the risk of having one's rights violated is not universal. Moreover, not every offense should be automatically classified as a human rights violation. Sticks and stones, we know, may break bones; and although it is not entirely true that "names will never hurt me," it is often unwise to take verbal violations as seriously as bodily ones.

Identity politics in the United States have indeed sought to extend the reach of rights language. But identity politics have remained parochial and national (indeed subnational) in this global era, and in a nation as affluent as our own, turning a human rights struggle into a bitter competition for a bigger slice of the pie results in the erasure of many linked to our affluence. It makes sense to distinguish between a struggle for access to power—breaking the gendered "glass ceiling" of transnational corporations, say—and a struggle for access to a basic good such as primary health care, especially if the same corporations that reluctantly open their boardrooms to a few women and minorities are involved in causing the deepening inequality between rich and poor. Should the frenzied quest for access to power and wealth be regarded as serving a social good simply because those who were historically underrepresented in the past are now filling roles that involve replicating inequality?

At the other end of the scale, moral relativism is similarly pernicious. Not all forms of suffering are equivalent. The public health and medical communities are accustomed to triage, to assessment of gravity, followed by action to address the problem at hand. It makes sense, in my view, to distinguish between the harm done by six lashes for vandalism—a tremendous cause célèbre when meted out to a U.S. citizen abroad, to judge by inches of newspaper copy—and the harm done to millions by a lifetime of institutionalized racism.[46] To make distinctions between committing genocide and censoring intellectuals is not to declare the latter trivial. But our job of telling the truth as best we can compels us to weight those wrongs differently.

The risk of stretching the concept of rights to cover every possible case is that obscene inequalities of risk will be drowned in a rising tide of petty complaint.[47] Only careful comparative analysis gives us a sense of scale; only careful analysis brings causal mechanisms into the light. We have seen brisk debate about a hierarchy of human rights abuses and about whether it makes sense to consider some rights "fundamental." The struggle for recognition of social and economic rights has engendered even more acrimony.[48] But this debate has been legal in nature—centered in and destined toward law, where it is customary to speak of inalienable rights and to wait decades or centuries to see them vindicated.

Merely telling the truth, of course, often calls for exhaustive research. In the current era, human rights violations are usually both local and global. Telling who did what to whom and when becomes a complicated affair. Take the case of Chouchou Louis, the young man tortured to death in Haiti in early 1992. I told his story in more detail in Chapter 1; here I will merely state that I was called to see him after he was cast out of police headquarters to die in the dirt. He did just that. I was too late, too unequipped, medically, to save his life. Documenting what had happened to him was the least I could do.

Was I to document only the "distal" events? Although all present were terrified, it was possible—in fact, quite easy—to obtain the names of those who had arrested and tortured Chouchou Louis. But the chain of complicity, I learned, kept reaching higher. At the time, U.S. officialdom's explanation of human rights abuses in Haiti, including the torture and murder of people like Chouchou Louis, focused almost exclusively on local actors and local factors. One heard of the "culture of violence" that rendered this and other similarly grisly deaths comprehensible. Such official analyses, constructed by conflating structural violence and cultural difference, were distancing tactics.

Innumerable immodest claims of causality—such as attributing a sudden upsurge in persons tortured while in police custody to longstanding local custom—play into the convenient alibi that refuses to follow the chain of events to their source, that keeps all the trouble local. Such alibis obscure the fact that the modern Haitian military was created by an act of the U.S. Congress during the twenty-year U.S. occupation of Haiti, from 1915 to 1934. Most official analyses around the time of Chouchou's death did not discuss generous U.S. assistance to the post-Duvalier military: more than $200 million in aid passed through the hands of the Haitian military in the eighteen months after Jean-Claude Duvalier left Haiti on a U.S. cargo plane in 1986. Bush administration statements, and their faithful echoes in the establishment press, failed to mention that many of the commanders who issued the orders to detain and torture civilians were trained by the U.S. military in Fort Benning, Georgia.[49] At this writing, human rights groups in the United States and Haiti have filed suit against the U.S. government in order to force the return of more than one hundred thousand pages of documents (taken away during the U.S. invasion of Haiti in the fall of 1994) revealing links between Washington and the paramilitary groups that held sway in Haiti between 1991 and 1994.[50]

Elsewhere, too the mechanisms of human rights violations have been masked. In El Salvador, the massacres of entire villages could not in good conscience be considered unrelated to U.S. foreign policy, since the U.S. government was the primary funder, adviser, and supporter of the Salvadoran government's war against its own people. Yet officialdom maintained precisely that fiction of deniability, even though the United States was also the primary purveyor of armaments, as physical evidence later showed.[51] It was years before we could read accounts such as that by Mark Danner, who, on investigating the slaughter of every man, woman, and child in one village, concluded: "Of the two hundred and forty-five cartridge cases that were studied—all but one from American M16 rifles—'184 had discernable headstamps, identifying the ammunition as having been manufactured for the United States Government at Lake City, Missouri.' "[52] The fiction of local struggles ("ethnic," "religious," "historical," or otherwise picturesque) is exploded by any honest attempt to understand. As Chapter 3 makes clear, paramilitary groups linked tightly with the Mexican government were and are responsible for the bulk of intimidation and violence in the villages of Chiapas.[53] But federal authorities have insisted that such violence results from "local intercommunity and interparty tension" or ethnic rivalries.[54]

Similarly inaccurate were claims that the U.S. military base on Guantánamo had become "an oasis" for Haitian refugees in the early 1990s and that Cuba's AIDS sanatoriums were "prison camps." Immodest claims of causality are not always so flagrantly self-serving as those proffered to explain Haiti's agony, the violence in El Salvador or Chiapas, or the contrasting AIDS dramas on the island of Cuba. But only careful analysis allows us to rebut them with any confidence. We cannot *merely* study human rights abuses, but we must not fail to study them.

What Can a Focus on Health Bring to the Struggle for Human Rights?

Medicine and public health, and also the social sciences relevant to these disciplines, have much to contribute to the great, often rancorous debates on human rights. But what might be our greatest contribution?

Rudolph Virchow saw doctors as "the natural attorneys of the poor."[55] A "health angle" can promote a broader human rights agenda in unique ways. In fact, the health part of the formula may prove critical to the success of the human rights movement. The esteem in which public health and medicine are held affords us openings—again, a space of privilege—enjoyed by few other professions. For example, it is unlikely that my colleagues and I would have been welcomed so warmly into Russian prisons if we had presented ourselves as social scientists or human rights investigators. We went, instead, as TB specialists, with the expectation that a visiting group of doctors might be able to do more for the rights of these prisoners than a delegation from a conventional human rights organization. It is important to get the story straight: the leading cause of death among young Russian detainees is tuberculosis, not torture or starvation. Prison officials were opening their facilities to us and asking for pragmatic solidarity. (In Haiti and Chiapas, by contrast, we were asked to leave when we openly espoused the cause of the oppressed.)

Medicine and public health benefit from an extraordinary symbolic capital that is, so far, sadly underutilized in human rights work. No one made this point more clearly and persistently than the late Jonathan Mann. In an essay written with Daniel Tarantola, Mann noted that AIDS "has helped catalyze the modern health and human rights movement, which leads far beyond AIDS, for it considers that promoting and protecting health and promoting and protecting human rights are inextricably connected."[56]

But have we gone far beyond AIDS? Is it not a human rights issue that Russian prisoners are exposed, often during illegally prolonged pre-trial detention, to epidemic MDRTB and then denied effective treatment? Is it not a human rights issue that international expert opinion has mistakenly informed Russian prison officials that treatment with second-line drugs is not cost-effective or is just plain unnecessary? Is it not a human rights issue that in relatively wealthy South Africa (where a glossy program reminded participants in the thirteenth annual AIDS meetings that "medical care is readily available in South Africa") the antiretroviral therapy that could prolong millions of (black) lives is declared "cost-ineffective"? Is it not a human rights issue that villagers in Chiapas lack access to the most basic medical services, even as government medical facilities stand idly by? Is it not a human rights issue that thousands of Haitian peasants displaced by a hydroelectric dam end up sick with HIV disease after working as servants in Port-au-Prince?

Standing on the shoulders of giants—from the authors of the Universal Declaration to Jonathan Mann—we can recognize the human rights abuses in each of these situations, including epidemic tuberculosis within prisons. But what, precisely, is to be done? Russian penal codes already prohibit overcrowding, long pre-trial detention, and undue risk from malnutrition and communicable disease. Prison officials already regard the tuberculosis problem as a top priority; that's why they let TB specialists in. In a 1998 interview, as noted, one high-ranking prison official told me that the ministry saw their chief problems as lack of resources, overcrowding, and tuberculosis.[57] And the pièce de résistance might be that Boris Yeltsin had already declared 1998 "the year of human rights."

Passing more human rights legislation is not a sufficient response to these human rights challenges, because those in charge already disregard many of those (clearly nonbinding) instruments. The Haitian military coup leaders were beyond the pale. But how about Chiapas? Instruments to which Mexico is already signatory include the Geneva Conventions of 1949; the International Covenant on Civil and Political Rights; the International Covenant on Economic, Social and Cultural Rights; the International Labor Organization Convention 169; the American Convention on Human Rights; the Maastricht Guidelines on Violations of Economic, Social and Cultural Rights; and the Convention on the Elimination of All Forms of Discrimination Against Women. Each one of these is flouted every day in Chiapas.

As the Haitians say, "Laws are made of paper; bayonets are made of steel." Law alone is not up to the task of relieving such immense suffering. Louis Henkin has reminded us that international law is fundamentally a set of rules and norms designed to protect the interests of states, not their citizens. "Until recently," he observed in 1989, "international law took no note of individual human beings."[58] And states, as we have seen, honor human rights law largely in the breach—sometimes intentionally and sometimes through sheer impotence. This chief irony of human rights work—that states will not or cannot obey the treaties they sign—can lead to despair or to cynicism, if all of one's eggs are in the international-law basket.

Laws are not science; they are normative ideology and are thus tightly tied to power.[59] Biomedicine and public health, though also vulnerable to being deformed by ideology, serve different imperatives, ask different questions. They do not ask whether an event or a process violates an existing rule; they ask whether that event or process has ill effects on a patient or a population. They ask whether such events can be prevented or remediated. A change of approach in that direction would have, I believe, a salutary effect on many human rights debates. And when medicine and public health are explicitly placed at the service of the poor, it provides even greater insurance against their perversion.

To return to the case of prisoners with MDRTB, the best way to protect their rights is to cure them of their disease. And the best way to protect the rights of other prisoners, and those who take care of them, is to prevent transmission by treating the sick. Thus, after years of hemming and hawing, all parties involved are being forced to admit that the right thing to do in Russia's prisons is also the human rights thing to do. A variety of strategies, from human rights arguments to epidemiologic scare tactics, have been used to make headway in raising the funds necessary to treat these and other prisoners. In the end, then, the health angle on human rights may prove more pragmatic than approaching the problem as one of penal reform alone. Previously closed institutions have opened their doors to international collaboration designed to halt prison epidemics. This approach—pragmatic solidarity—is, in the end, leading to penal reform as well. Similarly pragmatic approaches to addressing treatment and prevention of HIV also promise to reverse the scandalous inequalities of risk and access documented throughout this book.

In 1998, working in central Haiti, Partners In Health launched the "HIV Equity Initiative" in order to complement prevention efforts with antiretroviral treatment for those for whom prevention had failed. The care component includes an uninterrupted supply of antiretroviral agents, but only modest lab infrastructure. Use of these drugs is supervised, preferably by community-based health workers, called *accompagnateurs,* who visit patients each day. Between 10 and 12 percent—too small a proportion—of the more than 2,000 HIV-positive patients followed in the affiliated clinic receive such therapy. A clinical algorithm, described elsewhere, is used to identify those patients in greatest need.[60]

This project has been limited by an inability to find significant donor support for an integrated HIV-prevention-and-care project in a setting as poor as rural Haiti. Though we felt we had no choice but to move forward—years ago, HIV surpassed tuberculosis as the leading infectious cause of adult death in Haiti—we had to rely on private donations, support from patients in the United States, and the largesse of a major donor who has long supported our work in Haiti. In short, we would have much more to report in 2002 if we had been able to find pragmatic solidarity in the donor community. Instead, we encountered the argument that such projects were neither cost-effective nor feasible in a setting of such profound poverty.

As this book goes to press, all this could change: through the newly es-tablished Global Fund to Fight AIDS, Tuberculosis and Malaria, the United Nations has promised Haiti significant funds for HIV prevention and care. As we and other groups based in regions where poverty and HIV are the ranking threats to health contemplate the advent of new resources, we need to ask hard questions of ourselves and also of those who will evaluate their use. In seeking to promote accountability, will we develop yet another set of burdensome reporting requirements that will force us to hire expensive consultants from far beyond the boundaries of afflicted communities? Or will we seek innovative and realistic means of evaluating the impact of long-overdue investments? The point of bringing new funding to allay the suffering caused by AIDS, tuberculosis, and malaria was not merely to mimic existing transnational research projects, already struggling with se-rious ethical dilemmas, but rather to remediate inequalities of access to proven therapies. This goal should be embraced without apologies.

Embracing this goal, and embedding such actions in the rights frame-work, helps us to answer the question, What is the purpose of the research and evaluation that must certainly accompany such disbursements? Not merely to please skeptics, one hopes, since accountability should be to the afflicted rather than to the privileged. The purpose of this research should be to do a better job of bringing the fruits of science and public health to the poorest communities. If the purpose of the new funds is also to help us better promote access to health care as a fundamental human right, we will of course be called to address, in addition to nascent HIV projects, not only tuberculosis and malaria but also eclampsia, cervical cancer, and the long list of maladies transmitted by unsafe drinking water. This will mean making common cause with community health workers and others in the trenches. In the end, the burden of proof should lie on the shoulders of those who argue against making the elimination of inequalities of ac-cess to prevention and care our top priority in international public health.

I will return to the strategy of pragmatic solidarity in proposing a new agenda for health and human rights but will proceed under the as-sumption that any approach to human rights that regards research as an end in itself contains many pitfalls—moral, strategic, and analytic.[61]

A NEW AGENDA FOR HEALTH AND HUMAN RIGHTS

As I've argued thus far, we have a long way to go in the struggle for health and human rights. We cannot merely study this topic without proposing meaningful and pragmatic interventions; but to succeed, we must distinguish between our best analyses and our best strategies. The focus on health offers a critical new dimension to human rights work and is a largely untapped vein of resources, passion, and good will.

Is it grandiose to seek to define a new agenda? When one reads the powerfully worded statutes, conventions, treaties, and charters stemming from international revulsion over the crimes of the Third Reich, it might seem pointless to call for better instruments of this sort. Yet events in the former Yugoslavia and in Rwanda serve as a powerful rebuke to undue confidence in these approaches: "That it should nevertheless be possible for Nazi-like crimes to be repeated half a century later in full view of the whole world," remarks Neier, "points up the weakness of that system— and the need for fresh approaches."[62] Steiner and Alston, similarly, call for "heightened attention to the problems of implementation and enforcement of the new ideal norms. The old techniques," they conclude, "simply won't work."[63]

A corollary question is whether a coherent agenda springs from the critique inherent in the answers to the questions presented here. If so, is this agenda compatible with existing approaches and documents, including the Universal Declaration of Human Rights? To those who believe that social and economic rights must be central to the health and human rights agenda, the answers to these questions are yes. This agenda, inspired by the notion of a preferential option for the poor, is coherent, pragmatic, and informed by careful scholarship. Largely because it focuses on social and economic rights, this agenda, though novel, builds on five decades of work within the traditional human rights framework: Articles 25 and 27 of the Universal Declaration inspire the vision of this emerging agenda, which could rely on tighter links between universities, medical providers, and both nongovernmental and community-based organizations. The truly novel part of these alliances comes in subjugating these networks to the aspirations of oppressed and abused people.

How might we proceed with this effort, if most reviews of the effects of international laws and treaties designed to protect human rights raise serious questions of efficacy (to say the least)? What can we do to advance a new agenda of health and human rights? In concluding, I offer six suggestions, which are intended to complement ongoing efforts.

Make Health and Healing the Symbolic Core of the Agenda

If health and healing are the symbolic core of our new agenda, we tap into something truly universal—concern for the sick—and, at the same time, engage medicine, public health, and the allied health professions, including the basic sciences. Put another way, we need to throw the full weight of the medical and scientific communities behind a noble cause. Physicians and health researchers are not hostile to this cause; quite the contrary. What we lack, with some notable exceptions, are concerted efforts to engage health professionals in human rights work, broadly conceived. One of those notable exceptions is the recent AIDS initiative advanced by Physicians for Human Rights and partner organizations, which argues that access to care should be construed as a basic right.[64] It is tragic, surely, to note that such initiatives remain unusual within the mainstream human rights community.

Although many global health indicators show significant improvement, we still have endless work to do before we can claim to have made the slightest headway in ensuring the highest possible level of health for all. In fact, several studies suggest that inequalities in health outcomes are growing in many places.[65] From the human rights perspective advanced in this book, this growing outcome gap constitutes both a human rights violation and a means of tracking the efficacy of our interventions. That is, reduction of the outcome gap is the goal of our pragmatic solidarity with the destitute sick.

Make Provision of Services Central to the Agenda

We need to listen to the sick and abused and to those most likely to have their rights violated. Whether they are nearby or far away, we know, often enough, who they are. The abused offer, to those willing to listen, critiques far sharper than my own. They are not asking for new centers of study and reflection. They have not commissioned new studies of their suffering. That means we need new programs in addition to the traditional ventures of a university or a research center (the journals, books, articles, courses, conferences, research). Law schools have clinics, and so do medical schools. Programs promoting health and human rights should have not only legal clinics; in addition, a broad range of health professionals should help to establish, in every major medical center, referral clinics for those subjected to torture and other human rights abuses as classically defined.

But a far larger group calls for our pragmatic solidarity. We need programs designed to remediate inequalities of access to services that can help all humans to lead free and healthy lives. If everyone has a right "to share in scientific advancement and its benefits," where are our pragmatic efforts to improve the spread of these advances? Such efforts exist, but, again, the widening outcome gap stands as the sharpest rebuke to the health and human rights community. Even as our biomedical interventions become more effective, our capacity to distribute them equitably is further eroded. The world's poor and otherwise marginalized people currently constitute a vast control group of the untreated, and even cursory examination of the annual tally of victims reminds us that this sector also constitutes the group most likely to have their rights violated.

How can we make the rapid deployment of services to improve health—pragmatic solidarity—central to the work of health and human rights programs? Our own group, Partners In Health, has worked largely with community-based organizations in Haiti and Peru and Mexico whose expressed goal has been to remediate inequalities of access. This community of providers and scholars believes that "the vitality of practice" lends a corrective strength to our research and writing.[66] The possibilities for programmatic collaboration range, we have learned, from Russian prison officials to peasant collectives in the autonomous zones of Chiapas. Novel collaborations of this sort are certainly necessary if we are to address the increasing inequalities of access here in wealthy, inegalitarian countries such as the United States. Relying exclusively on nation-states' compliance with a social justice agenda is naïve at best. At the same time, it is important to respect the sovereignty of states, for experience shows that states, not "Western" human rights groups, are best placed to protect the basic social and economic rights of populations living in poverty. Ignatieff emphasizes precisely this point. "We are rediscovering," he notes, "the necessity of state order as a guarantee of rights. It can be said with certainty that the liberties of citizens are better protected by their own institutions than by the well-meaning interventions of outsiders. . . . State failure cannot be rectified by human rights activism on the part of NGOs."[67] We will not be excused from discernment.

These questions of new collaborations are raised at a time that is filled with contradiction: despite increasing globalization, our action agenda has remained parochial. We lag behind trade and finance, since we are still at the first steps in the press for universal rights while the Masters of the Universe are already "harmonizing" their own standards and practices. Fifteen years of work in the most difficult field conditions have taught our group that it is hard, perhaps impossible, to meet the highest standards of health care in every situation. But it is imperative that we try to do so. Projects striving for excellence and inclusiveness—rather than, say, "cost-effectiveness" or "sustainability," which are often at odds with social justice approaches to medicine and public health—are not merely misguided quests for personal efficacy. Such projects respond to widespread demands for equity in health care. The din around AIDS research in the Third World is merely the latest insistence that we reject low standards as official policy. That such standards are widely seen as violating human rights is no surprise for those interested in social and economic rights. Efficiency cannot trump equity in the field of health and human rights.

Establish New Research Agendas

We need to make room in the academy for serious scholarly work on the multiple dynamics of health and human rights, on the health effects of war and political-economic disruption, and on the pathogenic effects of social inequalities, including racism, gender inequality, and the growing gap between rich and poor. By what mechanisms do such noxious events and processes become embodied as adverse health outcomes? Why are some at risk and others spared?

Here again, we lag far behind. As Nancy Krieger notes, "epidemiologic research explicitly focused on discrimination as a determinant of population health is in its infancy."[68] To answer the questions posed earlier, we require a new level of cooperation between disciplines ranging from social anthropology to molecular epidemiology. We need a new sociology of knowledge that can pick apart a wide body of commentary and scholarship: complex international law; the claims and disclaimers of officialdom; postmodern relativist readings of suffering; clinical and epidemiologic studies of the long-term effects of, say, torture, and racism.[69] But remember that none of the victims of these events or processes are asking us to conduct research. For this reason alone, research in the arena of health and human rights is necessarily fraught with pitfalls:

> Imperiled populations in developing countries include extraordinarily vulnerable individuals ripped from their cultures and communities and victimized by myriad forms of abuse and violence. Public health research on violence and victimization among these groups must vigilantly guard against contributing to emotional and social harm.[70]

That research is and should remain a secondary concern does not mean that careful documentation is not critical to both our understanding of suffering and our ability to prevent or allay it. And because of its link to service, we need operational research by which we can gauge the efficacy of interventions that are quite different from those measured in the past.

Assume a Broader Educational Mandate

Human rights work usually has a suasive component. If the primary objective is to set things right, education is central to our task. But the educational mandate should not make two conventional mistakes: we must not limit ourselves to teaching only a select group of students who have an avowed interest in health and human rights, nor should we focus on trying to teach lessons to recalcitrant governments and international financial institutions. Jonathan Mann signaled the limitations of the latter approach: "Support for human rights-based action to promote health... at the level of declarations and speeches is welcome, and useful in some ways, but the limits of official organizational support for the call for societal transformation inherent in human rights promotion must be recognized."[71] A broader educational mandate would mean engaging students from all faculties—but also engaging the members of these faculties. Beyond the university and various governmental bodies lies the broader public within affluent societies, for whom the connections between health and human rights have not even been traced. It is doubtful that the destitute sick have much to learn from us about health and human rights, but there is little doubt that, as their students, we can learn to better convey the complexity and historicity of their messages.

Achieve Independence from Powerful
Governments and Bureaucracies

We need to be untrammeled by obligations to powerful states and international bureaucracies. A central irony of human rights law is that it consists largely of appeals to the perpetrators. After all, most crimes against humanity are committed by powerful states, not by rogue factions or gangs or cults or terrorists. That makes it difficult for institutions accountable to states to take their constituents to task. When in 1994 the United Nations created the post of High Commissioner for Human Rights, the $700,000 annual budget was paltry even by the standards of a nongovernmental organization. The results were predictable: "With denunciation of those responsible for abuses the only means available for carrying out his mission," the first commissioner "managed to go through his first year in his post without publicly criticizing a single government anywhere in the world."[72] It is not merely a problem of budgetary constraints. Many of the chief donor nations are themselves major violators of one or another of the international covenants discussed here. The United States and China are the world leaders in capital punishment, and the United States is implacably opposed, it would seem, to the creation of the International Criminal Court. The United States, Great Britain, and France are all major manufacturers of the weapons used to commit human rights abuses. And what about Mexico, partner with Canada and the United States in the world's largest "free trade" agreement? In Chiapas, numerous observers have documented the displacement and massacre of presumed Zapatista supporters by paramilitary groups tightly tied to the government: "State and federal authorities have permitted these groups to act with impunity, and state Public Security Police have not only failed to protect victims, but have sometimes participated in the evictions."[73]

None of this is to say that international organizations have little to offer to those seeking to prevent or assuage human rights abuses. It is rather to remind us that their supposed "neutrality" comes at a great cost, and that cost is usually paid by people who are not represented by ambassadors in places like New York, Paris, Geneva, Washington, London, or Tokyo. Along with nongovernmental organizations, university- and hospital-based programs have the potential to be independent, well-designed, pragmatic, and feasible. The imprimatur of medicine and public health would afford even more weight and independence. And only a failure of imagination has led us to ignore the potential of collaboration with community-based organizations and with communities in resistance to ongoing violations of human rights.

Secure More Resources for Health and Human Rights

In our own era, "growth is wildly uneven, inequality is immense, anxiety is endemic," says Todd Gitlin. "The state, as a result, is continually urged to do more but deprived of the means to do so."[74] The halting but ineluctable spread of the global economy is linked to an evolving human rights irony: states become less able to help their citizens attain social and economic rights, even though they often retain their ability to violate human rights. Even where reforms have led to the enjoyment of basic political rights, the implementation of neoliberal economic policies can erode the right to freedom from want. This is particularly true of many developing countries, as Steiner and Alston note:

Civil and political rights have been greatly strengthened in many countries. Nonetheless, related contemporary phenomena—including privatization, deregulation, the expanded provision of incentives to entrepreneurial behavior, and structural adjustment programs and related pressures from international financial institutions and developed countries—have had mixed, and sometimes seriously adverse, effects on the enjoyment of economic and social rights.[75]

Of course, it's easy to demand more resources; what's hard is to produce them. But if social and economic rights are acknowledged as such, then foundations, governments, businesses, and international financial institutions—many of them now awash in resources—may be called on to prioritize human rights endeavors that reflect the paradigm shift advocated here.

Regardless of where one stands on the process of globalization and its multiple engines, these processes have important implications for efforts to promote health and human rights. As states weaken, it's easy to discern an increasing role for nongovernmental institutions, including universities and medical centers. But it's also easy to discern a trap: *the withdrawal of states from the basic business of providing housing, education, and medical services usually means further erosion of the social and economic rights of the poor.* Our independent involvement must be quite different from current trends, which have nongovernmental organizations relieving the state of its duty to provide basic services. We must avoid becoming witting or unwitting abettors of neoliberal policies that declare every service and every thing to be for sale.

How will we live up to the challenge to promote the highest possible level of health for all? Universities and medical centers, I have argued, should conduct research, but the subject—health and human rights— demands complementary services. These services need to be provided urgently but must also be tied tightly to demands for social and economic rights for the poor. Linking research to service—and to social justice— costs money. An ambitious plan to redress injustice is what we need. "We could do more than we do," argues Ignatieff, "to stop unmerited suffering and gross physical cruelty. That I take to be the elemental priority of all human rights activism: to stop torture, beatings, killings, rape, and assault and to improve, as best we can, the security of ordinary people."[76] "Unmerited suffering" is what we encounter each day in clinics in Haiti, Chiapas, Siberia, the slums of Peru. This suffering can be prevented or, at the very least, alleviated. But if we lack ambition, we should expect the next fifty years to yield a harvest of shame.

The experience of Partners In Health suggests that ambitious goals can be met even without a large springboard. Over the past decade and against a steady current of nay-saying, we have channeled significant resources to the destitute sick in Haiti, Peru, Mexico, and Boston. We didn't argue that it was "cost-effective," nor did we promise that such efforts would be replicable. We argued that it was the right thing to do. It was also the human rights thing to do.

Some of the problems born of structural violence are so large that they have paralyzed many who want to do the right thing. But we can find more resources, and we can find them without sacrificing our independence and discernment. We will not do this by adopting defensive postures that are tantamount to simply managing inequality with the latest tools from economists and technocrats. Utopian ideals are the bedrock of human rights. By arguing that we must set standards high, we must also argue for redistribution of some of the world's vast wealth.

Claims that we live in an era of limited resources fail to mention that these resources happen to be less limited now than ever before in human history. Arguing that it is too expensive to treat MDRTB among prisoners in Russia, say, sounds nothing short of ludicrous when this world contains individuals worth more than $100 billion.[77] Arguments against treating HIV disease in precisely those areas in which it exacts its greatest toll warn us that misguided notions of cost-effectiveness have already trumped equity. Arguing that nominal civil and political rights are the best we can hope for means that members of the healing professions will have their hands tied, forced to stand by as the rights and dignity of the poor and marginalized undergo further sustained and deadly assault in what is essentially an undeclared war on the poor. Because it is undeclared, we need to declare against whom, for whose benefit, and how it is being waged. Naturally, prosecuting such a stealthy war requires a considerable investment in propaganda and "psy ops." Passivity and shortsightedness are invaluable to those who would keep the war undeclared. To argue that human rights abuses occurring in Haiti, Guatemala, or Rwanda are unrelated to our surfeit in the rich world requires that we erase history and turn a blind eye to the pathologies of power that transcend all borders. Perpetuating such fictions requires dishonest, desocialized analyses that mask—whether through naïveté or fecklessness or complicity—the origins and consequences of structural violence. The argument of this book has been that it is time to take health rights as seriously as other human rights, and that intellectual recognition is only a necessary first step toward pragmatic solidarity, that is, toward taking a stand by the side of those who suffer most from an increasingly harsh "new world order."

AFTERWORD

Apollo 2 cost more than Apollo 1
Apollo 1 cost plenty.

Apollo 3 cost more than Apollo 2
Apollo 2 cost more than Apollo 1
Apollo 1 cost plenty.

Apollo 4 cost more than Apollo 3
Apollo 3 cost more than Apollo 2
Apollo 2 cost more than Apollo 1
Apollo 1 cost plenty.

Apollo 8 cost a fortune, but no one minded
because the astronauts were Protestant
they read the Bible from the moon
astounding and delighting every Christian
and on their return Pope Paul VI gave them his blessing.

Apollo 9 cost more than all these put together
including Apollo 1 which cost plenty.

The great-grandparents of the people of Acahaulinca were less
     hungry than the grandparents.
The great-grandparents died of hunger.
The grandparents of the people of Acahaulinca were less
     hungry than the parents.
The grandparents died of hunger.
The parents of the people of Acahaulinca were less
     hungry than the children of the people there.
The parents died of hunger.
The people of Acahaulinca are less hungry than the children
     of the people there.
The children of the people of Acahaulinca, because of hunger,
     are not born
they hunger to be born, only to die of hunger.
Blessed are the poor for they shall inherit the moon.

                                    Leonel Rugama, Sandinista, 1949–70

HUMAN RIGHTS IN THE ERA OF MANAGED INEQUALITY

Progress is more plausibly judged by the reduction of
deprivation than by the further enrichment of the opulent. We cannot really have an adequate understanding
of the future without some view about how well the
lives of the poor can be expected to go. Is there, then,
hope for the poor?

> Amartya Sen, "Will There Be Any Hope for the Poor?"

History says, Don't hope
On this side of the grave,
But then, once in a lifetime
The longed-for tidal wave
Of justice can rise up
And hope and history rhyme.

> Seamus Heaney,
> "Voices from Lemnos"

Today's date—March 8, 2000—still seems futuristic. This in spite of the
fact that I'm writing between Moscow and Port-au-Prince. A long flight,
and so plenty of time, if not elbow room, for reading the complimentary
newspapers offered all passengers. Whether the dailies are from London
or New York or Paris, they share an editorial tone; the giant full-page
advertisements, many of them in color, are now overtly similar from capital to capital. And although I cannot read the Russian papers, I was able
to read the billboards en route to Sheremetyevo airport. They too are
adorned by familiar models, hawking perfumes. The alphabet is different, but the shapes of the bottles are spookily familiar—even to those
who do not wear or buy perfume.

Enough about form, though. What of the content of these papers?
Plenty of relevance, today, to those interested in human rights. "Pinochet
Flies Home a Free Man," reads the *Guardian*'s banner: "Although Spain,
Belgium, France and Switzerland—who all have outstanding extradition
warrants against him—could theoretically have launched last-minute
legal challenges to the decision, none was forthcoming."[1] The consensus
seems to be that Pinochet was just too old and sick for justice.[2] I skim
one of the U.S. papers; *USA Today* devotes little space to Pinochet. It
does, however, contain no shortage of detail (and even some editorial
heat) about a certain professional baseball player suspended briefly for

making racist and anti-immigrant comments during a locker-room interview.

But I do read the *International Herald Tribune*. Concocted from the *New York Times* and the *Washington Post*, it always offers a dependably mainstream kabob of U.S. journalism. The reporting on Pinochet is similar—too old, too sick for justice—and even more placatory than the *Guardian*. This was a sensible decision, in the eyes of the world press: leave the old dotard alone. Who wants to be cruel to the elderly? My head begins to ache a bit; perhaps it's this cramped middle seat? Better to read something else. After all, it's really none of my business. Perhaps it was a matter for the Chileans, in spite of all our helpfulness there in 1973 and after.

Looking for a new subject, I read on. "Boston is awash in wealth," explains another piece in the *Herald Tribune,* "so much disposable income that it seems like Monopoly money."[3] Impossible not to think of Haiti, where a bustling clinic full of sick and hungry people awaits me. Why is it so hard, I wonder, to raise money to treat these patients? Jostling the passengers on either side, I rip out page 15 ("Business/Finance") because it contains an article of interest to one traveling from Moscow to Port-au-Prince. Under the title "Now More Than Ever, Rich Nations Need the Cooperation of the Poorer States," a certain Reginald Dale holds forth:

> The rich countries have collectively never come close to meeting the target set in 1970 of devoting 0.7 percent of their annual gross national product to official aid.
>
> But a great deal has been learned. Paternalism has largely disappeared from the rich countries' approach, while developing countries have increasingly understood the need to help themselves. The importance of trade rather than aid is widely accepted.

On the back of page 15 is a full-page Chanel ad. Again, the model, whatever her name, has a spookily familiar face. So does the logic of Dale's essay. Developing countries have increasingly understood the need to help themselves. Trade rather than aid.[4]

How, precisely, do the leaders of developing countries "help themselves"? Why, they do it much the same way as political elites everywhere do: they help themselves, often enough, to whatever they can get their hands on. Or so it seems as one travels from Moscow, embroiled in transnational financial scandal,[5] to Port-au-Prince, home of the U.S.-enabled family dictatorship that made such skimming something of an art form. Even the U.S. General Accounting Office seemed to think that, during the Duvalier years in particular, the approach to U.S. aid was, "Hey, help yourself! Plenty more where that came from!"[6] The U.S. mission turned a blind eye to the massive diversions.[7] What Reginald Dale terms "paternalism" seemed a lot more like crime to those watching from rural Haiti who were trying desperately to raise funds for a clinic for the poor. As to the attitude of rich countries toward poor countries, "aid before trade" seemed legitimate enough if the goal was to prop up U.S.-friendly family dictatorships. But a free clinic seeking to serve the destitute sick had to fight against the logic of users' fees and had to endure scoldings from aid agencies and development specialists, since our approach, we were told, was neither "sustainable" nor "cost-effective." By which they meant that it's all right to treat poor people but only if they pay for it themselves.

And although official aid is now scant—far below 0.7 percent of rich countries' gross national products (GNPs), we are reminded—lending is not. These loans are made in order to increase trade, we're told. Who would argue with the proposition that a robust economy is preferable to handouts? But here, too, capital follows its familiar trajectory from public coffers to private pockets. In Peru, where anyone who insists that people with infectious multidrug-resistant tuberculosis have the right to treatment must labor against a riptide of "cost-effectiveness," we learn that the financing of offshore debt will this year consume the equivalent of some 40 percent of exported goods and services.[8] Thus does Peruvian public wealth vanish to private banks in New York and elsewhere. In Russia, where rates of tuberculosis have trebled in less than a decade and where merely straying into a prison often leads to infection with a deadly drug-resistant strain, it has become heresy to argue that the Soviet-era health infrastructure should not be dismantled in the name of "health care reform." Not enough money to rebuild the labs and diagnostic capacity, admonish the cheerleaders of such "reform," as billions of dollars pour out of the country into foreign banks.[9]

"Trade rather than aid"? How can medicine and public health, particularly when inspired by a nonprofit or social justice agenda, hope to compete with cash flows like this? How can we compete with interests that have the mass media on their side or in their pockets? We learn from Mr. Dale that "aid figures less prominently as a foreign-policy priority since the Cold War's end." I know I should stop reading, but my eyes are dragged, almost against my will, down the column: "The new consensus that is emerging is based on a less starry-eyed assessment of mutual interest. Rich countries increasingly recognize that they will need markets and investment outlets in today's developing countries..."

I realize, just now, that my teeth are on edge; my jaw clenched in fierce tetany. Why keep on reading? I decide to stop holding my nose, I forswear the other articles, such as the one about the new power vacuum at top of the International Monetary Fund. One can stomach only so much hypocrisy and chicanery about international cashflows. I reach instead for my headset. The feature presentation is about to begin, and the new James Bond film promises a bit more candor, especially if one sees taking care of the destitute sick as a realistic necessity rather than a "starry-eyed" fantasy. Perhaps, like Pinochet, I'm feeling too old and tired for justice.

.   .   .   .   .

The more there are suffering, then, the more natural
their sufferings appear. Who wants to prevent the fishes
in the sea from getting wet?

And the suffering themselves share this callousness
towards themselves and are lacking in kindness towards themselves. It is terrible that human beings so
easily put up with existing conditions, not only with
the sufferings of strangers but also with their own.

All those who have thought about the bad state of
things refuse to appeal to the compassion of one group
of people for another. But the compassion of the oppressed for the oppressed is indispensable.

It is the world's one hope.

Bertolt Brecht, "The World's One Hope"

It's now the fourth of March. I am back in the little hospital in rural Haiti, trying to help Manno, a young man I have known since his childhood, hobble back to his bed. He is whimpering, his left leg frozen in a foot-to-hip cast. His story is sad, but I can't really call it shocking; I've heard similar ones many times and had heard a good part of his while still in Moscow.

It all happened right here in the village, just yards from the clinic gate. A few days ago, a woman we both know was walking in the road not far from the clinic. It was shortly before dawn, and she was on her way to market. As she rounded a corner, she was struck and killed by a truck. The driver saw what he had done and panicked, fleeing the hue and cry raised by the villagers. Some of the passengers leapt from the truck, assuming that its brakes had failed.

The villagers gathered around the stricken woman. Her family began to wail inconsolably. The crowd decided to block the road with rocks and debris and to alert the officials at the closest town so that the driver could be apprehended. Another truck, coming from the opposite direction, stopped at the roadblock. The truck's occupants demanded to be let through, and when the villagers refused to dismantle the roadblock, an angry passenger got out and started shooting. Manno took a bullet in his left leg, just above the ankle.

The assailant was later arrested, but Manno's problems were just beginning. An X-ray taken in the clinic showed that both tibia and fibula were shattered. The bullet was still there, too. So Manno was taken to Port-au-Prince. In the general hospital—the national university's teaching hospital—he was told that they could not operate unless he could come up with the necessary hardware (pins, plates, an external fixator). While still in Moscow, I'd been told by the Haitian priest with whom I work that "one of the doctors said the leg might have to be cut off." An extreme course of action, from a medical point of view. But the reason for the assessment was really social: the doctors were pessimistic about Manno's chances of acquiring the requisite hardware, which would cost him six thousand dollars. Furthermore, the nurses in Port-au-Prince were on strike—the priest was not sure why—and Manno would be more likely to receive care, or at least not endure neglect, if he returned to our small, impoverished village of Cange. I argued from Moscow that he should not be transferred back to Cange, where there is no orthopedic surgeon. Instead, every effort should be made to secure the needed hardware.

Having made this suggestion, I headed back. For two days, I've been mostly on airplanes or driving a jeep. Now, as soon as I reach Cange, I come to see Manno, who, having seen not a single doctor or nurse for two days, returned home. The foot looks fine, and there is certainly no reason to amputate it. What did they do down there in Port-au-Prince, I wonder? To answer this question, I obtain a second film. Looking at the still-dripping film, I curse in English, to no one in particular. I thought they'd have done something, anything. But there's the damn bullet. There are the fractures, still out of line.

As I leave the ward, Manno is still whimpering, even though he's settled comfortably back into bed. More out of fear, I suspect, than pain. The outcome, here in Haiti, of a comminuted fracture resulting from roadside violence could indeed be the loss of his foot. That would be a crime. But what kind of crime? Manno's attacker is in jail; there's now less impunity in Haiti than there was a few years earlier. But that doesn't help Manno get his left leg fixed. The bullet is still there, still lodged in his flesh, the fractures unpinned. Haiti does not guarantee its citizenry access to orthopedic hardware, although most anything can be bought for the right price. The word "insurance" is unknown among the poor.

Is Manno's injury just hard luck, a freak accident? Of course not. If it were, I would not have seen anything like it before. But how, exactly, does one explain that what is violated, in Manno's case and in the case of all those denied decent medical care, are social and economic rights? Aren't we "starry-eyed" if we complain too much about the "new consensus" preaching "trade rather than aid"? Isn't Manno mostly a victim of the "inefficiencies" and "archaisms" of a "Third World" economy in need of thorough-going "reform"?

·   ·   ·   ·   ·

Things that go away never return—
everybody knows that.
And in the bright crowd of the winds
there's no use complaining!
                Federico García Lorca, "Weathervane"

The process of liberation brings with it a profound
conflict. Having the project be clear is not enough.
What is necessary is a spirituality of resistance and of
renewed hope to turn ever back to the struggle in the
face of the defeats of the oppressed.
                Leonardo Boff, "La originalidad de la
                      teología de la liberación"

I started this book with a reflection on liberal and neoliberal thought. The newspapers are full of that brand of preaching, as my glance at the *Herald Tribune* suggests. So are the universities. I know that the struggle for social and economic rights is often dismissed as a "radical" position, one held up as unreasonable even by some supporters of civil and political rights. I know, too, that much of the quarrel would sound like gobbledygook to most of my colleagues in medicine; they are unfamiliar with the terms of the debate, although it concerns them closely. It occurred to me, in editing these essays, that I should soften my stance a bit—one of my interlocutors, a friend, called it "principled, but extreme"—and I discussed this possibility with a couple of close friends. But as one of them, Jim Kim, noted, "The book isn't harsh; the realities it describes are harsh."

The spectacular aggressions I have witnessed are not accidents. Arising from complex social fields, these crimes are predictable and, indeed, ongoing. They are, I have tried to show here, pathologies of power. Looking through piles of notes and articles gathered to complete this book, I am reminded of many stories that are not told in these pages. I did not write about my patient who was the victim of a brutal gang rape inside military headquarters in Port-au-Prince. She told me that one of the most debasing moments of her experience was hearing the army's lawyer, a smartly dressed woman who spoke beautiful English, say on CNN that stories of political rapes were simply not true, that the alleged victims were lying to discredit the Haitian army.[10] To see these and similar claims subsequently taken up by reputable international print media was painful enough for me; I couldn't bear to discuss it with my patient.

Nothing is written in these pages of the thugs who in 1988 torched the church of Saint-Jean Bosco during mass or, even worse, of the paltry sum it cost the mayor of Port-au-Prince to have them do it.[11] Yes, the mayor (who is no doubt also getting on in years, although he has yet to reach the golden age of Pinochet). Even though one of my closest friends was among the survivors, and even though I have written about these events, I have never discussed them with this friend; and I never will.

And on and on. These events are added to a long list of things I wish I had not seen, or heard, or smelled. Indeed, staring at the X-ray image of the bullet in Manno's leg triggers recollection of many expediently forgotten bullets and their forgotten targets. I stop to recall, however briefly: in 1987, sewing up a child's gunshot wounds in the same general hospital from which Manno was just extruded; evaluating the surviving victims of a grenade pitched into a 1990 pro-Aristide rally; knowing what it looks like to watch, from the middle of a traffic jam, a crowd fired upon by automatic weapons, an anonymous ten-year-old boy caught in the crossfire; the death of Chouchou Louis in my presence; and the burning alive of secret police, killed by angry crowds. The even worse smells of morgues and prisons and deathbeds crowd my senses.

And the assaultive truths don't stop with the things that I have witnessed, since many of the stories I've heard from others elsewhere have a specific resonance for someone who has worked in Haiti. I think here of the exhumations in Guatemala, with which we did indeed help, and of the one unmarked grave that contained a young man, his wife, and their unborn infant (one bullet was within the fetus). I think of my friend "Julia's" martyred brother—a teenager, for God's sake—his body displayed like a hunting trophy; the disappearance of Armando Mazariegos; the terrible litany of others "disappeared" in Haiti and in Central America; the murder of Father Jean-Marie Vincent by the Haitian military. Father Vincent died, gasping like a fish, on the steps of the rectory.

What do all of these victims have in common? Not language or gender or political views; not religion or race or ethnicity. What they share, all of them, is poverty and, generally, an unwillingness to knuckle under. Pathologies of power damage all concerned—and who isn't concerned?—but kill chiefly the poor. These crimes are the symptoms and signs of structural violence. Indeed, when we regard the perpetrators of these crimes from any comfortable reserve, it is important to recall that with our comfort comes a loss of innocence, since we profit from a social and economic order that promises a body count. That is, surely there are direct and causal relationships between a protected minority enjoying great ease and those billions who go without the bare necessities of food, shelter, potable water, and medical services? Pathologies of power are also symptoms of surfeit—of the excess that I like as much as the next guy.

How do we, as the lingo would have it, "process" such abominable contiguity? Our best hope, it sometimes seems, is oblivion. Let the world's endless jeremiad be blotted out by action films and other entertainments, sport-utility vehicles, high irony, identity politics that erase the world's poor, or struggles for personal advancement within this or that institution. Choose your poison; choose your anesthesia. Help yourself. Soon we will all be too old for justice, anyway.

This is, I know, a plaintive book. It issues plaints and sides with the plaintiffs. In seeking to close it, I think of García Lorca's poem "Weathervane."[12] In it, he seeks approval of a claim—it's useless to complain—from a tree. "Am I right, poplar, teacher of the breeze?"

Most of these essays were written in Boston, on planes, or in hotels; it is hard to write here in Haiti. But I wanted to finish it here, with the sound of bamboo scratching on a tin roof, in order to ask a question. Is it really useless to complain? For my own amusement, perhaps, I ask the question out loud. The bamboo gives no answer. I hear only the faint sound of someone singing; a hoe striking the stony earth; a finch.

Writing about human suffering runs many risks, and most of these risks have been the subject of too much commentary. But there is also the artifice of packaging something so it offends the senses, but not too much. Surely this too is a marker of lost innocence. I have come to terms with the fact that here I will never be asked to write, or even to reflect overmuch on what is described in these pages, because in Haiti I am asked to do only one thing: to be a doctor, to serve the destitute sick. And since none of my patients can pay for my services, it is my job, my great privilege, to draw attention to the suffering of the poor and to bring resources to bear on the problems that are remediable. Most are. Manno's certainly is.

I contemplate my own loss of innocence with resentful, sometimes even tearful, silence. From whom can I demand it back? As García Lorca said, "Things that go away never return—everybody knows that."

Everybody knows that things that go away never return.

Cange, Haiti
March 8, 2000

NOTES

FOREWORD

1. This astounding figure is not a typographical error. See World Bank 1993, table A.3, and 1994b.

2. Wittgenstein 1958, p. 4.

3. Indeed, Farmer himself has made effective use of the concept of "structural violence" in earlier studies; see, for example, *Women, Poverty, and AIDS: Sex, Drugs, and Structural Violence* (Farmer, Connors, and Simmons 1996).

4. See, among other studies, Marmot, Smith, and Stansfeld 1991; Marmot, Bobak, and Smith 1995; Wilkinson 1996.

INTRODUCTION

1. The dimensions of the military presence in Chiapas have fluctuated widely over the past decade. In the days following the January 1994 uprising, fourteen thousand troops were dispatched to crush the Zapatista rebellion (see Womack 1999, p. 12). The number of troops deployed peaked at seventy thousand and waned after the Fox government pledged to demilitarize the state. For more on the federal military presence in Chiapas, see Global Exchange 1998. For an analysis of the tangled web of relations among the army, local police, and paramilitary groups, see Human Rights Watch/Americas 1997, whose title says it all: *Implausible Deniability: State Responsibility for Rural Violence in Mexico.*

2. Some forty-five thousand Guatemalan refugees were officially registered in United Nations refugee camps in southern Mexico in the early 1980s, with many remaining there for over a decade (Sawyer 1999).

3. Estimates of casualties vary widely, as ever. The two hundred thousand figure comes from Susanne Jonas (1991, p. 2). During the years of overt war in the highlands, it is estimated that one hundred thousand people were killed and

another forty thousand "disappeared" (Green 1999, p. 4). The exact figures are, of course, impossible to know, but the Argentine Forensic Anthropology Team wrote in 1996 that "more people have been forcibly disappeared in Guatemala during the past decade than in any other Latin American country" (Equipo Argentino de Antropología Forense 1996, p. 71; my translation). Note that disappearances have a permanent impact unlike other deaths: mourning and "closure" are impossible; trauma is ongoing and never becomes "post-trauma." Dead is dead, and "disappeared" is almost always dead, too, but on top of these outright deaths sits the grisly business of torture.

The Guatemalan Truth Commission has documented 42,275 separate human rights violations that occurred between 1962 and 1996, 85 percent of them committed by Guatemalan regular army troops. More than half of these were murders; the total number of dead and disappeared from this still-incomplete survey is estimated at more than ninety thousand. The number of documented violations peaked in the early 1980s—the years during which Julia lost her husband—climbing to more than ten thousand documented cases of arbitrary execution, nearly ten thousand cases of torture, and nearly four thousand cases of forced disappearance per year. Of the 669 documented massacres, 46 percent were committed in just one state on the border with Chiapas (Misión de Verificación de las Naciones Unidas en Guatemala 1999).

For raw data on numerous human rights violations that took place in Guatemala between 1960 and 1996, see the online Science and Human Rights Program of the American Association for the Advancement of Science (AAAS) and the International Center for Human Rights Research (CIIDH) (Ball 1999). This project contains information from both documents and testimonial sources and attempts to systematize known information about the violations that occurred. For a description of the database and the methods of gathering and analyzing the data as well as an extensive interpretation of the data, see Ball, Kobrak, and Spirer 1999 as well as CIIDH 1999. For other data and analyses of distribution of the massacres and genocide in Guatemala between 1977 and 1986, see Gulden 2002.

Elsewhere, I have tried to underline U.S. complicity in this officially blessed slaughter (Farmer 1994, pp. 237–46). It has deep roots. Even now, when there is supposedly peace, there is cause for shame, all too rare in such matters:

> One of the grandest of the Guatemalan killers, General Héctor Gramajo, was rewarded for his contributions to genocide in the highlands with a fellowship to Harvard's John F. Kennedy School of Government—not unreasonably, given Kennedy's decisive contributions to the vocation of counterinsurgency (one of the technical terms for international terrorism conducted by the powerful) (Chomsky 1993, p. 29).

Noam Chomsky cites a long interview that Gramajo accorded to anthropologist Jennifer Schirmer, who notes that the former Minister of Defense "granted me many hours of taped interviews." In the spring 1991 *Harvard International Review,* the general, then a Mason Fellow at Harvard, goes on record regarding the national-security doctrine he helped to put into practice:

We aren't renouncing the use of force. If we have to use it, we have to use it, but in a more sophisticated manner. You needn't kill everyone to complete the job. [You can use] more sophisticated means: we aren't going to return to the large-scale massacres.... We have created a more humanitarian, less costly strategy, to be more compatible with the democratic system. We instituted Civil Affairs (in 1982) which provides development for 70 percent of the population while we kill 30 percent. Before, the strategy was to kill 100 percent (Schirmer 1991, p. 11).

Others credit Efraín Ríos Montt, dictator between 1982 and 1983, with initiating the scorched-earth campaign against the highland poor. As this book goes to press, Ríos Montt has again taken control of the Guatemalan Congress, a move that has heightened fear among the survivors: " 'The problem is that the same actors trying to resolve the peace process' errors are the ones who committed them,' said Héctor Rosada, a former press secretary. 'The last word on important questions lies with Efraín Ríos Montt, a man who does not believe in the peace accords' " ("Guatemalan Peace Vows Unfulfilled" 2000).

4. The efforts to shed light on the extent of human rights violations by the Guatemalan military during the counterinsurgency campaign and the bloody thirty-six-year civil war include exhumations of clandestine mass graves of victims massacred during this period. These exhumations are being conducted by several nongovernmental organizations—as there is no official government program. Scientists involved in these efforts have given testimony against government officials accused of human rights violations; some of the scientists have received threats, and their work has been disrupted. For more on such threats during the first half of 2002, see Elton 2002 and two recent alerts from the Human Rights Action Network of the American Association for the Advancement of Science (2002a, 2002b).

5. The bishop delivered his speech on the occasion of the presentation of the Recuperación de la Memoria Histórica report, Guatemala City, April 24, 1998; see Human Rights Office of the Archdiocese of Guatemala 1999, p. xxiv (my translation). This publication is an abridged version of the original four-volume document published as *Guatemala: Nunca Más* (Oficina los Derechos Humanos del Arzobispado de Guatemala 1998).

6. An extensive discussion of the terms "liberalism" and "neoliberalism" is beyond the scope of this book, but these terms, as used in much of the world, refer to policies and ideologies that advance the market as the solution to most problems. They thus have a meaning more or less the opposite of that implied by the term "liberalism" as it is used in U.S. political and popular discourses, where liberals are perceived as favoring an interventionist state. There is a tradition of *obrerista* or workers' Liberalism that did favor the poor and that was significant in parts of Latin America, most notably Colombia and Nicaragua (where, in both cases, radical Liberals were associated with revolutionary movements and allied, at times, with the communist left). On the importance of these movements in Nicaragua, see Gould 1990; on Colombia, see Bergquist, Penaranda, and Sánchez 1992.

Elsewhere, we have explored in some detail the impact of neoliberal economic policies on the health of the Haitian poor (e.g., Farmer and Bertrand 2000). More generally, however, my understanding of the social structures of economies has been most influenced by Pierre Bourdieu, many of whose works are cited in the bibliography. He terms globalization—*mondialisation,* in French—a "pseudo-concept that is at once descriptive and prescriptive." Bourdieu has written bitingly of "neoliberal utopias" and their false promise for the poor:

> Integration into the global economic field through free trade, free circulation of capital, and export-oriented growth as now proposed to dominated countries as either destiny or ideal (as opposed to a more nationalist orientation seeking to develop domestic production for national markets) presents the same ambiguity that integration into a national economy once did: while giving all of the appearances of a limitless universalism, [this integration] serves the interests of the dominant—that is, the big investors who in situating themselves above the State, can nonetheless count on powerful States (and especially the most politically and militarily powerful United States) to assure favorable conditions for the conduct of their economic activities (2000b, pp. 277–78; my translation).

The impact of these policies and ideologies has been experienced most keenly in Latin America. Roberto Briceño-León and Verónica Zubillaga note the link between rising rates of violence and the triumph of neoliberal policies in the region:

> The new violence in Latin America is a consequence of the convergence of global transformations and local transformations in urban society since the 1980s. It is, thus, a violence born of a process of global mutation which fosters changes and interacts with local trends in countries having dependent economies. At the global level, we allude to the hegemony of a free market economy, the definition of consumption as a form of social participation and the weakening of the nation-states. At the local level, we make reference to the advance and perpetuation of economic recession. The weakening of the nation-state in the Latin American countries has taken the form of a dismantling of the welfare state, and at the local level that trend has resulted in a steady deterioration of public services and a devaluation of social rights among the most vulnerable populations (housing, education, employment, health care, personal security) (2002, pp. 21–22).

7. These themes are explored in Kim, Millen, Irwin, and Gershman 2000. See also the review by David Coburn (2000). For a more specific critique of how the laws of supply and demand are structuring growing inequalities in U.S. health care delivery, see Farmer and Rylko-Bauer 2001; Rylko-Bauer and Farmer 2002.

8. This moral blindness is hardly accidental; as one Peruvian economist puts it, "ethical obligations disappear from consideration" under a neoliberal paradigm—"or are subjugated before a fate considered practically inevitable" (Iguíñiz 1995, p. 59).

9. Wallerstein 1995a, p. 2. Wallerstein has done a great deal to constitute what he calls the "historical sociology of liberalism." As he notes:

> Liberalism was never a doctrine of the Left; it was always the quintessential centrist doctrine. Its advocates were sure of their moderation, their wisdom, and their humanity. They arrayed themselves simultaneously against an archaic past of unjustified privilege (which they considered to be represented by conservative ideology) and a reckless leveling that took no account of either virtue or merit (which they considered to be represented by socialist/radical ideology). Liberals have always sought to define the rest of the political scene as made up of two extremes between which they fall (pp. 1–2).

10. Sobrino 1988, p. 159.

11. Samantha Power (2002) speaks to this disingenuous surprise in her recent book on U.S. responses to genocide: "The forward-looking, consoling refrain of 'never again,' a testament to America's can-do spirit, never grappled with the fact that the country had done nothing, practically or politically, to prepare itself to respond to genocide. The commitment proved hollow in the face of actual slaughter" (p. xxi). Power interviewed more than three hundred persons, most of them U.S. officials and many a part of what she refers to as the "world of bystanders" (p. xviii). Some of them were certainly on the sidelines, although it is not clear that they were completely innocent bystanders. She continues:

> Before I began exploring America's relationship with genocide, I used to refer to U.S. policy toward Bosnia as a "failure." I have changed my mind. It is daunting to acknowledge, but this country's consistent policy of nonintervention in the face of genocide offers sad testimony not to a broken American political system but to one that is ruthlessly effective. The system, as it stands now, is working. No U.S. president has ever made genocide prevention a priority, and no U.S. president has ever suffered politically for his indifference to its occurrence. It is thus no coincidence that genocide rages on (p. xxi).

Writing of the apparent indifference not only of officials but also of U.S. society at large, Power raises disturbing issues in her study. On April 30, 1994, for example, "Representative Patricia Schroeder (D.-Colo.) described the relative silence in her district. 'There are some groups terribly concerned about the gorillas,' she said, noting that Colorado was home to a research organization that studied Rwanda's imperiled gorilla population. 'But—it sounds terrible—people just don't know what can be done about the people'" (p. 375).

12. In his classic work *The Power of the Poor in History,* Gustavo Gutiérrez makes sure that there is no confusion on this point, using the section heading "Injustice Is Not an Accident" (Gutiérrez 1983, p. 117).

13. For more on earlier uses of the term "structural violence," see Galtung 1969; see also the proceedings of the meetings of the Latin American bishops in Medellín in 1968 and Puebla in 1978. The preparatory documents and the theological underpinnings of these meetings are explored in Gutiérrez 1983.

Briceño-León and Zubillaga offer a compelling synthesis of both the causes and the consequences of structural violence in Latin America:

> Latin America underwent a process of impoverishment in the last 20 years of the 20th century, turning it into a breeding ground for violence. The minimum wage earned by workers in 1998 was lower than that of 1980 in 13 of the region's 18 countries, but expectations for consumption have not gone down; rather, they have risen in the urban areas, to levels comparable to those prevailing in the USA.... The cultural processes at work have been similar, advertising has achieved increasing penetration, the mass media make tastes increasingly uniform and the consumption of prestige brands has become a way of life. The ubiquitous presence of television, in even the poorest of urban homes (86 percent of Brazilian households and 89 percent of Venezuelan households have colour television), causes cultural patterns of consumption to spread massively. Hence, to the more traditional shortcomings of life are now added the desire to acquire the new products associated with the comfortable urban life and to display the outward signs of distinction, transmitted by fashionable brands (2002, p. 22).

14. Sobrino 1988, p. 107.

15. Sen 1999, pp. 3–4. Amartya Sen (e.g., 1981, 1985a, 1985b, 1987, 1992a, 1992b, 1993, 1998) has written extensively about the reticulated relationships between social and economic rights and well-being. Because he is an economist, Sen has to argue for the relevance of mortality, especially premature mortality among the poor, as a critical indicator of economic success or failure—a point that would strike most in public health and medicine as self-evident. Sen underlines the disjuncture between standard economic indices, such as GNP per capita, and mortality in order to draw attention to the importance of social entitlements and equity:

> In contrast with the "growth-mediated" mechanism, the "support-led" process does not operate through fast economic growth. It is well exemplified by countries such as Sri Lanka, pre-reform China, Costa Rica, or the Indian state of Kerala, which have had very rapid reductions in mortality rates, without much economic growth. This is a process that does not wait for dramatic increases in per-capita levels of real income, and it works through priority being given to providing social services (particularly health care and basic education) that reduce mortality and enhance the quality of life (Sen 1998, p. 9).

Because mortality is a well-accepted indicator of success or failure in medicine and public health, this book moves against a different undertow of opinion. Here, I emphasize the importance of poverty, inequality, and other forms of structural violence in considerations of human rights. As Chapter 1 makes clear, these arguments are consonant with those of Sen as outlined in the publications cited earlier. Throughout this book, people living in poverty are also cited as experts on structural violence. Indeed, much of their analysis is resonant with that of Sen. For example, Mexico's Zapatistas offer the following commentary: "The serious poverty that we share with our fellow citizens has a common cause: the lack of freedom and democracy. We think that authentic respect for the liberties and democratic will of the people are the indispensable prerequisites for the improvement of the economic and social conditions of the dispossessed of our country" ("Communiqué from the CCRI-CG of the EZLN, January 6, 1994," in Marcos and the Zapatista Army of National Liberation 1995, pp. 55–56).

16. Kirkpatrick 1981. See also Wronka 1997. Jeane Kirkpatrick was, of course, the U.S. ambassador to the United Nations during the Reagan administration.

17. Note that the Universal Declaration of Human Rights is regarded by many as a rather timid document, as far as social and economic rights go:

> Freedom of speech and opinion, the right of peaceful assembly and association, the ability to freely practice one's religion, and ownership of *private* property are among the rights enshrined in the Universal Declaration while economic rights, such as the right to food, which comprise only 4 of its 30 articles, are essentially neglected and the notion of the group, rather than the individual—a notion that is the basis of most Third World cultures—is given short shrift (Schwab 1999, p. 3).

These observations call for some remarks. It's not at all clear that the "notion of the group" is the basis of "most Third World cultures." Social and economic rights are undervalued in most cultures in which social inequalities figure prominently—that is, in the global era, most cultures, period. Cuba's opposition to the U.S.-sponsored focus on individual rights—the focus of Schwab's excellent book—is a *principled* stance and has little to do with Cuba's "Third World culture," which is not all that different from the cultures of other Latin American societies that care little, it would seem, about social and economic rights.

18. The contradictions encountered within the human rights movement are described by Michael Ignatieff:

> The worldwide spread of human rights norms is often seen as a moral consequence of economic globalization. The U.S. State Department's annual report for 1999 on human rights practice around the world describes the constellation of human rights and democracy—along with "money and the Internet"—as one of the three universal languages of globalization. This implies too easily that human rights is a style of moral individualism that has some elective affinity with the economic individualism of the global market, and that the two advance hand in hand. Actually, the relation between human rights and money, between moral and economic globalization, is more antagonistic, as can be seen, for example, in the campaigns by human rights activists against the labor and environmental practices of the large global corporations. Human rights has gone global not because it serves the interests of the powerful but primarily because it has advanced the interests of the powerless. Human rights has gone global by going local, imbedding itself in the soil of cultures and worldviews independent of the West, in order to sustain ordinary people's struggles against unjust states and oppressive social practices (2001, p. 7).

19. Galeano 1991, p. 108.
20. Gutiérrez 1983, p. 29.
21. Uvin 1998, p. 3. Since I am not an Africanist, I will not review here the long history of structural violence in the lacrustine region, but I feel obligated to note that the very notion of ethnicity in Rwanda is of fairly recent vintage. The Hutu and the Tutsi are ethnically similar people, and the rigid codifications that structured the genocide became entrenched only in the last century—the colonial and neocolonial periods. As ever, symbolic violence is a necessary component of structural violence, just as racism is a necessary component of genocide. As Claudine Vidal has noted:

> Historical myths concerning the categories "Hutu" and "Tutsi" were critical to the construction of hate, because they lent to these categories an imagined historical depth. They bolstered the ideology which suggested that these collective ethnic identities had been forged within communities forever at odds with each other, an ideology continuously invoked in the calls to violence which began in the 1950s, the beginning of the political conflict between Tutsi and Hutu leaders (1996, pp. 334–35; my translation).

These myths were purveyed more often in print than in oral tradition. That is, they were myths buttressed by colonial elites and their protégés. Philip Gourevitch gets close to the absurd horror and also its colonial roots:

> The Belgians could hardly have pretended they were needed to bring order to Rwanda. Instead, they sought out those features of the existing civilization that fit their own ideas of mastery and subjugation and bent them to fit their purposes. Colonization is violence, and there are many ways to carry out that violence. In addition to military and administrative chiefs, and a veritable army of

churchmen, the Belgians dispatched scientists to Rwanda. The scientists brought scales and measuring tapes and calipers, and they went about weighing Rwandans, measuring Rwandan cranial capacities, and conducting comparative analyses of the relative protuberance of Rwandan noses. Sure enough, the scientists found what they had believed all along. Tutsis had "nobler," more "naturally" aristocratic dimensions than the "coarse" and "bestial" Hutus. On the "nasal index," for instance, the median Tutsi nose was found to be two and a half millimeters longer and nearly five millimeters narrower than the Hutu nose (1998, pp. 55–56).

These same analyses are echoed by René Lemarchand (1997), who notes that while stratification and inequality existed in precolonial Rwanda, "nonetheless, Hutu and Tutsi shared the same language and culture, the same clan names, and the same customs, and the symbols of kingship served as a powerful unifying bond between them."

> ...Although the potential for conflict existed long before the advent of European rule, it was the Belgian colonial state that provided the crucible within which ethnic identities were reshaped and mythologized.... It was the colonial state that destroyed the countervailing mechanisms built around the different categories of chiefs and subchiefs, thus adding significantly to the oppressiveness of Tutsi rule. It was the colonial state that insisted that each individual carry an identity card specifying his/her ethnic background, a practice perpetuated until 1994, when "tribal cards" often spelled the difference between life and death; and it was with the blessings of the colonial state that Christian missionaries began to speculate about the "Hamitic" origins of the kingdom, drawing attention to the distinctively Ethiopian features, and hence the foreign origins, of the Tutsi "caste" (pp. 409–10).

22. Uvin 1998, p. 5.

23. Starn 1992, p. 168.

24. See, for example, the special issue of the Andean studies journal *Allpanchis* (no. 39, 1992) entitled "La guerra en los Andes," which reprinted Starn's piece in Spanish translation along with a number of indignant responses. See also Mayer 1992. Ellen Messer reviewed "anthropology and human rights" in a 1993 essay. It is not as easy to make the argument that anthropologists of highland Guatemala were able to divert their gaze from violence, as Leigh Binford (1996) points out in discussing anthropology's longstanding fascination with Guatemala (and lack thereof in El Salvador); for more on this, see note 25, below. Others have also noted anthropology's more complex engagement with historical and political realities in Guatemala and its "long heritage of writing in solidarity with the oppressed, however much uneasy conscience over U.S. complicity in that oppression obliges solidarity" (Watanabe 2002, p. 331).

25. Green 1999, pp. 57–58. She later adds, "Anthropologists for the most part have tended to report but not to analyze the effects and meanings of suffering on people's everyday lives, neglecting how racism, cultural imperialism, marginalization, exploitation, and powerlessness shape people's identities" (p. 169). Elsewhere (Farmer 1999b), I have written of "visual-field defects in anthropology and medicine," and several others have made similar commentaries: "To date," noted Carole Nagengast in 1994, "anthropology has not been in the forefront of the study of collective violence, terrorism, and especially violence in

state societies" (p. 112). In discussing the paucity of work on these topics, Alexander Laban Hinton asks why anthropologists have "failed to engage with the topic of genocide" and notes that it wasn't until the 1980s that "anthropologists began to more actively study war and political violence..., a trend that eventually contributed to a small body of work on genocide—particularly in the aftermath of Bosnia and Rwanda" (2002a, pp. 2, 3). For recent examples of such work, see Hinton 2002b and 2002c.

The genocide in Rwanda might not have surprised all scholars—Catherine Newbury's 1988 study was called *The Cohesion of Oppression: Clientship and Ethnicity in Rwanda, 1860–1960*—but almost all scholarly commentaries, including those from anthropologists, were written well after the journalists (e.g., Gourevitch 1998) published their accounts. John and Reinhild Janzen discuss the "advantages of hindsight" in their collection of testimonials from Rwanda and Burundi and note that their work there was on behalf of the Mennonite Central Committee rather than a university (Janzen and Janzen 2000, p. ix). Even within medical anthropology, which should, after all, concern itself primarily with sickness and suffering, similar critiques may be leveled even at this late date:

> While cultural factors are crucial, a major role of medical anthropology, whether directly related to medicine and public health or not...is also to direct our focus to the total context of people's lives—to the wider "social roots of disease"—and particularly to the deleterious elements in most societies of violence, inequity, and marginalization, pointing to issues such as power, dominance, paternalism and racism, and their implication for how diseases are created, distributed and treated (Heggenhougen 2000, p. 1171).

Similar pleas, and substantive empirical work, have come from a group of scholars who term themselves "critical medical anthropologists." (See, for example, the work of Hans Baer and Merrill Singer, including Baer and Singer 1997, Singer and Baer 1995, Singer 1994, and Singer 1998.) The March 1998 issue of *Medical Anthropology Quarterly* (vol. 12, no. 1) was entitled "The Embodiment of Violence"; and several anthropologists contributed to a special issue of *Daedalus* examining the topic of "social suffering" (Winter 1996, vol. 25, no. 1). Nancy Scheper-Hughes, Carolyn Nordstrom, Philippe Bourgois, Arthur Kleinman, Kris Heggenhougen, Alisse Waterston, Marcelo Suárez-Orozco, Jean and John Comaroff and several other anthropologists have focused their research and writing on structural violence—and thus we will eventually have to stop saying that there is too little focus on the topic. At this writing, however, each of these scholars has commented on our discipline's inattention to structural violence.

See also the essay by P. J. Magnarella (1994), who concludes with the following admonition: "As anthropologists we have benefited personally from the rich cultures that minority societies around the world have willingly shared with us. We, as members of more technologically advanced, more affluent societies, must not turn a blind eye to the sufferings of these and other peoples at the hands of insensitive or brutal governments" (p. 7). Binford (1996) makes a similar appeal, although, writing from El Salvador, he is pessimistic:

> The majority of anthropologists only object when imperialist intervention threatens the physical existence of the subjects who are the bearers of the ideas and

practices that they study. In El Salvador those prospective subjects—"exotic" Native Americans—were mostly killed off during the 1932 mantanza, with the results that El Salvador never developed a reputation in the United States or Europe as a desirable field site for anthropological work. With notable exceptions few U.S. anthropologists protested in print the slaughter perpetrated by their government and the Salvadoran military on tens of thousands of mestizo peasants, workers, and students. On the other hand, more anthropologists responded to the Guatemalan military's scorched-earth policies that were wiping out thousands of highland Mayans who had for decades served up the ethnographic "raw material" for the molding of academic reputations. But even in Guatemala, the response was muted; only a handful of dozens of anthropologists who had carried out research there got involved (p. 197).

While the majority of U.S. anthropologists can be accused of a "diverted gaze," Latin American scholars have a long tradition of studying structural violence and inequality. See, for example, Rodolfo Stavenhagen's delineation of the relationship between ethnicity and class for indigenous peoples in Mexico (1996b) (also the subject of Chapter 3 of this book); see also his more extended consideration of ethnic conflicts and the nation-state (1996a). There was also significant involvement by U.S. anthropologists in analyzing and denouncing the Guatemalan situation. See, for example, *Harvest of Violence,* the excellent volume edited by Robert Carmack (1988). The closing chapter is by Richard Adams, whose own 1970 volume *Crucifixion by Power* was something of a repentance for his role in the notorious political prisoners interview project reported in 1957 in a pseudonymously authored article by "Stokes Newbold" (the title: "Receptivity to Communist Fomented Agitation in Rural Guatemala"). Other anthropologists who did not fail to examine the workings of structural violence in Guatemala include, for example, June Nash (1995), Carol Smith (1990), and Ricardo Falla (1992). Finally, quite a few U.S. anthropologists participated, although not always as anthropologists, in Central America–related human rights and solidarity activities in the 1970s and 1980s. A thoughtful reflection on this, germane to a number of other discussions in this book, is offered by Philippe Bourgois (1990).

For more on anthropology and human rights, see the compendium edited by Theodore Downing and Gilbert Kushner, who attribute the "relative paucity of anthropological literature specifically focused on human rights" to "(1) the small number of anthropologists, (2) disciplinary tradition and (3) lack of funding for human rights research" (1988, p. 3). Binford agrees that, since Vietnam, "most anthropologists [have] demonstrated little public concern over violations of their subjects' human rights." But he takes issue with the explanation offered by Downing and Kushner:

> There are several reasons for this, but they don't appear among those listed by Theodore Downing and Gilbert Kushner.... These explanations strike me as less than satisfactory. First, their "small number" has not prevented anthropologists from devoting a great deal of attention to indigenous conceptions of time, Australian aboriginal kinship systems, Native American religion, or a host of other issues. Second, to attribute the lack of interest in human rights to anthropology's "disciplinary tradition" begs the question. Anthropology's historic subjects have, as defined by that "tradition," been among the oppressed, so why haven't the

various dimensions of oppression (social, economic, political) assumed a more prominent role within the anthropological discourse? And more importantly, why haven't more anthropologists committed themselves to political *engagement* on behalf of their subjects, rather than confining most of their energies to sharing materials with like-minded colleagues through specialist books and journals? Finally, one might ask how many funding proposals have anthropologists really introduced to carry out human rights research? Must all research wait on the largesse of a benevolent patron before being undertaken? (1996, pp. 198–99)

Since all sweeping generalizations about a large and complex field of inquiry will be incorrect, a careful examination of the anthropology (or lack thereof) of structural violence will demand a much more in-depth survey of the field. I would add, however, that such a survey should include a close reading of French and francophone anthropologists, several of whom have taken these topics seriously. For example, Françoise Héritier has collected a two-volume set of essays entitled *De la violence* (1996 and 1999); such works are too rarely read in North America. Didier Fassin has made great contributions to the anthropology of social inequalities; see Fassin 1996; Dozon and Fassin 2001; Leclerc, Fassin, Grandjean, et al. 2000.

26. The term "macrologics of power" is borrowed from Cindi Katz (1992). Anyone who can write an entire chapter on weaving—see "The Dialectics of Cloth" (Green 1999)—can hardly be accused of shirking her responsibility as an ethnographer. But Green's exploration of weaving is grounded not in foggy or nostalgic mysticism but in the harsh realities of her informants' lives.

27. Most anthropologists would argue that cultural relativism as a "metaethical theory" has its role and, contrary to popular belief, is not incompatible with universal values. The strengths and limitations—and especially the limitations—of cultural relativism are discussed throughout this book. Although I cannot review the topic here, my thinking on these matters has been informed most by my fieldwork in Haiti but also by colleagues in and outside anthropology. See, for example, Downing and Kushner 1992, Campbell 1972, Geertz 1984, Gellner 1985, Hatch 1983, Renteln 1988, and Schmidt 1955.

For an anthropologic perspective on the debates regarding universality versus cultural relativity in human rights, see the series of articles on this topic in the *Journal of Anthropological Research* (Messer 1997, Nagengast 1997, Nagengast and Turner 1997, Turner 1997, Zechenter 1997). For an ethnographically grounded discussion of culture and universalism in human rights discourse, see Adams 1998, an important study from Tibet.

28. Raoul Cédras delivered this address on Radio Nationale, December 13, 1991.

29. Constable 1991, p. 2.

30. The international context in which the minor dramas (e.g., Honorat's rise to power) were played out within the major tragedy that was the coup d'état of 1991 is discussed in greater detail in Farmer 1994.

31. Cited in Marcos and the Zapatista Army of National Liberation 1995, p. 81. This is a collection of the letters and communiqués of Subcomandante Marcos and the EZLN.

32. Ibid., p. 43. It is doubtful that scabies is ever lethal, but surely the point is well taken. "Breakbone fever" is a common term for dengue, now epidemic in much of Latin America.

33. Ibid., p. 38.

34. Hernández Castillo 1998a, p. 1.

35. Chomsky 1998, p. 25.

36. Schoultz 1979, p. 599.

37. This observation is quoted from Wisława Szymborska's poem "In Praise of Self-Deprecation" (Szymborska 1981).

38. It is a mistake to assume that globalization is associated with a weakening of all states. Some states have positioned themselves quite well over the past century or so. As Jacqueline Bhabha notes in writing of European polities, "Globalization does not necessarily weaken the national state; rather it alters its terms of reference and the temporal and spatial context within which it is embedded" (Bhabha 1998a, p. 699). Some states remain as powerful as ever, even when they are linked through emerging processes of globalization. As Bhabha notes of the European Union: "The philosophy underlying the early development of the [European] Union was that economic recovery and collaborative growth would of themselves fuel political cohesion and social progress by ensuring an improved standard of living and reducing the risk of social discontent or military conflict. Prosperity rather than justice or equality was the prime concern" (ibid., p. 698). See also Ignatieff 2001.

39. Galbraith 2002, p. 25.

40. For a broad overview of the health and human rights field, see Mann, Gruskin, Grodin, and Annas 1999. More recently, the British Medical Association (2001) has published a volume that looks specifically at the medical profession and its role on both sides of the human rights equation—the abuse, as well as the promotion and support, of human rights.

41. These outcomes range from increased handgun violence, as Briceño-León and Zubillaga (2002) argue, to coups d'état. In fact, the link between these policies and violent outcomes is regarded as determinant by James Galbraith, whose analysis is worth citing at length:

> After honing [neoliberal] policies in Latin America, they were applied after 1989 in Russia and Eastern Europe, and then in Asia.
>
> Everywhere, crisis ensued. Only where countries successfully resisted the neoliberal policy prescriptions—most notably in China, in Northern Europe, and in the United States itself after the mid-1990s—did growth continue and pay inequality remain under reasonable control.
>
> It is not, then, by accident that the effects of neoliberalism at a global level resemble those of a coup d'état at a national level.
>
> In an early analysis using UTIP's data set, George Purcell and I calculated the average effects of twenty-seven coups d'état on our measurements of pay inequality. We found a pattern of striking consistency. After rising four and five years before the coup, inequality would decline sharply in the two years immediately beforehand. In the year of the coup itself, the decline in inequality would stop. And in the five repressive years that followed (coups, as distinct from revolutions, are almost invariably right-wing), rising inequality would occur systematically in each year, until overall inequality stood far higher than in the period before the coup (2002, pp. 24–25).

PART I. THOUGHTS ON BEARING WITNESS

1. Bourgois 1995, p. 18. In her classic essay on "studying up," Nader (1972) notes that, "unfortunately, our findings have often served to help manipulate rather than aid those we study" (p. 294). Bourgois also examines some of the dilemmas inherent in publicly exposing details of the lives of the poor and the powerless when writing about them. In discussing his research on street life and the underground economy of East Harlem, he observes that, on the one hand, it is "imperative from a personal and ethical perspective, as well as from an analytic and theoretical one, to expose the horrors I witnessed among the people I befriended, without censoring even the goriest details. The depth and overwhelming pain and terror of the experience of poverty and racism in the United States needs to be talked about openly and confronted squarely, even if that makes us uncomfortable" (1995, p. 18). On the other hand, in line with Nader's admonition that what we write about the poor will be used against them, Bourgois reflects on his own concern and worry about the political consequences of exposing the lives of these vulnerable people to public scrutiny. In her 1972 essay, Nader provides a countervailing method for at least balancing out both what we know and who we scrutinize, by urging us to also "study up":

> The study of man is confronted with an unprecedented situation: never before have so few, by their actions and inactions, had the power of life and death over so many members of the species.... Studying "up" as well as "down" would lead us to ask many "common sense" questions in reverse. Instead of asking why some people are poor, we would ask why other people are so affluent? How on earth would a social scientist explain the hoarding patterns of the American rich and middle class? How can we explain the fantastic resistance to change among those whose options "appear to be many"? How has it come to be, we might ask, that anthropologists are more interested in why peasants don't change than why the auto industry doesn't innovate, or why the Pentagon or universities cannot be more organizationally creative? The conservatism of such major institutions and bureaucratic organizations probably has wider implications for the species and for theories of change than does the conservatism of the peasantry (pp. 284, 289).

2. Indeed, Clifford Geertz (1988) has said that proof of "being there" is the primary function of many of the ethnographic nuggets that one finds strewn throughout the classic works of anthropology.

3. I'm ashamed, I mean, to be impressed by fashionable but shoddy thinking. As Christopher Norris notes in his devastating essay *Uncritical Theory:*

> It is a sad reflection on the currency of "advanced" intellectual debate in the human sciences that so much of what passes for radical theory is in fact quite incapable of mustering resistance to a downright conformist or consensus-based account of knowledge, truth, and reality... it is hard to envisage an escape-route from this relativist impasse if rhetoric is indeed the last court of appeal, if truth-claims are nothing more than a species of suasive utterance, and if questions of factual or argumentative validity can only be settled on the terms laid down by some existing communal discourse.... What this argument ignores is the simple point: that *getting things right* as regards the historical record is the only adequate means of counteracting the various myths, pseudo-histories, propaganda ploys or strong revisionist narratives that can otherwise be invented pretty much

to order by those with the power to intervene in the production of socially-acceptable truth (1992, pp. 126, 129–30).

Nicole Polier and William Roseberry explore the impact of postmodernism in anthropology in a 1989 essay, "Tristes Tropes."
4. Scheper-Hughes 2000b, pp. xvi–xvii.

CHAPTER 1. ON SUFFERING AND STRUCTURAL VIOLENCE

1. The embodiment paradigm, for which we are to some extent indebted to Merleau-Ponty (e.g., 1945), has been used widely in medical anthropology. For a helpful review, see Csordas 1990 and 1994.

2. Sidney Mintz reminds us of the non-newness of many of the global phenomena under study today. More specifically, the history of Haiti and much of the Caribbean presages current critiques concerning transnationalism:

> Why, then, has the vocabulary of those events become so handy for today's transnationalists? Is one entitled to wonder whether this means that the world has now become a macrocosm of what the Caribbean region was, in the 16th century? If so, should we not ask what took the world so long to catch up—especially since what is happening now is supposed to be qualitatively so different from the recent past? Or is it rather that the Caribbean experience was merely one chapter of a book being written, before the name of the book—world capitalism—became known to its authors? (Mintz 1997, p. 120).

3. Weise 1971, p. 38.
4. Galeano 1973, p. 112. It's worth noting that those with miserable jobs are nonetheless considered fortunate in a country where unemployment is estimated, by the omniscient Central Intelligence Agency, at about 70 percent (U.S. Central Intelligence Agency 2001). It's no wonder that the CIA is interested in the matter: Haiti was, until quite recently, one of the world's leading assemblers of U.S. goods. For more on the conditions of Haitian workers in U.S.-owned offshore assembly plants, see Kernaghan 1993. Of course, U.S. industries are not alone in exploiting cheap Haitian labor, as evidenced by a recent report on labor conditions on the orange plantations that lend Grand Marnier liqueur its distinctive tang; see Butler 2000.

5. In addition to standard indices of well-being and development, the "human suffering index" takes into account such factors as access to clean drinking water, daily caloric intake, religious and political freedom, respect for civil rights, and degree of gender inequality. For information about the human suffering index and how it was derived, see the Web site at *http://www.basics.org/programs /basics1/haiti.html.*

6. Depending on the source, the demographic statistics vary. According to the World Health Organization's *World Health Report 2000,* life expectancy at birth is 52.8 years, while the mortality rate for children under five is 115.5 per 1,000 births (World Health Organization 2000c). The CIA, which should know, reports even grimmer statistics: life expectancy of 47.5 years for men and 49.2 years for women (U.S. Central Intelligence Agency 2000b). Life expectancy is likely lower and mortality rates are likely higher in the Central Plateau than elsewhere in Haiti. See also United Nations Development Programme 2001.

7. For reviews of morbidity and mortality in Haiti, see the reports from the World Health Organization (WHO) and the United Nations Development Programme (UNDP) mentioned in note 6. The Pan American Health Organization (PAHO) regularly updates its data on Haiti (see Pan American Health Organization 2001). For a review of health trends in central Haiti, see Farmer and Bertrand 2000 as well as Farmer 1999b; the latter volume also presents pertinent information on HIV and tuberculosis in Haiti. Those seeking the latest available data on HIV should consult UNAIDS/World Health Organization 2000, with updated information on the Web. Underreporting, in large part a result of weak surveillance, is a major hindrance to those seeking to interpret official data and its echoes by the PAHO or the WHO. For example, the PAHO noted that Haiti reported 10,237 cases of tuberculosis in 1991, giving an estimated incidence of 154.7 per 100,000 population. In that same period (May 1990 to August 1992), Desormeaux and colleagues performed a house-to-house survey in Cité Soleil, an urban slum, and came up with a figure of 2,281 per 100,000 population. Among the HIV-infected, TB prevalence exceeded 5,770 per 100,000 population. See Pan American Health Organization 2001; Desormeaux, Johnson, Coberly, et al. 1996.

8. It's hard to think of a more compelling example than the 1981 massacre of all the inhabitants of El Mozote, El Salvador, by U.S.-trained and U.S.-funded troops. Leigh Binford lays out the challenges faced by those who would bring such events to broader attention:

> From January 1983 through December 1989, "El Mozote" was cited in a mere fifteen articles published in major U.S. and Canadian newspapers. (During this same period the U.S. government provided the Salvadoran military with more than $500 million in direct military assistance.)...The coverage of El Mozote shows us that for the journalists, no less than for most people of the West, the daily lives of billions of people in the rest of the world do not exist outside the parameters of crisis or scandal: hurricanes, earthquakes, volcanic eruptions, droughts, crop failures, and civil wars (1996, p. 4).

9. The names of the Haitians cited here have been changed, as have the names of their home villages.

10. There is a large literature concerning the impact of dams on the lives of those displaced. In anthropology, a classic example would be the 1971 study by Elizabeth Colson. Alaka Wali (1989) charts the fate of those displaced by a hydroelectric dam in eastern Panama. Two different, more recent books on this subject provide poignant examples of the consequences of building big dams: Arundhati Roy's *Cost of Living* (1999) includes a passionate protest against the Sardar Samovar Dam in the Narmada Valley of India; Patrick McCully's *Silenced Rivers: The Ecology and Politics of Large Dams* (1996) details the specific effects of big dams on the health of the displaced (see esp. McCully's chapter "Dams and Disease," pp. 86–100). Michael Ignatieff outlines the links between human rights and dam projects in specific terms:

> A human rights perspective on development, for example, would be critical of any macroeconomic strategy that purchased aggregate economic growth at the price of the rights of significant groups of individuals. A dam project that boosts

electro-generation capacity at the price of flooding the lands of poor people without compensation and redress is an injustice, even if the aggregate economic benefit of such a measure is clear (2001, p. 167).

11. Chapter 2 discusses this matter in greater detail. For a comprehensive and well-documented overview of the plight of Haitian refugees, see "Symposium: The Haitian Refugee Crisis: A Closer Look" 1993, a special issue of the *Georgetown Immigration Law Journal.* In an excellent overview of the roots of human rights violations in Haiti, an essay in that issue describes the Reagan-Duvalier pact (Executive Order 12,324 issued by Ronald Reagan on September 29, 1981) as follows:

> The Interdiction Program worked with grim efficiency during the Duvalier era. From its inception in late 1981, thousands of Haitians have been stopped and forcibly repatriated to Haiti. In every case, the Coast Guard destroyed the Haitian vessel and the Coast Guard cutter returned crowded with Haitian asylum-seekers to Port-au-Prince. Despite well-documented evidence of gross and systematic human rights abuses during the Duvalier era and under the succeeding military governments, all but eight of the approximately 23,000 interdicted Haitians were returned to Haiti from October 1981 to September 1991 when President Aristide was overthrown in a military coup. Interviews conducted on the Coast Guard cutters were inherently flawed and help explain the blanket finding that all those interdicted were "economic refugees" (O'Neill 1993, p. 96).

O'Neill also provides a figure of 24,559 Haitian refugees applying for asylum during this period.

12. For more on U.S. aid to the military "governments" of post-Duvalier Haiti, see Farmer 1994 and Ridgeway 1994. Hancock (1989) also discusses the impact of U.S. aid to the Duvalier regimes.

13. This topic is discussed, at greater length and in general terms, in Farmer, Connors, and Simmons 1996. Concerning the expanding epidemic of HIV in Haiti and its relationship to structural violence, see Farmer 1992a and 1999b. For more on the situation currently confronted by Haitian women, most of whom live in poverty, see the review by Neptune-Anglade (1986) and the testimonies collected by Racine (1999). More recently, Beverly Bell (2001) documents stories of Haitian women's struggles for survival as well as resistance against tyranny and terror.

14. For an overview of the human rights situation after the 1991 coup, see Americas Watch and the National Coalition for Haitian Refugees 1993 and O'Neill 1993. For a review of these and other reports, see Farmer 1994. Additional reports include Inter-American Commission on Human Rights 1994 and United Nations Human Rights Commission 1995 as well as the report on internal displacement issued in 1994 by Human Rights Watch/Americas, Jesuit Refugee Service/USA, and the National Coalition for Haitian Refugees.

Toward the end of the Cédras-led coup, which led to thousands of outright murders, the army and paramilitary began a campaign of politically motivated rape. One survey terms this campaign "arguably the greatest crime against womankind in the Caribbean since slavery" (Rey 1999, p. 74). See also Human Rights Watch/Americas and National Coalition for Haitian Refugees 1994. It was during these years that our clinic received its first rape victims (Farmer 1996a); one of my patients went on to testify about politically motivated rapes in a hearing on this topic held by the Organization of American States.

15. Some would argue that the relationship between individual agency and supraindividual structures forms the central problematic of contemporary social theory. I have tried, in this discussion, to avoid what Pierre Bourdieu has termed "the absurd opposition between individual and society," and here acknowledge the influence of Bourdieu, who has contributed enormously to the debate on structure and agency. For a concise statement of his (often revised) views on this subject, see Bourdieu 1990. That a supple and fundamentally nondeterministic model of agency would have such a deterministic—and pessimistic—"feel" is largely a reflection of my topic, suffering, and my "fieldwork site," which is Haiti. The relationship between agency and human rights is traced by Ignatieff, among others:

> We know from historical experience that when human beings have defensible rights—when their agency as individuals is protected and enhanced—they are less likely to be abused and oppressed. On these grounds, we count the diffusion of human rights instruments as progress even if there remains an unconscionable gap between the instruments and the actual practices of states charged to comply with them (2001, p. 4).

16. Chopp 1986, p. 2.

17. I have made this argument at greater length elsewhere; see Farmer 1992a, chap. 22. The term "historical system" is used following Immanuel Wallerstein, who for many years has argued that even the most far-flung locales—Haiti's Central Plateau, for example—are part of the same social and economic nexus: "By the late nineteenth century, for the first time ever, there existed only one historical system on the globe. We are still in that situation today" (Wallerstein 1987, p. 318). See also his initial, magisterial formulation, *The Modern World-System: Capitalist Agriculture and the Origins of the European World-Economy in the Sixteenth Century* (1974).

18. Chopp 1986, p. 2. See also the works of Gustavo Gutiérrez (1973 and 1983, for example), who has written a great deal about the meaning of suffering in the twentieth century. (These books are cited more extensively in Chapter 5.) For anthropological studies of liberation theology in social context, see Burdick 1993 and Lancaster 1988.

19. Boff 1989, p. 20.

20. Brown 1993, p. 44.

21. The connections between the fecklessness of the powerful and the fates of the fragile have been well traced. The political economy of genocide is explored in Simpson 1993; see also Aly, Chroust, and Pross 1994. On the transnational political economy of human rights abuses, see Chomsky and Herman 1979a and 1979c, a two-volume study. When Mike Davis explores "late Victorian holocausts," which led to some fifty million deaths, he concludes that "we are not dealing, in other words, with 'lands of famine' becalmed in stagnant backwaters of world history, but with the fate of tropical humanity at the precise moment (1870–1914) when its labor and products were being dynamically conscripted into a London-centered world economy. Millions died, not outside

the 'modern world system,' but in the very process of being forcibly incorporated into its economic and political structures" (2001, p. 9).

22. For historical background on Haiti, see James 1980, Mintz 1974, and Trouillot 1990.

23. Sen 1998, p. 2.

24. Rosaldo and Lamphere 1974. For differing views, see Leacock 1981.

25. Koss, Koss, and Woodruff 1991, p. 342. From November 1995 to May 1996, the National Institute of Justice and the Centers for Disease Control jointly conducted a national telephone survey that confirmed the high rates of assault against U.S. women (Tjaden and Thoennes 1998). See also Bachman and Saltzman 1995.

26. It is important to note, however, that in many societies upper-class or upper-caste women are also subject to laws that virtually efface marital rape. The study by Koss, Koss, and Woodruff (1991) includes this crime with other forms of criminal victimization, but such information is collected only through community-based surveys.

27. Ward 1993, p. 414.

28. A recent joint report by WHO, UNICEF, and UNFPA on estimated maternal mortality for 1995 notes that of the 515,000 estimated maternal deaths worldwide, only 0.2 percent, or 1,200, occurred in industrialized countries. The lifetime risk of maternal death for women in such countries is calculated at 1:4,085, whereas for women in developing nations, the risk is much higher, at 1:61. In fact, for the subgroup of countries characterized as "least developed"— of which Haiti is one—the estimated risk of maternal death is, tragically, even higher, at 1:16 (World Health Organization, United Nations Children's Fund, United Nations Population Fund 2001, p. 48).

29. The maternal mortality rate (MMR) of 523 deaths is for the year 2000 and is based on reports from the national health authority to PAHO; see Pan American Health Organization 2001. The much higher rate of 1,100 maternal deaths per 100,000 live births comes from the joint report published by WHO, UNICEF, and UNFPA; see World Health Organization, United Nations Children's Fund, United Nations Population Fund 2001 (p. 44). These numbers are likely to be even higher if one measures maternal mortality at the community level. The only community-based survey done in Haiti, conducted in 1985 around the town of Jacmel in southern Haiti, found that maternal mortality was 1,400 per 100,000 live births (Jean-Louis 1989). During that same period, "official" statistics reported much lower rates for Haiti, ranging from an MMR of 230 for the years 1980–87 (United Nations Development Programme 1990, p. 148) and an MMR of 340 for 1980–85 to a higher estimate in the years that followed, 1987–92, of 600 maternal deaths per 100,000 live births (World Bank 1994a, p. 148). For additional maternal mortality data from that period, see World Health Organization 1985.

30. Sen 1998, p. 13. For an in-depth discussion of the population-based impact of gender bias in poor countries, see Sen's classic essay on "missing women" (Sen 1992b).

Sen summarizes the potential impact of public action in poor regions by examining Kerala state:

Kerala's experience suggests that "gender bias" against females can be radically changed by public action—involving both the government and the public itself—especially through female education, opportunities for women to have responsible jobs, women's legal rights on property, and by enlightened egalitarian politics. Correspondingly, the problem of "missing women" can also be largely solved through social policy and political radicalism. Women's movements can play a very important part in bringing about this type of change, and in making the political process in poor countries pay serious attention to the deep inequalities from which women suffer. It is also interesting to note, in this context, that the narrowly economic variables, such as GNP or GDP per head, on which so much of standard development economics concentrates, give a very misleading picture of economic and social progress (1998, p. 15).

31. Nightingale, Hannibal, Geiger, et al. 1990, p. 2098; emphasis added. For a more in-depth account, and a more complicated view of the mechanisms by which apartheid and the South African economy are related to disease causation, see Packard 1989.

32. Although HIV is said to have recently "taken off" among South Africa's black population, it has been, from the beginning, an epidemic disproportionately affecting black people in that country. South African data indicate that in 1994, when seventeen white women were diagnosed with AIDS, almost fifteen hundred black women—nearly one hundred times as many—had the disease (Department of Health, Republic of South Africa 1995, p. 67).

Even after the dismantling of the apartheid system, HIV continues to disproportionately affect black South Africans (Lurie, Harrison, Wilkinson, et al. 1997). As Chapman and Rubenstein (1998) note in a report for the American Association for the Advancement of Science and Physicians for Human Rights, "the epidemiology of the HIV/AIDS epidemic...demonstrates the link between poverty, low status and vulnerability to infection" (p. 20). They report the "rigid segregation of health facilities; grossly disproportionate spending on the health of whites as compared to blacks, resulting in world-class medical care for whites while blacks were usually relegated to overcrowded and filthy facilities; public health policies that ignored diseases primarily affecting black people; and the denial of basic sanitation, clean water supply, and other components of public health to homelands and townships" (p. xix). Along with being denied medical services, many black South Africans were forced to relocate to townships and were later forced, by economic conditions, to live in squatter settlements on the outskirts of cities, creating a culture of migration and disrupted family ties (pp. 18–20). As Lurie and colleagues note, "migrant labour was a central tenet of apartheid, which sought to create a steady flow of cheap black labour to South Africa's mines, industries and farms. A myriad of laws prohibited black South Africans from settling permanently in 'whites only' areas, and as a result, migration patterns in South Africa tend to be circular, with men maintaining close links with their rural homesteads" (1997, p. 18).

This forced system of migration has had a distinct impact on the shaping of the AIDS epidemic. As Carol Kaufman explains, "the system of labor migration remains deeply entrenched, and women who have partners involved in labor circulation are especially vulnerable to unprotected sexual intercourse as well as STDs and HIV/AIDS transmission" (1998, p. 432). Quarraisha and Salim Abdool-Karim cite a 1998 study conducted in rural South Africa which found that "women whose partners spent 10 or fewer nights per month at home had an HIV prevalence of 13.7% compared with 0% in women who spent more than 10 nights in a month with their partners" (1999, p. 139). See Lurie, Harrison, Wilkinson, et al. 1997 for further documentation of this link. Furthermore, data from 1994 reveal that poverty is rampant in South Africa, with close to two-thirds of black households surviving below the minimum subsistence level (Chapman and Rubenstein 1998, p. 20).

33. The National Center for Health Statistics (1998) reported life expectancies at birth in 1996 as 76.8 years for whites and 70.2 years for blacks. Two years later, the same sources suggest a heartening trend: reported life expectancies increased to 77.3 for whites and 71.3 for blacks (National Center for Health Statistics 2000). But the discrepancy is still on the order of 9 to 10 percent of lifespan. For a detailed discussion of recent health status disparities and leading causes of death for African Americans, see Byrd and Clayton 2002, pp. 519–45.

34. Navarro 1990, p. 1238.

35. Ibid., p. 1240.

36. Wilson 1980, p. 178.

37. McCord and Freeman 1990.

38. Sen 1998, p. 17.

39. Although class differences between physicians and university students are not as significant as others examined here, it is notable that a study reported in the *American Journal of Psychiatry* (Klein, Sullivan, Wolcott, et al. 1987) observed that gay psychiatrists were much more likely than students to adopt effective risk reduction. Clearly, many factors—age, educational level, and so on—may be significant here. In the United States, we still lack economically informed studies of risky behavior among gay men; for gay men in France, one study (Pollak 1988) suggests that economic status is important in determining access to information and services.

40. These data are reviewed in Farmer, Walton, and Furin 2000. See also Aalen, Farewell, De Angelis, et al. 1999.

41. Forster 1971, p. 255.

42. See the studies by Hatch (1983) and Gellner (1985). Of course, the discussion of violence and cultural difference is vastly more complicated than that presented here. One consideration is that anthropological confidence in cultural relativism failed not only as part of the shift to studying "complex societies" but also as a result of shifting demographics within anthropology itself. Following World War II, the entrance into U.S. professional anthropology of large numbers of veterans, some of working-class origins and with more radical political orientations, served to significantly undermine the extreme cultural relativist position. By the 1990s, it was no longer unusual to hear comments such as that made by Nancy Scheper-Hughes: "Anthropological relativism is no longer appropriate to the violent, vexed and contested political world in which we now live" (1994, p. 991). At the same time, however, argues William Roseberry, the "profoundly conservative reaction in politics and culture, marked politically by the Reagan victory in 1980," has had its echoes within anthropology: "What

has fallen out of favor? In practice, it seems to be any work that is too ethnographic, too sociological, too structural, too political, too economic, or too processual" (1996, pp. 17, 21).

43. Asad 1975, p. 17.

44. Wagner 1975, p. 2.

45. Johannes Fabian (1983) has argued that this "denial of coevalness" is much ingrained in our discipline. Not to be dismissed as an issue of style, such a denial contributes to the blindness of the anthropologist: "Either he submits to the condition of coevalness and produces ethnographic knowledge, or he deludes himself into temporal distance and *misses the object of his search*" (p. 32; emphasis added). See also Starn 1992.

46. For a penetrating examination of the appropriation of identity politics by big business, see Kauffman 1993. Naomi Klein's more recent work (2000) is a sophisticated study of the same topic.

47. Again, this chapter's discussion necessarily gives short shrift to the complexities of these debates. For a revealing example, see Amede Obiora's 1997 exploration of "polemics and intransigence in the campaign against female circumcision."

48. One recent example of the conflation of structural violence and cultural difference is found in the long lists of reasons given by those who do not believe that AIDS treatment is possible in Africa. One U.S. Treasury Department official—who wisely declined to be identified—observed that "Africa lacked the basic medical and physical infrastructure that would make it possible to deploy effectively the complex cocktail of drugs to fight AIDS. He said Africans lacked a requisite 'concept of time,' implying that they would not benefit from drugs that must be administered on tight time schedules" (Kahn 2001, p. 10).

Officially sanctioned justifications and explanations for structural violence come most often, however, from the reading and writing classes—that is, us. Guatemalan poet Otto René Castillo, who was killed by the Guatemalan army on March 19, 1967, avers that the "apolitical intellectuals" of his country will one day be judged harshly by the poor:

What did you do when the poor
suffered, when tenderness and life
were dangerously burning out in them?

Apolitical intellectuals
of my sweet country,
you will have nothing to say.

A vulture of silence
will eat your guts.
Your own misery
will gnaw at your souls.
And you will be mute
in your shame.

49. Boff and Boff 1987, p. 29.

50. World Health Organization 1995, p. 5.

51. Richard is cited in Nelson-Pallmeyer 1992, p. 14.

CHAPTER 2. PESTILENCE AND RESTRAINT

1. For more on U.S. folk models of Haitians, see Lawless 1992. George Black's wonderful 1988 collection of cartoons, photographs, movie stills, and travel brochures helps reveal the mechanisms by which folk models of Haiti (and other "banana republics") are born and sustained. I have also explored American notions of Haitians in earlier works, Farmer 1992a and 1994.

2. Schmitt 1991.

3. The words of Yolande Jean and of other Haitians quoted in this chapter derive from interviews conducted by the author in 1993. Ms. Jean's name has not been changed, at her own request.

4. In 1912, the annual rent was raised to five thousand dollars. For the text of the Platt Amendment, which formalized these arrangements, see Williams 1970, pp. 420–21.

5. Annas 1993, p. 592.

6. Scheper-Hughes 1994, p. 999.

7. Scheper-Hughes n.d., p. 29. (The page numbers cited are those of the manuscript, which is unpublished.) A similar view is offered by Julie Feinsilver (1993). See also Scheper-Hughes 1993 and 1994.

8. For more on the logic of quarantine and other punitive measures seeking to prevent the spread of sexually transmitted diseases, see Allan Brandt's classic study (1987).

9. O'Neill 1993.

10. Americas Watch, National Coalition for Haitian Refugees, and Physicians for Human Rights 1991.

11. O'Neill 1993, p. 115.

12. Johnson 1993, p. 37.

13. Schmitt 1991. Increasingly, the U.S. military is engaged in what it terms "humanitarian missions." The contradictions of such missions, and of U.S. foreign policy vis-à-vis human rights, are the subject of a powerful essay by Noam Chomsky (1999). See also Michael Ignatieff's pointed discussion of the lessons that "human rights activists from Western liberal democracies may need to learn." Ignatieff continues:

> It is inconsistent to impose international human rights constraints on other states unless we accept the jurisdiction of these instruments on our own. Anglo-Canadians have no business telling Latvia, Lithuania, and Estonia what to do about Russian minority rights unless they accept an obligation to subscribe to OSCE standards in their own treatment of French and aboriginal minorities. Americans have no business lecturing other countries about their human rights performance unless they are prepared to at least enter into dialogue with international rights bodies about sensitive areas—capital punishment and the conditions in American prisons, for example—that may be in contravention of international rights norms. The obligation to at least engage in dialogue is clear, and the obligation that nations actually practice what they preach is the minimum requirement for a legitimate and effective human rights policy (2001, pp. 36–37).

14. Arnesen 1993, p. 5.

15. Powell 1993, p. 59.

16. The half-hearted trade embargo declared against the Haitian military regime had its primary impact among the poor and vulnerable, since it leaked, among other goods, petroleum products; see Farmer 1994 for details. For more information about the impact of these sanctions on health and human rights in Haiti, see Gibbons 1999 as well as Gibbons and Garfield 1999. It is impossible not to discuss the hypocrisy of sanctions as currently used without mentioning the case of Iraq: see Harvard Study Team 1991, Cortright and Lopez 1999. Stephen Marks (1999) has summarized the case against economic sanctions from a human rights perspective. U.S. sanctions against Cuba are as impermeable as the 1992–94 sanctions against Haiti were leaky: "The U.S. sanctions against Cuba are the harshest in the world, much harsher than the sanctions against Iraq" (N. Chomsky 2000, p. 82). I will return to the legitimacy of the U.S. block- ade of Cuba later in this chapter.

17. Schoenholtz 1993, p. 71.

18. McCormick 1993, p. 157.

19. Ibid., p. 159.

20. Annas 1993, p. 590.

21. Cited in ibid.

22. Ibid.

23. And yet, in the United States, this practice has been part of the judicial- punitive process. As Steinbock notes: "Since 1966, there have been at least twenty cases in which judges [in the United States] have ordered criminal defendants to be sterilized, to practice contraception, or to refrain from becoming pregnant" (1996, p. 54).

24. Powell 1993, p. 64. As noted earlier, forced treatment fulfills the legal criteria for the crime of assault.

25. Clinton and Gore 1992, pp. 119–20.

26. Ibid., p. 119.

27. USA Today (magazine), vol. 121, no. 2568; see also the accompanying article, "Making Sense of America's Refugee Policy" (Stein 1992).

28. Take, for example, an editorial that appeared in the Boston Globe de- crying the "political leadership" of the United States for sending so many refugees back to Haiti ("Haitians Abused and Abandoned" 1992). Another editorial in the St. Louis Post-Dispatch bluntly stated that "the U.S. return of the Haitian refugees is an outrage" ("History Repeating by Haitian Return" 1992).

29. Cited in Arnesen 1993, p. 5.

30. See "South Florida Braces for Haitian Time Bomb" 1993.

31. Hilts 1993.

32. Powell 1993, p. 60.

33. Friedman 1993.

34. Cited in Powell 1993, p. 68.

35. For a more in-depth exploration of this folk model, and its relation to AIDS, see Farmer 1992a.

36. McCormick 1993, p. 151.

37. O'Neill 1993, p. 117.

38. Powell 1993, p. 58. Actually, Cuban nationals who reach U.S. soil enjoy a fast, third track, which entitles them to apply for U.S. residency based on the

"wet foot/dry foot" policy (whereas those caught while on the water—"wet foot"—are sent back).

39. McCormick 1993, p. 160.

40. Turque, Reiss, Liu, et al. 1993.

41. Annas 1993, p. 590.

42. Powell 1993, p. 65.

43. All quotations are from interviews I conducted in Cuba. Again, names have not been changed, by request of the interviewees.

44. The scandal of "tainted blood," which has devastated hemophiliacs and others dependent on blood products, was one of the largest political debacles of modern French history and landed several of the nation's highest-ranking health officials in prison; see, for example, the discussion in the volume edited by Feldman and Bayer (1999). Less well known, however, is the fact that U.S. officials were also slow to take decisive action to protect American hemophiliacs; see Keshavjee, Weiser, and Kleinman 2001. Recent reports from the popular press suggest the transfusion of HIV-infected blood is a growing problem in China; see, for example, "Cientos de miles de chinos han contraído el sida por vender su sangre al gobierno" 2001.

45. Personal communication to the author from Dr. José Joanes Fiol, Department of Epidemiology, Santiago de las Vegas, Havana, Cuba (ssida@infomed.sld.cu). At this writing, Cuba still continues to have the lowest HIV incidence in the hemisphere and since September 30, 2001, has registered only two more cases, with a total now of twelve cases of transfusion-associated HIV, with only two of these being hemophiliacs. As of April 2002, all 556 patients with advanced HIV disease receive highly active antiretroviral therapy with drugs that began to be produced in Cuba in 2001 (Castro, Farmer, and Barberia 2002).

46. Both Feinsilver (1993) and A. Chomsky (2000) underline this point; see also MacDonald 1999. Adds Scheper-Hughes, "AIDS was never treated in Cuba (as it was in virtually all western democracies) as a 'special case,' one to be treated gingerly by public officials for fear of offending or stigmatizing high risk populations. Instead, it was viewed and treated as any other threat to public health following a model of socialist rational planning that flies in the face of the global neo-liberal political spirit of the times" (1994, p. 997).

47. Scheper-Hughes described the clash of cultures as follows:

> By the end of the first year in the sanatorium, military doctors were perplexed by the growing number of ordinary civilians—most of them self defined homosexuals or bisexuals—who tested positive in their neighborhood clinics and began arriving at the sanatorium. Problems initially erupted between this new population and the defensively homophobic "internationalists," and the first dozen homosexuals were segregated from "the soldiers." The civilians were also discriminated against in terms of access to facilities and to recreation and other privileges. During this first phase of the sanatorium, medicalized prison camp is a good enough description of the institution and the international human rights community had reason for alarm (1994, p. 999).

The topic of Cuban attitudes toward homosexuality, and their relation to the country's AIDS policies, has been explored by Marvin Leiner (1994).

48. Scheper-Hughes 1994, p. 1000. She further notes that "a gay Cuban film-maker has produced a critical documentary, 'Beyond Outcasts,' that explores the feelings of those small number of sanatorium residents who have been denied the status, personal liberty, and autonomy of 'guaranteed' patients. Their anger and humiliation over the alternative 'chaperone' system is vividly documented" (ibid.).

49. As is often the case with all things Cuban, there is a great deal of documentation of trends during this period. I base my description on data from the Cuban Ministry of Public Health, but a very similar picture emerges in external studies as well. See, for example, the exhaustive review by the Comisión Económica para América Latina y el Caribe (1997).

50. On the wall opposite the portrait is a modernistic painting of Christ on the cross, looking sorrowfully down on legions of boat people. Although the U.S. press paints Cuba as anti-religious, even a brief visit to the island suggests that expressions of religious faith are welcome in modern Cuba. Many of the patients I've visited have Bibles by their bedside. Another subtle hint is found in the giant statue of Christ overlooking old Havana. Illuminated at night by what one assumes is state electric power, the towering icon was completed just before the revolution and is locally termed *Cristo Libertador*. For more on Cuban official-dom's views on religion, see *Fidel and Religion* (Castro 1987), a series of conversations between Castro and a Dominican monk.

51. A. Chomsky 2000, p. 340. A perusal of national headlines from the late 1980s offers a number of examples of the bias that characterized much of the popular reporting on the Cuban AIDS program: "Cuba's AIDS Center Resembles Prison" (Rowley 1989); "Cuba's Callous War on AIDS" (Betancourt 1988); "Cuba's AIDS Quarantine Center Called 'Frightening'" (Zonana 1988). Later reports tended to provide more balanced views but were still often skewed toward presenting a negative image: for example, "Patients Pay High Price in Cuba's War on AIDS" (Golden 1995).

52. As Peter Schwab has noted, "Economic and social human rights are fundamental to Cuba. The state, according to the Cuban constitution, is obligated to provide the essential elements required by any people for survival (such as medical care and employment), while the population in turn is obligated to accept that 'The Republic of Cuba is a Socialist State'" (1999, p. 9).

53. Molinert's statement is from an interview accorded Karen Wald in 1989; cited in A. Chomsky 2000, pp. 339–40.

54. See Betancourt 1988, Golden 1995. Nancy Scheper-Hughes was criticized bitterly by some of her peers when she attempted to reflect on the different approaches to responding to HIV taken in Brazil and Cuba and the United States:

> What critics in the west call "quarantine," if they are being delicate, or "concentration or prison camps" if they are not, Cubans call "sanatoriums" intended for the evaluation, monitoring, and treatment of seropositive people. The point of the sanatorium, Cuban health officials argue, was never "quarantine" since HIV is not an air borne virus. However, HIV is viewed as a transmissible condition and as the dangerously latent phase of the AIDS syndrome. The purpose of the sanatorium is aggressive medical treatment, research and experimental testing of new drugs, and close epidemiological surveillance (1994, p. 998).

55. The World Health Organization official is cited in A. Chomsky 2000, p. 338.

56. Taubes 1997, p. 174. The article further accused the Cuban government of violating the human rights of a physician who had been denouncing an official cover-up of the outbreak. The director of Cuba's infectious-disease institute, wounded by an attack from within the scientific community, was proven correct when he predicted, "I doubt they will run my rebuttal."

57. Chelala 2000.

58. Mittal and Rosset 1999, p. viii.

59. World Health Organization 2000c, pp. 188–89.

60. Although Cubans have generally remained healthy despite the economic crisis, Hansen and Groce (2001) suggest that current conditions have led the Cuban government to promote tourism, and, as in other settings where tourism functions across steep social gradients, commercial sex work has again emerged. Since HIV is so much rarer in Cuba than in expatriate visitors, the risk of contracting HIV from foreigners will no doubt rise. The authors argue that a condom promotion campaign is thus timely and could be accomplished within Cuba's health care infrastructure.

61. For evidence of a viral etiology for the outbreak of optic neuritis, see Mas, Pelegrino, Guzman, et al. 1997; Ito, Nishibe, and Inoue 1998.

62. Dirección Nacional de Estadísticas del Ministerio de Salud Pública, de la República de Cuba 1998. See also Comisión Económica para América Latina y el Caribe 1997.

63. The infant mortality rate (IMR) for Haiti for the year 2000 is 80.3 per 1,000 live births (Pan American Health Organization 2001). As this book goes to press, Cuba reports an IMR of 6.2 per 1,000 live births, thus sharing, along with Canada, the lowest rate in this hemisphere (*Boletín de la Organización Panamericana de la Salud-Cuba* 2002, p. 4). Compare this to the IMR for the United States, which is 7.1 per 1,000 live births. The discrepancies are even greater when one looks at this statistic by race, since the U.S. IMR for white infants is 5.8 per 1,000 live births, whereas that for black infants is 14.6 per 1,000 (Kaiser Family Foundation 1999). Statistics are similar for the city of Boston, where in 1999 the IMR was 7.4 deaths per 1,000 live births. Racial disparities are also evident at this local level: black infants have a mortality rate of 13.1 per 1,000 live births, compared to the IMR of 5.6 per 1,000 live births among whites. Part of this discrepancy is a result of the increasing proportion of extremely low birthweight black babies. In the neighborhood of Roxbury, where Mission Hill is located, 11.9 percent of all babies born have a low birthweight—the second highest rate of all Boston neighborhoods (Boston Public Health Commission 2001, pp. 53–54).

64. Representative Alcee Hastings, Democrat of Fort Lauderdale, quoted in a *Boston Globe* interview (A. Walker 2000).

65. Ibid.

66. Coatsworth 2000.

67. Peter Schwab's assessment of the real purpose of the embargo rings true, as the U.S. government has taken pains to tighten sanctions in spite of clear evidence that their only victims are among the vulnerable:

The real goal of many of the embargo's supporters is not the achievement of better relations with Cuba that might lead to increased political rights for its citizens, but the overthrow of Fidel Castro. In profiling the inconsistency of America's embargo war against Cuba, [Jimmy] Carter developed for all who cared to notice perspective as to the reasons why the embargo has been a conspicuous failure: Written in the lofty language of trying to move Cuba toward democracy, its real purposes are treacherous and violent and have nothing at all to do with achieving that goal. Its unstated but obvious effort is the violation of the human rights of Cubans by trying to destroy and eliminate the only leader in contemporary times who has tried to stand up for the Cuban people (1999, pp. 17–18).

In an essay subtitled "David vs. Goliath," Noam Chomsky summarizes the long history of U.S. sanctions against Cuba, reaching a conclusion similar to Schwab's:

The real problem of Cuba remains what it has always been. It remains the threat of "the Castro idea of taking matters into [your] own hands," which continues to be a stimulus to poor and underprivileged people who can't get it driven into their heads that they have no right to seek opportunities for a decent living. And Cuba, unfortunately, keeps making that clear, for example, by sending doctors all over the world at a rate way beyond any other country despite its current straits, which are severe, and by maintaining, unimaginably, a health system that is a deep embarrassment to the United States. Because of concerns such as these, and because of the fanaticism that goes way back in American history, the U.S. government, for the moment, at least, is continuing the hysterical attack, and will do so until it is deterred (2000, p. 92).

68. Some have worried that Taliban and al-Qaeda prisoners held on Guantánamo are being mistreated—one physician recently described their living conditions as "bordering on torture." See Dyer 2002.

69. Concannon 2001a, p. 641.

70. Ibid., p. 642.

71. Ibid., p. 645.

72. Ibid., p. 644.

73. On Earth Day in April 2000, the year of the Raboteau trial, the Philadelphia municipal incinerator ash was finally removed from Gonaïves. This was a result of significant collaborative efforts by the Haitian government, Greenpeace, Essential Action, and a coalition of Haitian environmental groups, along with the New York Trade Waste Commission. These efforts culminated in the removal of the ash to a barge for temporary storage in the United States. See Karshan 2000.

74. Concannon 2001a, p. 647.

75. United Nations 2000.

76. Hayner 2001, p. 204.

77. Ibid., pp. 203–4.

78. Both men had settled comfortably in Florida—Valmond is a church pastor, and Dorélien won $3.2 million in the lottery. Former army major general Jean-Claude Duperval is also living in Florida, where he worked at Disney World until a story in *Newsweek* publicized his conviction in the Raboteau massacre. He has thus far avoided deportation, although the INS is currently appealing an

immigration judge's decision in Duperval's favor. See Lush 2002; Fainaru 1999; Contreras 2002; Lambert, Tauber, and Tresinowski 2002. See also Amnesty International 2002 for numerous other case studies of torturers living within the United States.

79. Grann 2001.

80. This complex process has been described concisely by Lovinsky Pierre-Antoine, who contends not only that the "intellectual branch of the failed coup" is to be found among the Convergence leaders but also that among their supporters are unlikely bedfellows, including "certain human rights organizations" (2002, p. 13).

81. Dame Eugenia Charles, the former prime minister of Dominica, who was recently appointed Caricom representative to the Organization of American States/Caricom mission to Haiti, remarked in an interview: "After listening to the members of Convergence, I had to ask them why they called themselves 'Convergence.' They were not converging on anything. They were not agreeing on anything. They cannot get together to form a plan. No one in Convergence was talking about what the Haitian people themselves want" (in Ross-Robinson 2001, p. 1).

82. According to a U.S.-sponsored Gallup poll conducted in 2000, the groups composing the convergence had a 4 percent credibility rating (CID/Gallup 2000); their electoral support was around 12 percent in this same year. See Brian Concannon's essay dealing with the subject, available online at *http://www.uchastings.edu/boswell_01/Brian%20on%20Dec%2017.htm*.

83. Amy Wilentz wrote a wonderful account of these years: "As Namphy's regime became weaker and more violent, such groundless rumors against Aristide—which you could hear from the mouths of bishops and ambassadors... grew wilder and more fantastic. Eventually, whisperers would accuse him of involvement in the attack on the [1987] presidential elections, would say that he had invented out of whole cloth various Church orders against himself, would even go so far as to claim that Aristide himself had paid a band of men to feign an assassination attempt against him. In other words, every action of the right-wing forces was accompanied by a rumor blaming Aristide for the thing. The campaign seemed organized—each rumor popped up whole and was reiterated each time by the same bunch of people" (1989, p. 115).

84. In one of the few sensible editorial commentaries to appear in the past few months, Larry Birns and Michael McCarthy (2001) put it clearly: "The Convergence appears to many as a bad-faith negotiator intent on fueling local and international anti-Aristide sentiment by sabotaging his as well as Haiti's prospects. Essentially, Convergence's negotiating position is non-negotiation. While Convergence is Washington's and the publicly funded International Republican Institute's faithful legate on the island, it is held in contempt by most Haitians who cannot understand why the United States views Aristide as a rogue radical, rather than a precious asset in whom the majority of Haitians believe." Another editorial commentary, by Joseph E. Baptiste and Bob Maguire (2001), concurs: "The recent approval by the Organization of American States of a carefully worded resolution endorsing Haitian President Jean-Bertrand Aristide's proposals aimed at breaking his country's political impasse is encouraging news to all who desire progress in Haiti. The immediate negative response to the OAS action by the Democratic Con-

vergence, a coalition of small political groups whose unyielding opposition to Aristide is virtually all they have in common, is very discouraging.... Sadly, this response of Haiti's so-called 'democratic opposition' has become predictable."

85. See the Web site for the National Endowment for Democracy at *http://www.ned.org/about/faq.html.*

86. Burns 2001.

87. An example closer to home is Nicaragua, where Arnoldo Alemán of the Liberal Constitutionalist Party (PLC) was elected president in 1996. Despite Alemán's record as head of what was possibly the most corrupt executive branch in Latin America, the PLC retained power in the elections of November 2001. Many attribute the victory of PLC candidate Enrique Bolanos to U.S. support and intimidation. The pro-Sandinista daily *El Nuevo Diario* reported that U.S. Ambassador Oliver Garza spoke in "a threatening tone" when discussing the repercussions of a possible win by Sandinista candidate Daniel Ortega. In the month before the election, Governor Jeb Bush of Florida (2001) wrote an editorial in the *Miami Herald* attacking Ortega: "It would seem inconceivable that a people would choose to return to a totalitarian past.... [Daniel Ortega] is a foe of the values for which the United States stands." This article was translated and run in the conservative Nicaraguan daily *La Prensa* and may have reversed the lead that Ortega—not without his own checkered past—had built in the polls. See Council on Hemispheric Affairs 2001; Campbell 2001, p. 17.

88. See Gibbons 1999. The author has qualms about all sanctions, including the leaky ones against the military regimes. I would only add that surely it is even worse to enforce sanctions against a democratically elected government.

89. See the IDB's country assessment on Haiti (Robert and Machado 2001).

90. Lee 2002. Congresswoman Lee introduced House Congressional Resolution 382, titled "Urging the President to end any embargo against Haiti and to no longer require, as a condition of providing humanitarian and development assistance to Haiti, the resolution of the political impasse in Haiti, and for other purposes"; see U.S. House 2002.

91. Norton 2002.

92. In 2000 and 2001, there were thirteen laboratory-confirmed cases of polio in the Dominican Republic and eight in Haiti (Centers for Disease Control and Prevention 2001).

93. Cited in Schmidt 1971, p. 28.

94. Birns and McCarthy 2001.

95. The events of September 11 and their aftermath have dominated the popular press in recent months. Although the scope of the debate is too large to address here, see Wright 2002 and Dowd 2002 for coverage that calls into question recent U.S. government actions.

96. Concannon 2001b, p. 24.

CHAPTER 3. LESSONS FROM CHIAPAS

1. Modern liberation theologians, who claim Las Casas as one of their own precursors, assert that his metanoia followed his reflections, in the setting of a Hispaniola *encomienda,* on Ecclesiastes 34:18–22:

Bread is life to the destitute,
and to deprive them of it is murder.
To rob your neighbor of his livelihood is to kill him,
And he who defrauds a worker of his wages sheds blood.

2. Gustavo Gutiérrez, cited often in these pages, believes that accusations of Las Casas's involvement in the African slave trade are inaccurate. For more on the life and example of Fray Bartolomé, see Gutiérrez's important study (1993). Some have held that, in order to spare the Indians, Las Casas suggested to King Charles V of Spain that each white settler be issued a license to import twelve African slaves (see, for example, James 1980). Given the precedents, however, Rout is probably correct when he suggests that "it is more than likely that this decision would have been made even if Charles's friend, Las Casas, [had] never suggested the importation of blacks to Hispaniola" (1976, p. 24). See also Patterson 1979 and Mintz 1977.

3. Ross 1995, p. 15.

4. John Womack Jr.'s wonderful biography of Zapata, published in 1968, remains the classic account of this remarkable life. It's our good fortune that Womack has also published a historical reader on the rebellion in Chiapas (1999). This chapter is much informed by Womack's understanding of modern Mexico.

5. Comandancia General del EZLN 1993; my translation. Other similar translations can be found in Womack 1999 and in Marcos and the Zapatista Army of National Liberation 1995.

6. Whether or not the revolt was scheduled to coincide with the signing of NAFTA is the subject of some debate. When Subcomandante Marcos was asked about the timing of the uprising, he reportedly remarked, "It's like the myth of the facemasks. We used facemasks because of the cold. But suddenly the facemasks caught on with the people, and so now we keep them on. We had not planned to rise up on January 1" (Collier 1994, p. 86; Collier quotes from Subcomandante Marcos's interviews with journalists, e.g., *Tiempo*, February 26, 1994, p. 3). At other times, Marcos seemed to contradict this assertion. John Ross notes that "Marcos and other EZLN officers suggest that the Zapatistas, sensing they were being discounted by the Mexican government because passage of NAFTA by the U.S. Congress was [President] Salinas's abiding consideration, selected January 1st, the very day his pet treaty took effect, to retaliate for being ignored for so long" (1995, p. 35). Selected writings of Subcomandante Marcos were published in 2001 under the title *Our Word Is Our Weapon*.

7. For more on this topic, see Womack 1999 and Ross 1995.

8. For more on representations of the Chiapas struggle, see Hellman 2000. The Zapatistas have concentrated a good deal of their efforts on the war of words, as Womack suggests:

> In military terms the EZLN offensive was a wonderful success on the first day, a pitiful calamity on the second....But politically the Zapatistas had thrown the country into a tremendous uproar. Their first "Declaration from the Lacandón Jungle" resounded nationally like the trumpets of Jericho. And their "Revolutionary Legislation" broadcast a radical egalitarianism deeply dreadful to some, but deeply appealing to many others. A public hoping through NAFTA to estab-

lish itself in "the First World" suddenly had to recognize how deeply a part of "the Third World" it also remained. To their immense credit, within a few days, amid stupefying confusion and bewildering denunciations left, right, and center, most Mexicans outside Chiapas formed two clear, simple opinions: they were for the poor Indians in Chiapas, and they were against war (1999, pp. 43–44; paragraphing altered).

The poignancy of this conditional support was not lost on Zapatista leadership, as the following letter (Marcos and the Zapatista Army of National Liberation 1995, pp. 118–19) to schoolchildren in the northern border town of Jalisco suggests:

To the Solidarity Committee of Elementary Boarding School #4,
"Beatriz Hernández," Guadalajara, Jalisco

Boys and girls,
We received your letter of February 19, 1994, and the poem "Prayer for Peace" that came with it. It makes us very happy to know that boys and girls who live so far away from our mountains and our misery are concerned that peace should come to Chiapan lands. We thank you very much for your brief letter.

We would like you (and your noble teachers) to know that we did not take up arms for the pleasure of fighting and dying; it is not because we don't want peace that we look for war. We were living without peace already. Our boys and girls are like you, but infinitely poorer. For our children there are no schools or medicines, no clothes or food, not even a dignified roof under which we can store our poverty. For our boys and girls there is only work, ignorance, and death. The land that we have is worthless, and in order to get something for our children we have to leave home and look for work on land that belongs to others, powerful people, who pay us very little for our labor. Our children have to begin working at a very young age in order to be able to get food, clothing, and medicine. Our children's toys are the machete, the ax, and the hoe; from the time they are barely able to walk, playing and suffering they go out looking for wood, cleaning brush, and planting. They eat the same as we do: corn, beans, and chile. They cannot go to school to learn Spanish because work kills the days and sickness kills the nights. This is how our children have lived and died for 501 years.

We, their fathers, mothers, sisters, and brothers, no longer want to carry the guilt of not doing anything to help our children. We look for peaceful roads to justice and we find only mockery, imprisonment, blows, and death; we always find pain and sorrow. We couldn't take it anymore, boys and girls of Jalisco, it was too much pain and sorrow. And then we were forced to take the road to war, because our voices had not been heard.

Boys and girls of Jalisco, we do not ask for handouts or charity, we ask for justice: a fair wage, a piece of good land, a decent house, an honest school, medicine that cures, bread on our tables, respect for what is ours, the liberty to say what is on our minds and to open our mouths so that our words can unite with others in peace and without death. This is what we have always asked for, boys and girls of Jalisco, and they didn't listen. And it was then that we took a weapon in our hands, it was then that we made our work tools into tools of struggle. We then turned the war that they had made on us, the war that was killing us—without you, boys and girls of Jalisco, knowing anything about it— we turned that war against them, the rich and the powerful, those who have everything and deserve nothing.

That is why, boys and girls of Jalisco, we began our war. That is why the peace that we want is not the peace that we had before, because that wasn't peace, it was death and contempt, it was pain and suffering, it was disgrace. That is why we are telling you, with respect and love, boys and girls of Jalisco, to raise high the dignified flag of peace, to write poems that are "Prayers for a Dignified Life," and to search, above all, for equal justice for everyone.

Salud, boys and girls of Jalisco.

From the mountains of the Mexican Southeast
Subcomandante Insurgente Marcos
February 1994

9. "It became apparent that the government had known about the guerilla army in Chiapas for over a year. Rumors flew that Salinas had done nothing for fear of jeopardizing U.S. congressional approval of NAFTA, or that hard-liners in the ruling party and in the military had lent support to the rebels in protest against Salinas's policies" (Collier 1994, p. 5).

10. For more on "what Washington knew," see Ross 1995, pp. 37–51.

11. Letter from Subcomandante Marcos, January 18, 1994 (Marcos and the Zapatista Army of National Liberation 1995, pp. 81–82).

12. See, for example, Physicians for Human Rights 1999 and Human Rights Watch/Americas 1997.

13. Virtually every comprehensive report on human rights violations in rural Mexico discusses the *guardias blancas* in detail. For more on this topic, see Human Rights Watch/Americas 1997, pp. 38–72; Physicians for Human Rights 1999; Global Exchange 1998. The role of the *guardias* in the 1997 massacre in Acteal is discussed at the end of this chapter.

14. For more on the logic behind these areas seceding as "autonomous zones" and their relationship to the EZLN, see Womack 1999, pp. 48–59.

15. Collier 1994, p. 10.

16. See, for example, pre-uprising ethnographies such as Gossen 1974, Tedlock 1982, Tedlock 1993, and Wasserstrom 1983.

17. A similar "liberation of the word" occurred during the original Zapatista revolt, decades earlier; and that flurry of popular commentary grated on the ears of privileged people just as it did seventy years later. Womack writes of the events of 1909: "What increasingly struck observers as dangerous was not the planters' arrogance, which they took for granted, but the revival of bitterness and open sarcasm among the common people" (1968, p. 31).

18. For a gender perspective on the Zapatista movement, see Hernández Castillo 1998b.

19. Declaration of Moisés Gandhi, First Forum of Health Promoters and Agents, Moisés Gandhi, February 24, 1997. This is an unpublished document written by the attendees at this meeting; my translation.

20. As elsewhere, self-identification of ethnicity is something of a crapshoot and may not square with official reports. The Mexican population census uses linguistic criteria in its definition of ethnicity—a person whose first language is a Mesoamerican language is classified as indigenous (Gall 1998). Both official government data and that collected by scholars and observers put the indigenous population of Chiapas at about 30 percent. (The Ministry of Social Development in Mexico estimates 27 percent; Olivia Gall posits the figure of 26 percent.) The indigenous population of Mexico as a whole is much lower: 7.5 percent, according to Gall. See also Collier 1997 as well as Stephen and Collier 1997.

21. Marcos and the Zapatista Army of National Liberation 1995, p. 36. Ross (1995) reports similarly dire statistics. Chiapas is also among the group of Mexican states with the highest rates of maternal mortality (Reyes-Frausto, Lezana-Fernández, Garcia Peña, et al. 1998).

22. Ross (1995) reports that, in Chiapas, 63 percent of homes do not have electricity, 90 percent of indigenous homes do not have potable water, and 30 percent of the state's people are illiterate, the highest proportion in the country.

23. Letter from Subcomandante Marcos, January 13, 1994 (Marcos and the Zapatista Army of National Liberation 1995, p. 73).

24. Collier 1994, p. 16. Womack makes a similar point:

> As Mexico has grown and modernized, Chiapas has not been an isolated corner. In the country's economic development it has had an integral, important part. It has produced the most coffee and bananas of all the states in the country, accounting for a notable fraction of the national income from exports. Its cacao and beef production each figure second nationally. Its corn farms ordinarily make the third largest contribution to the domestic supply of Mexico's daily staff of life. Its great dams provide half of the country's hydroelectric power. Its gas fields yield a quarter of the country's natural gas (or did, until Cactus Petrochemical exploded) (Womack 1999, p. 10).

With his characteristic eloquence, Subcomandante Marcos writes of the Mexican petroleum interests:

> In Chiapas there are eighty-six fangs of Pemex sunk into the municipalities of Estación Juaréz, Reforma, Ostuacán, Pichucalco, and Ocosingo. Every day they suck out 92,000 barrels of petroleum and 516.7 million cubic feet of natural gas. They take the gas and oil and leave the trademark of capitalism: ecological destruction, agricultural waste, hyper-inflation, alcoholism, prostitution, and poverty. The beast is not satisfied, and extends its tentacles to the Lacandón jungle: eight oil fields are now under exploration. The jungle is opened with machetes, opened by the very same campesinos whose land has been taken away by the insatiable beast (Marcos and the Zapatista Army of National Liberation 1995, p. 33).

25. Womack 1999, p. 5. He continues:

> The Spanish conquerors did not bring stability. They brought war and epidemic diseases that destroyed most villages. They uprooted many others to concentrate their populations, the better to control them; in these operations, they nearly depopulated the Lacandón. And they institutionalized migratory labor in official, periodic conscriptions of Indians for work as farm laborers or two-footed beasts of burden. This was the exploitation against which the first bishop of Chiapas, Bartolomé de Las Casas, raised hell in 1545, in vain. It still beset the conquerors' heirs in the 1620s. It was the burden the Indians hoped to overthrow in a great rebellion in 1712, again in vain. It remained a force well into the 1800s (ibid.).

26. Womack writes of the impact of the original Zapatista land reform. Villagers, once workers on sugarcane plantations, became *ejidatarios* on communal lands and "did not regret the ruin of the old industry. 'What was called prosperity for the state,' they recalled, 'was misery for us.' As *ejidatarios* told [an American journalist], 'We are [now] growing what we want to grow and for our

own use' " (1968, pp. 373–74; Womack is quoting from Ernest Gruening [1928, p. 162]).

27. It is possible to exaggerate the degree to which Chiapans hopeful for land supported PRI candidates even before 1992, when President Salinas backed away from land reform promises. Although election results suggest that Salinas won by a landslide and captured most municipalities, some residents insisted they had not voted at all: " 'We have never voted here,' a Tzeltal farmer on the Morelia *ejido* outside Altamirano" told U.S. journalist John Ross shortly after the 1994 rebellion (Ross 1995, p. 74). For more in-depth considerations of the roots of the rebellion and the history of land reform in Chiapas, see Wasserstrom 1983 and Rus 1994. Neil Harvey's study of the Chiapas rebellion (1998) offers a comprehensive and readable overview of peasant movements and their relation to the struggle for land and democracy.

28. Womack 1999, p. 8. He adds: "Chiapas became Mexico's Mississippi not because the economy had not developed, or because it did not go through the Revolution, but because of the sort of development and the sort of Revolution it suffered" (p. 9).

29. "By the mid-1960s the population had so increased in the northern valleys around Ocosingo, Altamirano, and Las Margaritas, that many of their young men had no land, for corn or coffee. And by then these communities had reached a limit on their number. This was not for lack of peons wanting land, but for lack of grantable land in the vicinity. Because the agrarian law gave the widest exemption to ranches, many landlords in the 1950s and '60s quit growing sugar and coffee, expelled their peons before they could file for status as a community, and opened their fields to cattle" (ibid., p. 15).

30. Stea, Elguea, and Pérez Bustillo (1997) explore the uprising as a response to, among other problems, growing environmental degradation.

31. Womack 1999, pp. 6–7.

32. Womack estimates that small farmers who had invested in coffee trees lost 65 to 70 percent of their income after the 1989 drop in coffee prices (ibid., p. 21).

33. Collier 1994, p. 8. Womack also describes the complex processes by which "these villages were transformed from closed, internally bonded communities into broken, bourgeois-ridden, mistrustful bossdoms" (1999, p. 13).

34. Cited in Collier 1994, p. 45. Collier agrees with the analysis of Subcomandante Marcos: "When, in 1992, the government of President Salinas de Gortari brought land reform—the issue on which his party had originally risen to power—to a halt, he signaled an abrupt end to a traditional government covenant with the peasantry and deprived many peasants not just of the possibility of improving their livelihoods, but of their power as a constituency. The Zapatistas are trying to reclaim that constituency" (ibid., p. 8). Womack adds important context:

> In the thick of this pauperization, in November 1991, news spread across the state of Salinas's plan to reform the constitutional article on agrarian reform. For landless youngsters in the central highlands, still stuck in Los Altos but hoping to migrate, or struggling in the jungle to claim an ejido, the central and outrageous aim was to end the government's obligation to grant lands to any more landless

communities. Myriad earnest and honest explanations of the plan—that hardly any land remained to give away, agrarian reform for the last 25 years had been only on paper, a trick on poor country people, a racket, existing ejidos could stay as they were or receive titles to their grant as their property, the central aim of the new reform was to undermine traditional national bosses and break local bossdoms, an antipoverty program would save the disentitled, and so on—made no difference. In this plan the poorest of the poor Chols, Tzotzils, Tzeltals, and Tojolabals heard the national government's final judgment on them: fend for yourselves. In January 1992 Mexico's Congress passed the reform. In February the new agrarian code went into effect (1999, p. 21).

35. According to *Forbes* magazine, Mexico was a "hot spot" in 1994, as the number of billionaires rose from fourteen to twenty-four; this placed it fourth in the world in total number of billionaires, after the United States, Japan, and Germany. In December 1994, the number of billionaires dropped to ten as a result of the devaluation of the Mexican peso ("A Decade of Global Wealth" 1999). By late 1996, however, that number had grown again, to fifteen—even as millions of Mexicans were unable to find work or feed their families (Serrill 1996).

36. For a penetrating exploration of the impact of large-scale social and economic changes on the emotional well-being of highland Maya, see Collier, Farías Campero, Pérez, and White 2000. This is further explored by Roberto Briceño-León and Verónica Zubillaga, who trace the links between rising inequality, globalization of desires, and violence: "The social process is a two-directional encounter in which individuals' expectations increase but their real chances of satisfying those aspirations diminish. The friction between the two processes provokes tensions which are unprecedented and very difficult to bear" (2002, p. 23). The association between unequal growth and human rights violations has been underlined by Ana Luisa Liguori, who notes that "in Mexico, it is paradoxical that the more wealth is generated by industrial development and the greater the potential becomes for improved living conditions for all, the greater the distance from full realization of the Universal Declaration of Human Rights" (1995, p. 303).

37. For more on ethnic identity in rural Mexico, see Hewitt de Alcántara 1984 and Hindley 1996.

38. Collier 1994, p. xiv.

39. Ibid., p. 7. It is useful to compare Collier's analysis, on which I rely heavily, with that of other anthropologists of the region. As was the case with the Andeanists who "missed the revolution" in Peru (see Starn 1992), some ethnographers working with the Maya seemed taken by surprise by the Zapatista uprising. Gossen's appositely named *Telling Maya Tales* brings some of these interpretive complexities to light:

> It is therefore not surprising that the composition of EZLN, although generally Maya, is actually fairly diverse in terms of ethnic, linguistic, and religious backgrounds that are represented. Tzotzil, Tzeltal, Zoque, Chol, and Tojolabal speakers, as well as Mexican mestizos and ethnically "white" Mexicans, are all united in pursuit of common political and social goals. What is Maya about the Zapatista movement must therefore be sought not in particular variants of Maya or other Indian cultural identity but rather in general principles of values and con-

duct that all might share, be they Tzotzils, Chols, or Zoques. This common
ground is what I have tried to identify here.

While the immediate goals of the Maya Zapatistas appear to outside observers to be primarily of an economic or political nature, I believe that the pan-
Indian nature of this enterprise has a powerful component of post-colonial ethnic
affirmation that goes well beyond political action (1999, p. 262).

40. Bishop Vasco de Quiroga represented, as did Las Casas, a utopian tendency within the early colonial church. For more on the role of the church in the
European colonization of Latin America, see Rivera 1992; for an account specific
to Mexico, see Tangeman 1995.

41. See Graham Greene's 1939 report from Mexico, *Another Mexico,* and
also his 1940 novelization of this era, *The Power and the Glory.*

42. The principle of making a "preferential option for the poor" has been a
part of Catholic social teaching for several decades. It was initially introduced
in Pope Paul VI's encyclical Populorum Progresio (On the Development of Peoples), issued in March 1967, which decried the great inequalities of modern times
and called on individuals, nations, and the Church to foster true development
of human potential:

> It is not just a matter of eliminating hunger, nor even of reducing poverty. The
> struggle against destitution, though urgent and necessary, is not enough. It is a
> question, rather, of building a world where every man, no matter what his race,
> religion or nationality, can live a fully human life, freed from servitude imposed
> on him by other men or by natural forces over which he has not sufficient con-
> trol; a world where freedom is not an empty word and where the poor man
> Lazarus can sit down at the same table with the rich man.... We must repeat
> once more that the superfluous wealth of rich countries should be placed at the
> service of poor nations. The rule which up to now held good for the benefit of
> those nearest to us, must today be applied to all the needy of this world (Paul VI
> 1967).

This principle was further elaborated and politicized within the Latin American context by liberation theologians. Chapter 5 provides additional discussion
of this topic.

43. Womack 1999, p. 27. By the time of the Medellín bishops' conference in
1968, Ruíz's metanoia was complete. He presented a paper there, one of only
seven bishops to do so: "The poor cannot be evangelized if we own vast estates.
The weak and the oppressed withdraw from Christ if we appear as allies of the
powerful. The illiterate cannot be evangelized if our religious institutions continue looking for paradise in the big cities, and not on the poor edges of town
and out in the disinherited hamlets" (ibid., p. 30).

44. Collier (1994, pp. 53–66) discusses Catholic responses to Protestant
evangelization, and also the impact of the 1974 Indigenous Congress, at length.
He compares, point by point, the concerns of the Congress and the later Zapatistas, noting that "during the Indigenous Congress, the delegates talked about
the same bread and butter issues the Zapatistas have: land, food, education, and
health" (p. 63) and that the documents issued during the 1974 Congress are "almost identical" to those published twenty years later in the early days of the Zapatista rebellion. Womack's historical reader contains a translation of the text

issued at the end of the Congress (Womack 1999, pp. 148–61). His summary of the Congress:

> For two days they recounted the misery and indignity of their lives, denounced particular injustices in vivid detail, analyzed the causes of their poverty, torments, and frustration, and discussed strategies for action, including a union of canyon communities. On the third day, in their customary way, but not quickly, they reached their own accords: the need for land to belong to the man who worked it, more land, good land, honest counselors to teach them their rights under the agrarian code; the need for doctors, effective programs of public health, proper medications, and an end to traffic in government-dispensed medicines; the need for basic services, like running water; the need for more and better schools, and for Indian priests; the need for fair wages and enforcement of the labor law; the need for Indian markets, to avoid "merchants and monopolists [who] are A GREAT PLAGUE" (pp. 31–32).

45. Relations between the local elite and Ruíz have been strained since before the 1974 Congress, but they were nothing short of poisoned by 1981, when a Columbus Day sitdown strike in Tuxtla clearly had the support of the bishop:

> San Cristóbal's bourgeoisie led the irate reaction. It published demands for the government to restore order, "or must we take action into our own hands?" Locally and in Mexico City the press speculated that "since communists had killed Archbishop Romero" in El Salvador, to make a martyr for their cause, they might kill Bishop Ruíz too. One columnist had the bishop running a guerrilla training center at the San Cristóbal seminary, which in hours could bring 300,000 Indians into guerrilla warfare. The death threats began, and police terrorist operations, to create a climate of intimidation (Womack 1999, p. 35).

46. Womack again underlines the antipathy of local elites toward Ruíz:

> San Cristóbal's own bourgeoisie, in the full flush of its traditional ladino presumption and bigotry, contributed a particular malevolence to the strife. Aided by the local PRI, abetted by conservative nationalists throughout the country (including Mexico's Lyndon Larouchers!), the city's self-styled true "San Cristóbalites" publicly and repeatedly vilified the bishop. He was "the Anti-Christ of San Cristóbal, the enemy of the people, Satan's son, the devil's bishop, a communist, the reason for the Zapatistas." Among the graffiti on a downtown wall was "Vote for Peace—Kill Samuel" (1999, p. 46).

For more on the demonization of the Catholic Church in Chiapas, see Human Rights Watch/Americas 1997, pp. 73–88.

47. "Communiqué from the CCRI-CG of the EZLN, January 6, 1994," in Marcos and the Zapatista Army of National Liberation 1995, p. 57.

48. During the parleys brokered by Ruíz and church officials, the Zapatista negotiators were offered sanctuary in the cathedral, in keeping with an agreement with the federal government. Their presence enraged local elites. Womack reports the comments of "a diplomatic and smiling tour guide" addressing American reporters:

> "The bishop has created this controversy. There is no injustice here. . . . We have lived peacefully with the Indians for over 500 years [sic] and never had a problem. The bishop is all mixed up in politics, and we want our religion to be a comfort, the way it used to be before he came." Some excellent Catholics, he

explained, were so discomfited that they would no longer set foot in the cathedral. "It was desecrated by the presence of those filthy Zapatista Indians who
lived there like animals during the bishop's so-called dialogues for peace. The
cathedral must now be reconsecrated" (1999, p. 46).

49. Human Rights Watch/Americas 1997.
50. Ibid., p. 46.
51. Womack 1968, p. ix.
52. Marcos and the Zapatista Army of National Liberation 1995, p. 38.
53. The massacre occurred on December 22, 1997. According to press accounts, those killed included twenty-one women and fifteen children (Moore and
Anderson 1997, Smith 1997). For an in-depth account of the attack, see Womack 1999; his reading, "The Civil War in the Highlands: Acteal, December 22,
1997" (pp. 340–54), includes letters from both Subcomandante Marcos and
Bishop Samuel Ruíz. See also Ross 2000, pp. 239–55; as well as the account of
Hernández Castillo (1998b).

54. Shortly after the massacre, the Mexican federal attorney general's office
claimed the killings were the product of family feuds and arrested sixteen Maya
Indians and charged them with the slaughter. The international press published
the claims of the Mexican government; see, for example, "Sixteen Charged in
Chiapas Massacre" 1997. But the responsibility of local and federal authorities
could not be overlooked (which is why Human Rights Watch/Americas could
title its 1997 report on human rights violations in rural Mexico *Implausible Deniability*). The EZLN high command issued a press release the following day. It
contained ten points, including the following:

> First. In accord with the information obtained so far, some 60 paramilitaries
> from the PRI (sponsored by the federal and state governments) were those
> who attacked with high-powered firearms the dislocated Indians taking refuge
> in Acteal.
>
> Second. As a result of this attack, which lasted up to four hours, at least 45 Indi-
> ans were murdered, among them nine men, twenty-one women, and fifteen
> children (one of them less than a year old). Besides the dead, seven males were
> wounded (four of them children), and ten females (four of them children).
>
> Third. In accord with radio transmissions from the Chiapas state government
> (intercepted by the EZLN), police from the Chiapas Public Security force on
> the outskirts of Acteal and at the time the massacre was being committed
> backed the attack, and during the evening and night collected bodies to hide
> the massacre's magnitude. Homero Tovilla Cristiani and Uriel Jarquín, Chia-
> pas's state secretary and undersecretary of government, respectively, commis-
> sioned the police to back the crime. Governor Julio César Ruíz Ferro was
> constantly informed as the "operation" developed (at least from noon on
> December 22, when the massacre has already been going on for an hour).
> Approved by the federal and state governments, plans for the attacks were
> refined on December 21 in a meeting of paramilitaries that the PRIista munic-
> ipal president, Jacinto Arias, convened from the communities of Los Chorros,
> Puebla, La Esperanza, and Quextic, all in the Chenalhó township.
>
> Fourth. The direct responsibility for these bloody acts falls on Ernesto Zedillo
> Ponce de León and the Interior Ministry, who for the last two years have
> given a green light to the counter-insurgency project proposed by the army.
> *This project is an attempt to turn the Zapatista war into a conflict between*

> *Indians, motivated by religious, political, or ethnic differences.* To accomplish it, the government has committed itself to pay for the equipment and arms (with funds from the Ministry of Social Development) and to give military training (by army officers) to Indians recruited by the PRI. To allow time for these death squads to get ready, the federal government designed a parallel strategy of feigned dialogue, consisting in a process of negotiation without any intention of fulfilling its agreements and at the same time increasing the military presence in Zapatista zones. The state government was left in charge of guaranteeing the impunity of the paramilitary groups and facilitating their operation in the principal rebel zones, Chiapas's north, the jungle, and the highlands (cited in Womack 1999, p. 350; emphasis added. For the complete communiqué, see *http://www.ezln.org*, December 23, 1997).

It is important to note that independent observers from Mexican and international human rights groups have since confirmed almost all of these allegations. Jorge Castañeda (1998) wrote in the *Washington Post:* "The Acteal massacre was the saddest example of state violence.... There is no longer much doubt that the perpetrators of the massacre were paramilitary groups armed and organized by local authorities, with some degree of complicity from the state government and the responsibility, at least by inaction, of the federal government."

55. Even in the international press, such eyewitness accounts are clearly presented. See, for example, Walker 1997, Kleist 1997, and "Death in Chiapas" 1997.

56. Global Exchange 1998, p. 6.

57. Physicians for Human Rights 1999, p. 57.

58. Womack 1999, p. 59.

59. Enlace Civil, A.D., Chiapas Community Defenders Network, Alianza Cívica, et al., Urgent action letter sent to Mexico Solidarity Network (*msn@mexicosolidarity.org*), entitled "Paramilitary Attack in Yajalón, Chiapas," on August 7, 2000.

60. See Global Exchange 2000.

61. Mexico Solidarity Network 2000.

62. The Mexican government's response to the massacre at Acteal was not to address the underlying social and economic causes of the atrocities but rather to bring six thousand troops, within a week of the attack, to the previously unoccupied region (Global Exchange 1998, p. 5). As stated in Global Exchange 1998: "The government has justified the invasion of indigenous areas as an attempt to disarm pro-government paramilitary groups, bring humanitarian aid to vulnerable communities, and introduce a peace-keeping force to prevent further massacres. Six months of military operations, however, have not resulted in major arms finds, nor the disarmament of paramilitary groups—which continue to act with full impunity in areas of army occupation. Despite the army's social labor campaign, the well-being of occupied communities has gone into sharp decline as people are displaced and normal economic activity disrupted" (p. 4). Furthermore, "ironically, the Mexican government's use of militarization as a response to a conflict with roots in economic and social problems has actually exacerbated the underlying injustices from which the Zapatistas draw their significant community support" (p. 5).

63. Womack 1999, p. 59.

CHAPTER 4. A PLAGUE ON ALL OUR HOUSES?

1. As Juviler (2000, p. 119) notes: "The Ministry of Justice took control of prison facilities from the Interior Ministry (in charge of police and special forces) in September 1998. The head of the Ministry of Justice may openly deplore conditions, a Duma committee may investigate them, and a president's commission may propose reforms, but they all lack the means to carry them out."

2. For more on the complex impact of Russia's social and economic transformations on the quality of tuberculosis care, see Farmer, Kononets, Borisov, et al. 1999. Chapter 7 of this volume also discusses this subject further.

3. In much of Siberia, case notifications have gone from 30 per 100,000 population to more than 100 per 100,000. Rates are forty to fifty times higher within prisons. For a review of tuberculosis epidemiology in Russia, see Farmer, Kononets, Borisov, et al. 1999.

4. For more on the collapse of the Russian health care system and the deteriorating health of its citizens over the past decade or so, see Laurie Garrett's informative *Newsday* series, "Crumbled Empire, Shattered Health" (1997). Garrett further elaborates in her book on the decline of global public health (2000); see her chapter "Bourgeois Physiology: The Collapse of All Semblances of Public Health in the Former Soviet Socialist Republics," which details such topics as childhood disease, tuberculosis in the general population and in prisons, abortion rates, rising rates of HIV and hepatitis, drug addiction, and alcoholism. See also the following newspaper articles: Goldberg and Kishkovsky 2000; "Russian Population to Continue to Decline" 2000; Specter 1998; Specter 1994; Wines 2000a and 2000b; Wines and Zuger 2000; Zuger 2000. Murray Feshbach (1995) and Martin McKee (Walberg, McKee, Shkolnikov, et al. 1998) are among those who have written about the Russian "mortality crisis."

5. This seemed to be the case even in the nineteenth century, if Fyodor Dostoyevsky's *House of the Dead*—based on his four years in a convict prison in Omsk, Siberia—is to be believed:

> The way the common people see it is that they are to be given treatment by their masters, for the doctors belong to a higher social class than they. However, when they get to know the doctors better (though there are exceptions, this is mostly true) all these terrors disappear, a fact which to my mind redounds to the honour of our medical men, most of whom are quite young. The majority of them know how to win the respect and even the love of the common people (1985, p. 224).

6. Karel Styblo and others have estimated that a smear-positive patient infects ten to fourteen susceptible contacts with *M. tuberculosis* each year (Styblo 1984; see also Sutherland and Fayers 1975).

7. Recent estimates of this figure vary. Alexander Borodulin, the deputy head of the penitentiary department at Russia's Justice Ministry, estimates that approximately 20 percent of those prisoners with active tuberculosis have MDRTB (Blagov 2002), while other estimates are less conservative. In a survey performed in Tomsk prison in 1998, more than half of prisoners with active TB had histories of previous treatment. None of the chronic patients were sick from fully sus-

ceptible strains. The majority (87 percent) had poly-drug-resistant tuberculosis. Among patients with newly diagnosed active TB, the majority (57 percent) had drug-resistant TB, and 46 percent had poly-drug-resistant TB (Mishustin 1999, cited in Farmer, Kononets, Borisov, et al. 1999, pp. 56–57).

8. Coninx, Eshaya-Chauvin, and Reyes 1995.

9. In the words of one high-ranking World Health Organization official, the Soviet victory over tuberculosis bred "a tremendous pride on the Russian side" (cited in Zuger 2000). Some have held this and similar attitudes—rather than the gutting of health budgets—at least partially responsible for ineffective responses to the later resurgence of tuberculosis.

10. Most surveys of drug-susceptibility profiles within prison populations show that a majority have drug-resistant disease; as many as two-thirds are resistant to streptomycin. This resistance suggests, of course, that novel strategies, and more than first-line drugs, will be required to arrest tuberculosis in the former Soviet Union. Given this context, it is disturbing to note that many experts have called for the universal use of short-course chemotherapy; some have even suggested fixed-dose combinations of these drugs. Either of these two prescriptions will fail to cure patients with MDRTB. For a review of this debate, see Coker 2000 and Farmer and Kim 2000.

11. For more on the recrudescence of drug-resistant tuberculosis in New York, see the review by Frieden, Fujiwara, Washko, et al. (1995).

12. Garrett 1994, p. 524.

13. Amnesty International 1997, p. 31.

14. As of January 2002, Russian prisons reportedly held 977,700 inmates (Sentencing Project 2002a).

15. Becerra, Freeman, Bayona, et al. 2000.

16. The exact costs of such regimens are in dispute. One report claimed that six months' worth of drugs costs only thirteen dollars (World Health Organization 1998). We have never been able to bring the cost lower than two hundred dollars in our clinic in Haiti and suspect that this is closer to the real cost of treating fully susceptible tuberculosis. A recent, honest accounting comes from Chicago, where it costs more than sixty thousand dollars to treat a single case of *drug-susceptible* tuberculosis (Wurtz and White 1999).

17. Portaels, Rigouts, and Bastian 1999.

18. For an example of such logic, see Alexander 1998, in which one World Bank official "defends non-treatment of MDR strains" (p. 53).

19. The number of new cases reported for the year 2000 was 134,000. However, the Russian government announced in February 2002 that this figure had dropped very slightly—the number of new tuberculosis cases in 2001 was around 133,000. But an Associated Press headline captured the proper response to this small decrease: "Experts Warn Russia's Fight Against TB Is Far from Over" (Engleman 2002). For more on the reemergence of TB in the Russian Federation, see Farmer, Kononets, Borisov, et al. 1999.

20. See Field and Twigg 2000.

21. It's even more felicitous in the original: *"la gestion policière et carcérale de la misère"* (Wacquant 1999, p. 63).

22. Juviler 2000, p. 132.

23. Löytönen and Maasilta 1998.

24. A CIA report released in 2000 warned of the threat posed by infectious diseases and biological warfare to U.S. security and interests abroad (U.S. Central Intelligence Agency 2000a). In remarks before Congress, a leading National Intelligence Council official warned that infectious diseases such as tuberculosis, malaria, and pneumonia pose a threat to U.S. security and will continue in the coming decades to harm economic and social development in those countries in which the U.S. has vested interests (Tang 2000). See Henry and Farmer 1999a for a discussion of emerging infectious diseases as "national security concerns"; Henry and Farmer 1999b contains a more thorough exploration of the topic. See also the preface to the second edition of *Infections and Inequalities* (Farmer 2001a).

25. Farmer, Kononets, Borisov, et al. 1999, pp. 56–57.

26. Frieden, Fujiwara, Washko, et al. 1995, p. 232; emphasis added.

27. In 2000, the Bill & Melinda Gates Foundation made an enormous commitment to tuberculosis control. The Foundation's support will permit the Lima project described in this book to be "scaled up" so that every Peruvian sick with TB may have hope of a cure—regardless of the drug-susceptibility pattern of the infecting strain. The generous support of Tom White, who paid for this project in its early years, has yielded important insights that are now having an impact throughout the former Soviet Union and in other settings in which a significant proportion of TB cases result from drug-resistant strains.

28. Farmer, Kim, Mitnick, et al. 1999.

29. By consolidating the market for quality-assured second-line drugs and collectively negotiating with manufacturers, Partners In Health and other organizations were able to lower per-patient treatment costs dramatically. Access to these concessionally priced drugs is regulated: the multi-institutional body known as the "Green Light Committee" (GLC) determines which tuberculosis programs have sufficient technical capacity and will adequately adhere to international treatment guidelines. The GLC has given way to a seemingly paradoxical outcome: decreased costs and increased control over the proper distribution of these drugs. For more on this collective effort, see Gupta, Kim, Espinal, et al. 2001.

CHAPTER 5. HEALTH, HEALING, AND SOCIAL JUSTICE

1. Boff 1989, p. 23.

2. The literature on the correlation between poverty, inequality, and increased morbidity and mortality is massive. For reviews, see, for example, Farmer 1999b; Kim, Millen, Irwin, and Gershman 2000; and Wilkinson 1996. Other major reviews include Leclerc, Fassin, Grandjean, et al. 2000; World Health Organization 1999d, 2000c;World Bank 2000a; Bartley, Blane, and Smith 1998; Sen 1998; Coburn 2000; and Fiscella, Franks, Gold, et al. 2000. Other articles review case studies of inequality in access to treatment of specific diseases; see, for example, Rathore, Berger, Weinfurt, et al. 2000; and of course the sizable body of literature on inequality of access to HIV therapy.

3. Gutiérrez 1983, p. 44.

4. For a concise history of liberation theology, its historical relevance, and an explanation of key themes and motivations, see Leonardo and Clodovis Boff's slim and helpful volume *Introducing Liberation Theology* (1987).

5. Base-community movements, also known as "basic ecclesial communities," are disparate and sociologically complex, and I do not aspire to review their idealized or actual impact. But, as this movement has been felt throughout Latin America, I would encourage further reading. For an insider account, see the volume by Father Álvaro Barreiro (1982). A study by John Burdick (1993) contains a complementary, scholarly examination of such communities in urban Brazil.

6. There are other clues that liberation theology might have something to offer the healing professions: for one, the more destructive forces hate it. In 1982, for example, advisers to U.S. President Ronald Reagan argued that "American foreign policy must begin to counterattack (and not just react against) liberation theology" (quoted from the Santa Fe Document, a Reagan administration working paper; cited in Boff and Boff 1987, p. 86).

7. Recent health care "reforms" in Latin America and other developing regions have followed a neoliberal framework that favors commercialization, corporatization, and privatization of health and social welfare services. Most notable is the enthusiastic exportation of the U.S. model of "managed care." As Neill notes in his critique of these developments, "managed health care is touted by many experts—usually found in USAID, the World Bank, and various havens of academia—as a tangible model which can be of immense value to developing countries if applied wisely and efficiently" (2001, p. 61). This position, of course, ignores the growing body of evidence challenging the unabashed claims that managed-care organizations (MCOs) provide quality care with efficiency and cost-effectiveness—evidence that also points to managed care's role in exacerbating the already large inequities that characterize health care in the United States (Anders 1996; Andrulis and Carrier 1999; Farmer and Rylko-Bauer 2001; Ginzberg 1999; Himmelstein, Woolhandler, and Hellander 2001; Lewin and Altman 2000; Maskovsky 2000; Pellegrino 1999; Peterson 1999; Schneider, Zaslavsky, and Epstein 2002).

In fact, Waitzkin and Iriart note that, as the U.S. market has become saturated and MCOs face growing criticism, these corporations

> have turned their eyes toward developing countries, especially those in Latin America. In the tradition of tobacco and pesticides, U.S. corporations are exporting to developing countries—in the form of managed care—products and practices that have come under heavy criticism domestically. The exportation of managed care is also receiving enthusiastic support from the World Bank, other multilateral lending agencies, and multinational corporations.... developing countries are experiencing strong pressure to accept managed care as the organizational framework for privatization of their health and social security systems.... this experience is serving as a model for the exportation of managed care to Africa and Asia (2001, p. 497).

There is, of course, much money to be made by tapping into the health care and social security funds of the public sector even in poorer developing nations, under the guise of rescuing these countries from inefficient bureaucracies and rising costs by importing neoliberal managed-care solutions. Large segments of the population in Latin America live in poverty and often have minimal or no access to formal health care. The consequences of such health care transformations for the poor and the oppressed in developing countries, as well as for the public health systems they might rely on, are dire, to say the least. "As public health systems are dismantled and privatized under the auspices of managed care, multinational corporations predictably will enter the field, reap vast profits, and exit within several years. Then developing countries will face the awesome prospect of reconstructing their public systems" (Waitzkin and Iriart 2001, p. 498). For more on health care reforms in Latin America, see Armada, Muntaner, and Navarro 2001; Barraza-Lloréns, Bertozzi, González-Pier, et al. 2002; Iriart, Merhy, and Waitzkin 2001; Laurell 2001; Pérez-Stable 1999; and Stocker, Waitzkin, and Iriart 1999.

8. Segundo 1980, p. 16; quoted from Segunda Conferencia General del Episcopado Latinoamericano, Medellín 1968.

9. Boff 1989, p. 20.

10. Eagleson and Sharper 1979, p. 128.

11. Gutiérrez 1983, p. 87.

12. Sobrino explains the link between structural violence and structural sin:

God's creation is being assaulted and vitiated.... because this reality is not simply natural, but historical—being the result of action taken by some human beings against others—this reality is sinful. As absolute negation of God's will, this sinfulness is very serious and fundamental (1988, p. 15).

13. Pixley and Boff 1989, p. 242.

14. In the English translation of *Pedagogy of the Oppressed,* the original Portuguese term is retained. In Freire's own words, *"Conscientização* is the deepening of the attitude of awareness characteristic of all emergence"—in other words, critical consciousness (1986, p. 101).

15. Brown 1993, p. 45.

16. Sobrino 1988, p. 31.

17. Ibid., pp. 13, 15.

18. Brown 1993, p. 45.

19. Sobrino 1988, p. 32.

20. "Communiqué from the CCRI-CG of the EZLN, January 6, 1994," in Marcos and the Zapatista Army of National Liberation 1995, p. 58.

21. See Farmer 1999b, chap. 1; and Farmer and Nardell 1998.

22. Even at the dawn of the era of antibiotics, when streptomycin was already available, class divisions were sharp inside Europe's sanatoriums. George Orwell's journal entries from the year before his death of tuberculosis are telling:

Curious effect, here in the sanatorium, on Easter Sunday, when the people in this (the most expensive) block of "chalets" mostly have visitors, of hearing large numbers of upper-class English voices. I have been almost out to the sound of them for two years, hearing them at most one or two at a time, my ears growing more & more used to working-class or lower-middle-class Scottish voices. In the hospital at Hairmyres, for instance, I literally never heard a "cultivated" accent except when I had a visitor. It is as though I were hearing these voices for the first time. And what voices! A sort of over-fedness, a fatuous self-confidence, a constant bah-bahing of laughter abt [*sic*] nothing, above all a sort of heaviness & richness combined with a fundamental ill-will—people who, one instinctively feels, without even being able to see them, are the enemies of anything intelligent or sensitive or beautiful. No wonder everyone hates us so (journal entry from April 17, 1949; Orwell 1968, p. 578).

For more on the history of tuberculosis in North America, see Georgina Feldberg's (1995) helpful review; see also the classic study by Dubos and Dubos (1952). Unfortunately, little has been written of the history of tuberculosis in the regions of the world where it has taken its greatest toll.

23. For an overview of the burden of disease and death caused by *M. tuberculosis,* see Farmer, Walton, and Becerra 2000.

24. These "twists" are reviewed in Farmer 1999b, chap. 9.

25. This story is told more fully in Farmer 1992a, chap. 2, pp. 19–27.

26. For a more detailed discussion of this study, see Farmer 1999b, pp. 217–25.

27. Farmer 1990.

28. Farmer, Robin, Ramilus, et al. 1991, p. 260. For more on this project, see Farmer 1999b, chap. 8.

29. Indeed, one does not need to ascribe directly to the religious tenets of liberation theology in order to make a "preferential option for the poor." Pixley and Boff summarize the widespread starvation, malnutrition, and poverty that are a daily reality for millions (remarking that one does not need "socio-scientific instruments" to prove this) and conclude that "this state of affairs is *morally intolerable,* for those who do not believe in the God of the Bible as much as for those who do" (1989, pp. 238, 239). They note the simple facts of the situation and what our response—whether one imbued with faith, or one relying solely on reason—must logically be:

> The energy to find the solution can come only from the oppressed themselves. Wherever there is oppression, there will be struggles to win life-sustaining conditions—struggles between classes, between races, between nations, between sexes. This is simply an observable fact, not a moral imperative or a scientific conclusion. We can see the just struggles of the oppressed going on around us, and we cannot see any other way out of the vast problems that afflict humanity at the close of the twentieth century (p. 242).

For a more in-depth discussion of these matters, refer to the full argument made by Pixley and Boff (1989, pp. 237–43).

30. Perhaps it goes without saying that no physician who bases his or her practice on clinical trials can in good faith buy into the postmodern argument that all claims to truth are merely "competing discourses." But, as Christopher Norris writes, in both the social sciences and the humanities, the conviction that we ought to find out what really happened is proof

> that we hadn't caught up with the "postmodern" rules of the game, the fact that nowadays things have moved on to the point where there is no last ground of appeal to those old, self-deluding "enlightenment" values that once possessed authority (or the semblance thereof), at least in some quarters. Anyone who

continues to invoke such standards is plainly in the grip of a nostalgic desire for some ultimate truth-telling discourse—whether Platonist, Kantian, Marxist or whatever—that would offer a delusory refuge from the knowledge that we are nowadays utterly without resources in the matter of distinguishing truth from falsehood (1992, p. 13).

Norris's devastating account of intellectuals and the Gulf War (1992) is one of the best critiques of the postmodern foolishness that has gained quite a foothold in universities on both sides of the Atlantic. See also Norris 1990.

31. West 1993, p. 4.

32. Freire 1986, p. 29.

33. Poppendieck 1998, p. 5.

34. Turshen 1986, p. 891.

35. Samuel Johnson once observed that "a decent provision for the poor is the true test of civilization." Surely this is true, and it serves as an indictment of affluent society. But liberation theology delivers an even more damning indictment, since its proponents argue that we should reserve our highest standards for the poor.

36. My critique of development is by no means original; it draws heavily on a very large literature reaching back almost thirty years. From André Gunder Frank to Immanuel Wallerstein, the more refined versions of dependency theory cannot be lightly dismissed. For more recent reviews of the limitations of development approaches to health care, see Meredeth Turshen's wonderful book *Privatizing Health Services in Africa* (1999).

37. Pixley and Boff 1989, pp. 6–7.

38. Boff and Boff 1987, p. 5.

39. Gutiérrez 1973, p. xiv.

40. Berryman 1987, p. 91.

41. For an introduction to the notion of health transition, see Caldwell, Findley, Caldwell, et al. 1990; Gutiérrez, Zielinski, and Kendall (2000) have more recently qualified this concept by placing it in broader social context. See also the discussion by Mosley, Bobadilla, and Jamison (1993) on the implications of this model for developing countries.

42. McCord and Freeman 1990.

43. Brown 1993, p. 44.

44. Carney is said to have been killed after being captured when he participated in an ill-fated guerrilla incursion from Nicaragua into Olancho Province, Honduras.

45. Carney 1987, p. xi. Carney goes on to criticize the United States directly, citing the U.S.-backed 1973 military coup d'état in Chile, in which tens of thousands were killed, as his own moment of realization about the extent of the often brutal U.S. involvement in the political and economic affairs of the region:

> After the bloody military coup of 1973 in Chile, *it was obvious that the United States would never allow a country that is economically dependent on it to make a revolution by means of elections*—through the democratic process directed by the majority—at least as long as the country has an army that obeys the capitalist bourgeoisie of the country (p. 311).

For an examination of U.S. policy toward progressive movements in Guatemala, El Salvador, and Haiti in a similar light, see Farmer 1994.

CHAPTER 6. LISTENING FOR PROPHETIC VOICES

1. A recent *New York Times* headline, reporting on national data and analyses from the 2000 U.S. census, captures the inequality that characterized the previous decade: "Gains of 90's Did Not Lift All, Census Shows." The article goes on to say, "Despite the surging economy of the 1990's that brought affluence to many Americans, the poor remained entrenched.... The bureau's statistics... show that 9.2 percent of families were deemed poor in 2000, a slight improvement from 10 percent in 1989" (Kilborn and Clemetson 2002). While the 2000 census may have noted a slight decrease in the official poverty rate, child poverty in particular is likely to grow in the United States as a result of recent welfare changes and a rising unemployment rate. According to one study, the U.S. child poverty rate is the highest among nineteen wealthy countries of the Organization for Economic Cooperation and Development. Even within the United States, the disparities between rich and poor are vast—a child whose family income is in the 90th percentile has an adjusted income five times higher than the child of a family whose income falls in the 10th percentile; the average gap for other nations varies by a factor of three (Madrick 2002; Smeeding, Rainwater, and Burtless 2001).

2. Jencks 2002, p. 64.

3. For an in-depth discussion of these issues, see Kim, Millen, Irwin, and Gershman 2000.

4. As James K. Galbraith observes: "When the global trend is isolated, we find that in the last two decades, inequality has increased throughout the world in a pattern that cuts across the effect of national income changes. During the decades that happen to coincide with the rise of neoliberal ideology, with the breakdown of national sovereignties, and with the end of Keynesian policies in the global debt crisis of the early 1980s, inequality rose worldwide" (2002, p. 220).

5. Jencks 2002, p. 64.

6. According to a report from *Fortune* magazine, in 1999 the profit margins of the pharmaceutical industry far exceeded those of all other U.S. industries. Pharmaceutical companies realized on average an 18.6 percent return on revenues; second was commercial banking, at 15.8 percent, while other industries ranged from 0.5 to 12.1 percent ("How the Industries Stack Up" 2000). The drug industry has continued this stellar performance, topping the Fortune 500 list of most profitable industries for both 2000 and 2001, while other industries have faltered to varying degrees. In 2000, pharmaceutical profits were again 18.6 percent of revenues, with commercial banks still holding second place despite dropping to 14.1 percent return on revenues ("How the Industries Stack Up" 2001); similar results were posted for 2001 ("How the Industries Stack Up" 2002). The disparities between the pharmaceutical industry and others widened

even further during the economic downturn of 2001, with the return on revenues for industries other than commercial banks ranging from 0.2 to 10.9 percent.

Meanwhile, spending on prescription drugs is skyrocketing (expenditures have nearly doubled since 1997, and in 2001 stood at $154.5 billion), in part a result of price increases, use of more expensive drugs, greater demand, and more aggressive marketing (National Institute for Health Care Management 2002b). In fact, relaxation of the U.S. Food and Drug Administration rules on mass media advertising for prescription drugs in 1997 has led to an explosion of direct-to-consumer advertising by drug companies, especially in TV ads, and a concomitant rise in spending on the most heavily advertised drugs (National Institute for Health Care Management 2001).

Noting that the top ten drug companies have a 30 percent profit margin, Marcia Angell observes, "An industry whose profits outstrip not only those of every other industry in the United States, but often its own research and development costs, simply cannot be considered very risky" (2000c, p. 1903). The pharmaceutical industry, on the other hand, "disputes the view that its profits are unconscionably high," arguing "that they are 'only slightly above the average for all industries,'" and that "'we need to be profitable in order to attract the capital to sustain innovation'" (McNeil 2000d, p. A14).

These corporate claims are easily refuted when one takes a closer look at where profits and spending are directed. A July 2001 report by Families USA finds that "all of the nine U.S. pharmaceutical companies that market the top-selling 50 drugs for seniors spent more money on marketing, advertising, and administration than they did on R&D" (Pollack and O'Rourke 2001, p. 3). And six of these companies made more money in net profits than they spent on research and development. A goodly portion of the money went to pad the pockets of chairpersons, CEOs, and vice-presidents. The twenty-five highest-paid executives for these nine companies garnered a total of $331.6 million in compensation—not counting unexercised stock options—during the year 2000 alone (ibid., p. 5).

7. For protests against the Human Genome Project, it is useful to consult the numerous Web pages and e-mail discussion groups that have sprung up surrounding the issue. See, for example, the Declaration of Indigenous People of the Western Hemisphere Regarding the Human Genome Diversity Project 1995; Cunningham and Scharper 1996, a commentary on the Human Genome Project and the issue of patenting DNA; and the Web site of the Indigenous Peoples Council on Biocolonialism (*http://www.ipcb.org*). These protests have also been extensively documented by the press; for a sampling, see Harry 2000, Monmaney 1997, and Rifkin 2000. The title chosen by journalist Philip Bereano for a 1995 *Seattle Times* piece sums up the problem nicely: "Patent Pending: The Race to Own DNA; Guaymi Tribe Was Surprised to Discover They Were Invented." See also the excellent consideration of "patenting the primitive" by Hilary Cunningham (1998).

The trade in organs has been followed most closely by anthropologist Nancy Scheper-Hughes (2000a, 1998, 1996b). I know that she does her own fieldwork, as I recently bumped into her in a Cuban morgue. (I consider it important to note that she wasn't finding evidence of organ peddling there.) Lawrence Cohen

(1999) has contributed further to this disturbing literature, which can also be found on the University of California's Organs Watch Web site at *http://sunsite.berkeley.edu/biotech/organswatch*. As this literature documents, organs too often move along social fault lines, from the poor to the rich. In her article "Theft of Life: The Globalization of Organ Stealing Rumours," Scheper-Hughes reports that "as poor people in shantytowns [in northeastern Brazil] see it, the ring of organ exchange proceeds from the bodies of the young, the poor, and the beautiful to the bodies of the old, the rich, and the ugly, and from poor nations in the South to rich nations in the North" (1996b, p. 7). In a world of overwhelming inequality, organs have become just another commodity, as evidenced by the newspaper advertisement run by a destitute shantytown dweller in the early 1980s: "I am willing to sell any organ of my body that is not vital to my survival and which could help save another person in exchange for an amount of money that will allow me to feed my family" (ibid.).

On "orphan drugs," see Ashbury 1991. An orphan drug is defined under the U.S. Orphan Drug Act as one that would not recoup development costs for domestic sales and affects fewer than two hundred thousand individuals in the United States ("Buying into the Orphan Drug Market" 1995). Placing tuberculosis drugs in this category is certainly ironic, considering that tuberculosis remains, along with AIDS, the leading infectious cause of adult death in the world today (Dye, Scheele, Dolin, et al. 1999; World Health Organization 2000a; Joint United Nations Programme on HIV/AIDS 2000). However, tuberculosis drugs have not been deemed profitable, since the poor are so disproportionately afflicted. One candid review of drug development notes that "few developments are need-driven." The average cost of bringing a new drug to market is said to be $224 million, costs that pharmaceutical companies argue would not be recouped for diseases endemic in poor countries, which have few resources and which lack property rights laws to prohibit far cheaper generic products from entering the market (Trouiller and Olliaro 1999). The market fails when it comes to research and development of drugs for diseases of the poor—in the case of tuberculosis, the last novel treatment was developed more than thirty years ago (t'Hoen 2000). For more on the extent to which pharmaceutical companies in the United States and elsewhere neglect diseases that plague the poor in developing regions, see Médecins Sans Frontières 2001.

8. For a more extensive critique of such commodification and the growing influence of market ideology in shaping health care access and delivery in the United States, see Farmer and Rylko-Bauer 2001; Rylko-Bauer and Farmer 2002.

9. Pellegrino 1999, p. 246.

10. Ibid., p. 252.

11. Ibid., p. 257. For more on the concerns regarding American health care and the moral dilemmas created as doctors attempt to straddle conflicting business and medical ethical codes, see Nutter 1984, AMA Council on Ethical and Judicial Affairs 1995, Relman 1991, Gunderman 1998, and Kaveny 1999. Two recent books provide a disturbing view of the issues surrounding "cost-effective" health care and the drive for increasing profit margins by HMOs despite loud protests from both doctors and patients. In *Health Against Wealth*, George Anders describes how the managed-care system used what it termed "Total Qual-

ity Management" (TQM) as its preferred analytic method for assessing the quality of health care, modeled after quality engineering methods employed by the American business community for years: "In the eyes of many managed-care enthusiasts, medicine wasn't that different from car-making or computer-chip fabrication—no matter what doctors or patients thought" (1996, p. 40). In this model, primary-care measures and prevention dominate, and, in the logic of managed care, an HMO could garner a high rating "without having the ability to deliver good care in a crisis" (ibid., p. 41)—in other words, without ever taking care of sick people. *Making a Killing: HMOs and the Threat to Your Health* provides disturbing stories and statistics about poor—and often deadly—management of patients (Court and Smith 1999).

12. The December 2000 decision by Aetna, Inc., to cut 2 million of its 19 million customers and close unprofitable Medicare HMOs in an attempt to increase profits highlights the disturbing trend of HMOs dumping "customers" deemed not profitable (Freudenheim 2000). Since January 1999, more than 1.6 million Medicare beneficiaries have been dropped by HMOs, who claimed that federal payments were too low to cover costs. And the industry's trade association predicts even further pull-outs by health plans in 2002, leaving almost another half million elderly and disabled people with fewer health care options. HMOs that remain in Medicare for the time being predict cuts in benefits or increases in premiums or co-payments to cover costs (Pear 2001).

Others argue that the current for-profit trend of the American health care system is simply not tenable. "Intentionally providing minimally acceptable care to some for the benefit of others in an arbitrary group—let alone for the benefit of the bottom line—is wrong," writes Jerome Kassirer (1998, p. 397). "When patients are sick and vulnerable, they expect their physicians to be their advocates for optimal care, not for some minimalist standard." Arnold Relman concurs: "Today's market-oriented, profit-driven health care industry therefore sends signals to physicians that are frustrating and profoundly disturbing to the majority of us who believe our primary commitment is to patients. Most of us believe we are parties to a social contract, not a business contract. We are not vendors, and we are not merely free economic agents in a free market" (1991, p. 858).

13. Engelhardt and Rie 1988, p. 1089.

14. Ibid., p. 1088.

15. Hasan 1996, p. 1055.

16. Pellegrino 1999, p. 253.

17. Engelhardt and Rie 1988, p. 1086. See also Engelhardt's 1998 comments on the lack of "global bioethics," in which he articulates "the blessings of inequality" (p. 646).

18. For example, in a study of anonymous HIV testing of U.S. women attending an urban prenatal clinic, researchers found that 43 percent of the women who tested positive for HIV reported no "traditional" risk behaviors (Barbacci, Repke, and Chaisson 1991). A different study performed in a gynecology emergency department found that 29 percent of HIV-positive women reported no risk factors for infection (Lindsay, Grant, Peterson, et al. 1993). In a study conducted among U.S. blood donors, nearly half of the women found to be seropositive for

HIV could not identify a risk factor for their infection (Ward, Kleinman, Douglas, et al. 1988).

19. Sontag and Richardson 1997. See also Farmer 1999b, chap. 10.

20. In her discussion of barriers to patient adherence (compliance), Esther Sumartojo cites research showing that "physicians' predictions of nonadherence are accurate in fewer than 50% of cases." In one study, "physicians identified only 32% of nonadherent patients and incorrectly identified 8% of adherent patients as nonadherent" (1993, p. 1312). See also reviews by Mushlin and Appel (1977) and Wardman, Knox, Muers, and Page (1988).

21. See Farmer 1999b and Farmer 2000. For a detailed look at the inequalities faced by one inner-city African American family seeking health care, see Abraham 1993; see also American College of Physicians 1997 for a discussion of inner-city health care problems and policy recommendations.

22. One prescient commentary from 1983 noted the untenable nature of unequal health care provided to rich and poor: "Care of the disadvantaged is a central problem in the health-care system, and it is getting worse. It may not be uppermost among the current concerns of the health professions, government, or industry, but it should be, because it could be the critical weakness in the whole structure. For all the skills that may be developed in the competitive environment, all the marketing, reorganizing, diversifying, and maneuvering of hospitals, unless some combination of the resources of hospitals, doctors, industry, and government can be used to accommodate the needs of the unserved and underserved, our health-care system will be overturned—no matter how efficiently it may serve those who can afford it" (Cunningham 1983, p. 1314).

23. Waldholz 1996.

24. Others, it seems, feel few qualms about making such a statement. George Sher, in detailing why health care options for some "may have to be restricted," observes: "Poverty may be said to be deserved because of past behavior. But one may also connect poverty with desert by invoking *present* behavior. Whatever his history, a person's poverty may be currently avoidable. There may be work available that would provide a decent income. If a poor person rejects such work, or makes only a half-hearted attempt to do it, then he may again be said to deserve his current status" (1983, p. 9).

25. McNeil 2000b. For a description of the processes by which HIV has become entrenched among the poor, see Farmer, Walton, and Furin 2000. The plight of the world's poor who are infected with HIV in the era of effective antiretroviral therapy is discussed in Farmer 2000. Our own efforts to provide such therapy to the destitute sick of Haiti are detailed in Farmer, Léandre, Mukherjee, Claude, et al. 2001 and in Farmer, Léandre, Mukherjee, Gupta, et al. 2001.

26. See Farmer 1999b, chap. 1, for a more detailed description of the clinic, which is in fact a community hospital.

27. World Health Organization 1998. In its 2000 report, the WHO reports that more than two million people died of tuberculosis in 1999, more than 98 percent of them in developing countries (World Health Organization 2000b). Note that HIV has recently overtaken tuberculosis as the leading single infectious killer of adults. But it is also true that many people living with poverty and HIV die of tuberculosis.

28. Reichman 1997, p. 4.

29. Anders 1994.

30. Freudenheim 1995.

31. For a discussion of the compensation of health care executives and HMO profits, see also Anders 1996, chap. 4.

32. Pollack, Woods, and O'Rourke 2001, p. 8.

33. Ibid.

34. Eisenberg 1999, pp. 2253–54.

35. Some have gone so far as to champion "the virtues of skimming and dumping": "Because medicine for profit leads to skimming, it also leads to moral candor, which is an element of good public policy" (Engelhardt and Rie 1988, p. 1088). In the era of managed care, doctors have found themselves in the role of gatekeepers, under pressure to practice "two-tier medicine." For example, patients with "generous" insurance plans can remain in the hospital for the complete maternity stay recommended by the medical panel, whereas those with less coverage are forced out earlier unless they are willing to pay the extra costs themselves (Anders 1996, p. 83). In her detailed study of one poor African American family's struggle for health care, Laurie Kaye Abraham remarks, "Perhaps the *only* time the uninsured have a good chance of getting timely, quality care is when they are damn near death" (Abraham 1993, p. 3).

36. Churchill 1999, p. 255.

37. The problem, according to one critic, lies in the approach of bioethics itself, which fails to acknowledge the experiences of patients and physicians: "Principle-oriented, applied-ethics bioethicists do, of course, use terms like 'empathy' and 'recognition' in their analyses. Yet they are usually pressing to get beyond these items to a formulation of 'the problem' or 'the issue' that will allow them to apply their principles. They tend to see empathy and recognition as preliminaries in the real work of ethics" (Churchill 1997, p. 318). Marcio Fabri dos Anjos, writing from the perspective of liberation theology, offers the following critique of medical ethics:

> If one focuses solely on individuals and relationships among individuals, one robs medicine of the capacity to reflect critically on the influence of social structures on illness and health, and condemns the discipline to a naivete.... In one way or another, social injustice permeates medicine. It is, therefore, impossible for medical ethics as a profession to continue to ignore the issues inherent in social injustice and still consider itself to be "ethical" or as interested in the fundamental moral equality of all persons (1996, p. 633).

This failure of medical ethics is the topic of Chapter 8.

38. Certainly there are other "global cultures," including those advancing one sort of human rights agenda or another. As Michael Ignatieff notes, "We can call this global diffusion of human rights culture a form of moral progress even while remaining skeptical of the motives of those who helped bring it about" (2001, p. 7). Many of the major players have been nongovernmental organizations: "The phrase 'global civil society' implies a cohesive moral movement when the reality is fierce and disputatious rivalry among nongovernmental organiza-

tions. These groups frequently claim that they represent human interests and human rights more effectively than governments, and while this is sometimes true, NGOs are not necessarily more representative or more accountable than *elected* governments" (ibid., pp. 8–9). Two decades in Haiti have certainly convinced me of the importance of this point.

39. Many have commented on what they perceive as a change for the worse in the doctor-patient relationship in this era of HMOs, noting that the cost-control aspect of managed care has the potential to undermine all aspects of the ideal physician-patient relationship, embodied in six tenets: "choice, competence, communication, compassion, continuity, and (no) conflict of interest" (Emanuel and Dubler 1995, p. 323). An estimated 40 million Americans are uninsured during the course of a year; the number almost doubles when you include those who are irregularly insured (lacking coverage during some part of the year) or underinsured (Institute of Medicine 2001, pp. 2–3; Lewin and Altman 2000, p. 91). When they do receive care, the often transitory nature of their interactions with providers means that, "for millions of uninsured Americans, impersonal care has all but displaced caring and enduring physician-patient relationships" (Emanuel and Dubler 1995, p. 325). In their race to cut costs, HMOs have largely ignored what many see as critical to effective medicine: the physician's relationship with the patient over time. Not only is a deeper understanding of the patient's social and medical history realizable only over time, but this relationship itself has a therapeutic value:

> When a physician truly knows a patient, a heartfelt caring and commitment can evolve, which then generates self-love and the motivation to change on the part of the patient. Health is not a state prescribed by the physician; rather, the therapeutic partnership can be the field in which healing takes place.... It therefore seems ironic that while we know the value of this relationship, the managed care mentality regards physicians and patients as faceless pieces of a health care machine that can be substituted without consequences. We hope wise plans will emerge that recognize the price for taking the heart out of healing and realize that, truly, compassion is cost-effective (Doner 1995, p. 609).

The need to argue that even compassion can be cost-effective shows how entrenched these processes of market ideology have become in U.S. medicine.

40. World Health Organization 2000c, p. 55.

41. Rudolf Virchow, along with making great advances in scientific medicine, fought tirelessly for equity and social justice. Virchow and his colleagues called for, among other social changes, the public provision of medical care. As Leon Eisenberg explains in his article "Rudolf Ludwig Karl Virchow, Where Are You Now That We Need You?" (1984, p. 526), Virchow argued that medicine should be reformed on the basis of four principles:

> First, that the health of the people is a matter of direct social concern; second, that social and economic conditions have an important effect on health and disease, and that these relations must be subjected to scientific investigation; third, that the measures taken to promote health and to combat disease must be social as well as medical...; fourth, that "medical statistics will be our standard of measurement."

CHAPTER 7. CRUEL AND UNUSUAL

1. Greifinger, Heywood, and Glaser 1993.

2. Although careful studies are lacking, tuberculosis incidence in prisons in Kazakhstan and other newly independent states of the former Soviet Union may well exceed one hundred times that in surrounding communities. (This estimate is based on data presented at the conference on Public Health Implications of Tuberculosis in Prisons and Jails in Eastern Europe and Central Asia, Budapest, Hungary, June 4–7, 1998. Many of the papers presented at the Budapest conference appear in Stern and Jones 1999.) See also Reyes and Coninx 1997; and Greifinger, Heywood, and Glaser 1993. It's important to add here that nameless millions live in a pre-antibiotic time warp, since they, whether in or out of detention, continue to die from this disease worldwide.

3. The term "geoculture" is after Immanuel Wallerstein: see, for example, Wallerstein 1994 and 1995a.

4. Farmer, Bayona, Becerra, et al. 1997. See also Farmer, Kim, Mitnick, et al. 1999.

5. The U.S. Department of Justice estimates that 13,980,297 arrests took place in the United States in 2000; of these, 625,132 were for violent offenses, and 1,620,928 were for property crimes (U.S. Department of Justice and Federal Bureau of Investigation 2000, p. 216).

6. Reyes and Coninx 1997, p. 1449.

7. The literature on tuberculosis and prisons is of mixed quality. The term "resistance," for example, is misused in several ways. Some social scientists pour resources, material and intellectual, into celebrating prisoners' refusal to take medications as acts of "resistance." For a review, see Farmer 1997d. Certain public health specialists and policymakers, in turn, often attempt to ignore drug resistance in the hope that it will go away.

8. Compare Reyes and Coninx 1997 (pp. 1447, 1449) to Greifinger, Heywood, and Glaser 1993 (p. 339). Note, of course, that the former study refers primarily to resource-poor countries, whereas the latter refers to U.S. institutions.

9. See, for example, Kimerling, Kluge, Vezhnina, et al. 1999; Portaels, Rigouts, and Bastian 1999.

10. According to the *Bureau of Justice Statistics Bulletin,* there were 705 white male inmates per 100,000 residents of this demographic group at mid-year 2001. The corresponding rate for black males was many times higher, at 4,848 per 100,000 (Beck, Karberg, and Harrison 2002).

11. According to the U.S. Bureau of Justice Statistics, 1,965,495 inmates were being held in federal and state prisons and in local jails as of June 30, 2001. In comparison, Russian prisons held 977,700 inmates, who face severe overcrowding and long periods of pre-trial detention (often, years). These statistics are taken from Sentencing Project 2001, 2002a. For a discussion of earlier trends, see Stern 1998. For detailed analyses of the politics and policies of sentencing and incarceration in the United States and a critique of the growing prison industry, see Hallinan 2001 and Wacquant 1999. For the English translation of

this latter volume, see Wacquant 2002; the Wacquant epigraph that opens this chapter is my translation.

12. See, for example, Garrett 1994: "Studies showed that some 80 percent of all MDR-TB index cases in 1989–90 (not including the secondary HIV-positive cases) were injecting drug and crack users, many of whom, as a result of federal and local crackdowns, drifted in and out of the jail and prison system" (p. 524).

13. Braun, Truman, Maguire, et al. 1989.

14. Centers for Disease Control and Prevention 1989; Centers for Disease Control and Prevention 1992b.

15. Laurie Garrett puts it best: "The emergence of novel strains of multiply drug-resistant TB came amid a host of clangs, whistles, and bells that should have served as ample warning to humanity. But the warning fell on unhearing ears" (1994, p. 508).

16. Skolnick 1992.

17. Greifinger, Heywood, and Glaser 1993, p. 335.

18. By 1992, it was being reported that "New York has had the highest reported prevalence of HIV infection among inmates: 12 percent of incoming males and 20 percent of incoming females" (Greifinger, Heywood, and Glaser 1993, p. 334). In 1997, 10.3 percent of the male population and 20.7 percent of the female population in New York prisons were HIV-positive—compared to national rates of 2.2 percent for males and 3.5 percent for females (Maruschak 1999).

19. For a penetrating analysis of the rise of incarceration as a key plank in the "neoliberal" agenda regnant in the United States, see Wacquant 1999. The "war on drugs" is interpreted in a similar light in Chien, Connors, and Fox 2000.

20. Mauer 1999, p. 183. The racial disparity in rates of incarceration increased dramatically between 1988 and 1996: whereas the incarceration rate among whites increased from 134 to 188 per 100,000 population, an increase of 28 percent, the rate among blacks jumped 67 percent, from 922 to 1,547 per 100,000 population (Human Rights Watch 2000). "For the first time, the number of persons admitted for drug offenses was greater than the number admitted for property offenses, violent offenses, or public-order offenses" (Greifinger, Heywood, and Glaser 1993, p. 333). For an important study of race and class in the U.S. criminal justice system, see David Cole's No Equal Justice (1999). "This downward spiral cannot go on forever," concludes Cole. "Unless we begin to think about what criminal justice policy would look like if we could not rely on double standards and disparate impacts, we will continue to be plagued by persistent crime. For pragmatic as well [as] moral reasons, the future of criminal justice depends upon reducing the race and class disparities that society has thus far found so 'useful' " (p. 178).

21. Wacquant 1999, p. 88. Note that the process of privatization Wacquant describes—increasingly, government prisons and holding facilities are transferring prisoners to private security corporations—is not unrelated to the processes of medical privatization described in other chapters. And in both cases, there is growing evidence that privatization has not resulted in the promised cost savings and efficiency and has, in some ways, exacerbated existing problems. (For

example, see Himmelstein, Woolhandler, and Hellander 2001 for a discussion of the impact of for-profit medicine on costs, access, quality, outcomes, and equity in U.S. health care.) In fact, there is a direct link between these two privatization trends. In an effort to cut costs, a number of prisons have hired managed-care organizations (MCOs) to provide health care to inmates. Although money may have been saved, numerous reports describe declining quality of care, including denial or delay of treatment, as well as use of less costly but ineffective treatment. "Since the primary goal of MCOs is enhancing the financial bottom line...[this] often results in treatment decisions that are based less on the inmates' needs and more on saving money" (Robbins 1999, pp. 202–203). A report by the Sentencing Project (2002b) notes that poor oversight has allowed severe mismanagement and even abuse to occur in privately operated prisons, and evidence suggests that private prison corporations have tried to influence sentencing legislation through political contributions.

22. Greifinger, Heywood, and Glaser 1993, p. 333.

23. For example, John Raba, formerly medical director of the Cook County jail, was quick to link the "war on drugs" to outbreaks of MDRTB: "The result is that we are now seeing outbreaks including a number of cases of highly lethal multidrug-resistant TB. We're continuing the nation's program of incarcerating drug users despite the absence of any demonstrated individual or social benefit" (cited in Skolnick 1992, p. 3177).

24. Many patients later shown to have HIV-associated active tuberculosis were smear-negative; many had atypical chest radiographs and disseminated disease.

25. Snider, Salinas, and Kelly 1989, p. 647.

26. Centers for Disease Control and Prevention 1991.

27. Bifani, Pjikaytis, Kapur, et al. 1996.

28. Garrett 1994, p. 520.

29. *New York Post* reporter Ann Bolinger was herself infected with *M. tuberculosis* while covering the Rikers Island outbreak; see Skolnick 1992.

30. Greifinger, Heywood, and Glaser 1993, p. 335.

31. Notes Robert Cohen, former medical director of the Rikers Island jail, "Court-ordered inmate population caps have been the only thing that has kept correctional institutions in many jurisdictions from collapsing into total chaos" (cited in Skolnick 1992, p. 3178).

32. Garrett 1994, p. 523.

33. Cohen is cited in Skolnick 1992, p. 3178.

34. Wacquant 1999, p. 12.

35. Taylor, Besse, and Healing 1994, p. 968.

36. See Garrett 1998.

37. In his remarkable review essay "A Perfect Crime," economist James K. Galbraith offers a view of "rising inequality in the age of globalization" by looking at global trends between 1988 and 1994. "The rise in Russia is extreme," he notes (2002, p. 21). See Figure 4 in his text.

38. Reyes and Coninx 1997, p. 1450; these authors cite A. Khomenko and Médecins Sans Frontières. Note that in the United States, in spite of the magnitude of the problem, deaths from tuberculosis remained relatively rare and did

not inflect the country's overall mortality curves. In a sense, the Russian patients have been transported to the "pre-antibiotic time warp" inhabited by the poor of the Southern hemisphere.

39. Interview by the author with Ivan Nikitovich Simonov, former Chief Inspector of Prisons and now with the Chief Board of Punishment Execution, Ministry of Internal Affairs, Russian Federation, Moscow, June 4, 1998.

40. See Kazionny, Wells, Kluge, et al. (2001) for a description of Russia's growing HIV rates and the potential impact on tuberculosis. According to this study, the seroprevalence of HIV-1 increased thirty-three-fold between 1997 and 2000 in Orel Oblast. The authors warn that if aggressive measures are not taken to halt the HIV epidemic, tuberculosis incidence will skyrocket, as it has in sub-Saharan Africa. Many others have expressed concern over Russia's burgeoning number of HIV cases. At the beginning of May 2002, a total of 193,400 cases were officially registered, up from 177,000 in December 2001, placing Russia right behind the Ukraine for the fastest rise of HIV incidence in the world. AIDS experts warn that the actual number may be much higher, since only a small percent of the Russian population has been tested ("World Bank Forecasts 5.4 Million HIV Cases in Russia by 2020" 2002). World Bank analysts and Russia's Federal AIDS Center have projected that by 2020 the country's economy (as measured by gross domestic product) could shrink by as much as 10.5 percent unless this trend is reversed (Rühl, Pokrovsky, and Vinogradov 2002).

41. Interview by the author with Valery Sergeyev of Penal Reform International, Moscow Bureau, Moscow, June 5, 1998. U.S. prisons are not as crowded as their Russian counterparts because of a meteoric rise in the construction of private prisons: privately owned facilities increased their holding capacities from 15,300 inmates in 1990 to 145,160 by December 1999 (Thomas 2000).

42. It is encouraging that reforms in the Russian penal system (e.g., placing the Department for Execution of Punishments—known as GUIN—under the Ministry of Justice) have led to a drop in the number of people waiting in pretrial detention centers. Just several years earlier, the number was up around 300,000 (GUIN 1999 data); it has since declined to 216,700 (Program in Infectious Disease and Social Change 1999; "Nearly 1,000,000 Locked Up in Russian Prisons" 2002).

43. See Stanley 1998.

44. Alexandra Stanley (1998) recounts a very similar story—that of teenager Dima Shagina, arrested for stealing a car along with other boys. It took almost three years for Shagina's case to come to trial, and by then he was sick with active tuberculosis. His mother hopes that his next stop will be a TB penal colony— she "hopes so" because many tuberculosis patients die in the Matrosskaya Tishina jail.

45. The prison also lacked syringes, masks, and other supplies. As a result, staff morale was low, if not as low as some would expect. "We regard this as an especially terrible problem," remarked the facility's medical director. "We have professionals who want to work but don't have the necessary resources."

46. Interview with Valery Sergeyev.

47. Stanley 1998.

48. The experience accumulated by Partners In Health in Peru shows that a majority of patients sick with even highly resistant strains of MDRTB can be cured; see Farmer, Bayona, Shin, et al. 1998. See also Turett, Telzak, Torian, et al. 1995.

49. "Cohorting" prisoners means that they are divided into groups based on whether or not they have drug-resistant tuberculosis. However, the prisoners are released at the end of their prison terms—if they have managed to survive. With permanent isolation, of course, there is no release (except through death).

50. Reyes and Coninx 1997, p. 1448.

51. Ibid. The irony here is that we're willing to go to war over gasoline prices or weapons inspections but throw our hands up in the face of relatively minor challenges, such as quality control in prison laboratories.

52. Ibid., p. 1449.

53. Cited in ibid., p. 1447; emphasis added.

54. "Since the outbreak in New York, other outbreaks have been reported in correctional systems in Connecticut, Washington, Ohio, Alabama and California. Following the reports of cases in these states, resources were provided for an appropriate public health response. *In contrast, there has been scant funding for TB control outside the prison walls.* This is unfortunate, because TB in prison is solely a symptom of a broader public health problem" (Greifinger, Heywood, and Glaser 1993, p. 336).

55. As this book goes to press, a rethinking of the DOTS strategy in order to account for the problems of HIV and MDRTB has just been published; see *The Global Plan to Stop Tuberculosis* (World Health Organization, Partners In Health, Open Society Institute, et al. 2002).

56. Reyes and Coninx 1997, p. 1447.

57. Foucault 1975, p. 22; my translation.

58. *Estelle v. Gamble*, 429 U.S. 97 (1976). See Robbins 1999 for a discussion of the legal cases since 1976 that have helped to establish the "deliberate indifference" standard for judging the medical treatment (or lack thereof) received by prisoners.

59. The court ruled that the " 'resulting threat to the well-being of the inmates is so serious, and the record so devoid of any justification for the defendants' policy that, under the standard of *Bell v. Wolfish*, this practice constitutes 'punishment' in violation of the Due Process Clause" (cited in Greifinger, Heywood, and Glaser 1993, p. 336).

60. *Austin v. Pennsylvania Department of Correction*, WL 277511, E.D.Pa. (1992).

61. For example, Abbott (1998) describes how a parolee sued a county jail, a prison, and the Colorado Department of Health in 1998 after developing tuberculosis while in prison for theft. This case was later dismissed.

CHAPTER 8. NEW MALAISE

1. For more on the Tuskegee study, including the role that racism played in its continuation, see Brandt 1978 and Jones 1993. The statements of some of those who conducted the study harmonize with the attitudes of their contem-

poraries, the Nazi doctors: "If we could find from 100 to 200 cases...we would not have to go do another Wasserman [test] on useless individuals" (cited in Brandt 1978, p. 23). In response to a suggestion that the study be continued post-1933, one physician initially wrote, "We have no further interest in these patients until they die" (Brandt 1978, p. 24). See also Rothman 1984 and Reverby 2000, a helpful and comprehensive volume.

2. Brandt 1978, p. 27.

3. "Criticized Research Quantifies the Risk of AIDS Infection" 2000.

4. Quinn, Wawer, Sewankambo, et al. 2000, pp. 921, 927, 928.

5. Cohen 2000, p. 972; emphasis added.

6. Shuger 2000. It should be noted that Ugandan government policy allows patients to decide whom to inform of their HIV status and that Quinn and colleagues report that they "strongly encouraged" participants to share their status with their partners (Gray, Quinn, Serwadda, et al. 2000, p. 361).

7. In her accompanying editorial, *New England Journal of Medicine* editor Marcia Angell voiced her hesitation about publishing the study and was quite pointed in her criticism: "It is important to be clear about what this study meant for the participants. It meant that for up to 30 months, several hundred people with HIV infection were observed but not treated." Furthermore, "the very condition that justified doing the study in Uganda in the first place—the lack of availability of antiretroviral treatment—will greatly limit the relevance of the results there" (Angell 2000b, pp. 967–68).

In a letter responding to criticisms from Angell and other researchers, Quinn and colleagues addressed a number of the critiques levied against their study. To those arguing that the study's findings were irrelevant to cash-strapped Uganda, Quinn and colleagues retorted: "Evaluating the control of STDs for the prevention of HIV infection was directly relevant to Ugandan policy. The secondary finding of reduced rates of HIV transmission with lower viral loads provides an impetus for the development of safe, effective, simple, and affordable strategies (use of antiretroviral agents or vaccines) to control the spread of HIV by reducing viremia" (Gray, Quinn, Serwadda, et al. 2000, pp. 361–62). As for the criticism that the care offered was substandard compared to care available in the United States and was therefore unethical, the authors contend that "in both study groups, the care provided far exceeded that available in rural Uganda and in many other states in this country" (ibid., p. 361).

While some argued that the study was important for establishing a "foundation for further research on low-cost, easily administered HIV therapies" (Cates and Coates 2000, p. 363), others were vehement in their criticism. Referring to the oft-used rationale that lack of services in resource-poor settings constitutes a "local standard of care," one researcher questioned the usefulness of the study to the participants: "In the study by Quinn et al., is there any hope that the information gleaned will benefit the population studied? Will members of the population be able to afford viral-load testing? Will adult circumcision be of any benefit? Will this information lead to a reduction in the cost of antiretroviral drugs, making them more affordable in developing countries?" (Mullings 2000, p. 362). Another researcher from the developing world, citing the standards established in the Declaration of Helsinki, wrote: "Clinical trials should be performed when use of the 'best proven' methods can be assured. This approach may delay access to trials for some countries but will be safer and ethical. If at the end of the trial the drug, vaccine, or procedure is found to be effective, it should be made available wherever it is needed.... The justification for different ethical standards for poor countries is based on economic, not on ethical or scientific grounds. Such trials should not be permitted" (Greco 2000, p. 362).

8. Yach and Bettcher comment positively on the effects globalization is having on health systems: "National health systems are becoming transnationalized: the ease and rapidity of communications have facilitated the diffusion of ideas, ideologies, and policy concerns relating to health care (as well as diseases), thereby fostering a global culture of reform" (1998a, p. 736). In calling for "the development of a transnational research agenda" (p. 737), they also note that although the potential health benefits of globalization are immense, "making these technologies available in the poorest communities of the world may require special government incentives, including incentives that could be at odds with norms governing liberalization of trade and removal of special subsidies" (p. 736). For further commentary, see also Yach and Bettcher 1998b; Navarro 1998; and Kim, Millen, Irwin, and Gershman 2000, which provides case studies from several countries on the often detrimental effects of globalization.

9. See Farmer 1996c; Farmer 1999b; Farmer, Bayona, Becerra, et al. 1998; and Garrett 2000. For details on transnational cases of drug-resistant tuberculosis, for example, see Becerra, Farmer, and Kim 1999.

10. In defending their decision not to treat HIV-infected study participants, Quinn and colleagues wrote, "Most importantly, neither we nor the Ugandan government had, or currently have, the clinical capacity to manage antiretroviral treatment, including side effects and compliance" (Gray, Quinn, Serwadda, et al. 2000, p. 361). It is precisely this attitude that I, and many of those who wrote letters voicing their objections to the study, argue is wrong. Critiquing the common argument that weak infrastructure makes treating the sick an impossibility in poor countries, Nguyen retorts, "Using the 'weak-infrastructure' excuse to not do anything is equivalent to refusing to offer someone CPR because cutbacks have closed the local intensive-care unit" (2000). Farmer, Léandre, Mukherjee, Claude, et al. 2001 describes an HIV-treatment project in Central Haiti that demonstrates the feasibility of complex antiretroviral treatments in resource-poor settings with minimal infrastructure. It can be done, if the will and the resources are there.

11. In 2000, South Africa and Namibia rejected the offer of a billion dollars in annual loans from the United States to purchase antiretrovirals, arguing that such measures would only burden their already struggling economies with more debt. Dr. Kalumbi Shangula, permanent secretary for the Namibian Ministry of Health, noted, "When you take loans, you are actually plunging the country deeply into debt. We are actually looking for ways to acquire the anti-retroviral drugs to improve the quality of life of our people, but this does not offer a solution" (Swarns 2000).

Pharmaceutical companies in the United States and other industrialized nations have protested vehemently when drugs, including antiretrovirals, are produced as generics in the developing world. Such competition, they argue, leaves them unable to recoup their research and development (R&D) costs. However, closer scrutiny of profits and spending shows that, in many cases, U.S. drug companies devote more money to marketing, advertising, and administration than to R&D (Pollack and O'Rourke 2001).

A recent study also challenges this oft-stated justification that high drug costs are needed to help fund the R&D of new drugs. Analysis of the 1,035 new drugs approved by the U.S. Food and Drug Administration in the twelve-year period from 1989 to 2000 found that only 15 percent were highly innovative drugs—containing new active ingredients and promising significant clinical advances. Most of the remaining approved drugs were incrementally modified (changed versions of older products) and often provided a high return on investment, since R&D costs were lower (National Institute for Health Care Management 2002a).

In addition, transnational pharmaceutical companies based in Europe, the United States, and Japan are coming under criticism for focusing all their R&D efforts on drugs for health problems that occur primarily in relatively wealthy industrialized countries, to the neglect of infectious diseases that largely affect the "bottom billion" and account for most premature deaths in the developing world today. Industry-sponsored surveys indicate that of the 137 new medicines under development in 2000, only one was intended to treat sleeping sickness and one to treat malaria; none were being developed for tuberculosis or leishmaniasis (Médecins San Frontières 2001, p. 12). Although almost twice as many drugs are being developed in 2002, according to the U.S. drug industry lobby group PhRMA, the R&D efforts aimed at neglected diseases remain negligible (Pharmaceutical Research and Manufacturers of America 2002).

The R&D protection argument is especially flawed when applied to anti-HIV drugs, since many antiretrovirals were developed in publicly funded laboratories and underwent clinical trials using public funds; public authorities hold the patents for antiretrovirals such as didanosine, stavudine, and zalcitabine, although private companies hold the commercial rights. For more on how U.S drug companies profit from public research funds, see Gerth and Stolberg 2000. One commentary notes: "Nothing explains why companies charge so much except that [the drugs] were initially put on the market in the USA, a rich country without price controls. Unfortunately for most of the world's 34 million people infected with HIV, pharmaceutical companies impose U.S. prices on the rest of the world" (Chirac, von Schoen-Angerer, Kasper, et al. 2000, p. 502).

Pharmaceutical giant Glaxo-Wellcome's attempt in 2000 to block the sale of cheaper generic AIDS drugs in Ghana is just one example of the high stakes and complicated legal battles surrounding patent rights versus patient rights in the developing world. The *Wall Street Journal* reported in December 2000 that when a Ghanaian pharmaceutical distributor purchased an Indian-made generic version of Glaxo-Wellcome's potent (and highly profitable) Combivir, Glaxo-Wellcome threatened retribution, charging that this violated its exclusive patent rights—an argument that, some noted, had no legal grounds. Estimated total worldwide sales of Combivir (and the two drugs forming the combination, AZT and 3TC) topped $1.1 billion in 2000 (Schoofs 2000). The pharmaceutical companies' offers to African governments to provide AIDS drugs for reduced cost prompted the following criticism from India's Minister of Health: " 'If they can offer an 80% discount, there was something wrong with the price they started off with' " (McNeil 2000d, p. A14).

The expanding debate around anti-HIV therapy in developing countries provides a hopeful sign that things may be changing. For example, in a letter to the journal *Health and Human Rights,* Chirac and colleagues argue that the increasing technology and outcome gap between AIDS patients in the developed world and those in the developing world is more than a medical concern: "This gap is also a social, economic, moral, and political issue. The question of AIDS treatment leads to a wider reflection of the balance between public and private interests, between patent rights and the rights of patients. Access to health care and to medical progress as a human right is a challenge that AIDS poses to humanity. It is no longer morally acceptable to debate if antiretrovirals should be provided. We should now concentrate on how quickly they can be provided" (Chirac, von Schoen-Angerer, Kasper, et al. 2000, p. 502).

The author of a series of *New York Times* articles about the global AIDS crisis concludes on a similar note: "The question is: How much would it cost to contain the global AIDS epidemic? The short answer is: Well, how much have you got? How much would it cost to banish ignorance, to deaden lust, to shame rape, to stop war, to enrich the poor, to empower women, to defend children, to make decent medical care as globally ubiquitous as Coca-Cola—in short, to get rid of all the underlying causes of the epidemic in the third world?" (McNeil 2000b, p. 1).

The growing awareness of the magnitude of the global AIDS crisis and its massive mortality, coupled with uproar over the high cost of AIDS drugs, has led some pharmaceutical companies to bow to public pressure and start reducing prices. In fact, PhRMA, on its Web site, touts the philanthropic efforts of its members in creating global partnerships aimed at improving public health; see, for example, the Web publication "Global Partnerships: Humanitarian Programs of the Pharmaceutical Industry in Developing Countries" (Pharmaceutical Research and Manufacturers of America 2001). What isn't evident from this public relations material, according to Pollack (2001), is that such efforts are sometimes aimed at protecting self-interests and preempting anti-patent actions on the part of developing countries.

Some critics argue that such efforts on the part of the drug industry are not enough and that the only moral and ethical step is to reduce the cost of AIDS drugs to zero in the settings most affected by both HIV and poverty. "These initial acts of generosity only set the stage for what the world really needs: a dramatic, unprecedented, and unequivocal decision by the boards and executives of several important pharmaceutical companies to make their anti-HIV drugs free. Not half a loaf—a whole loaf. If they did that, these leaders would change the face of the world" (Berwick 2002, p. 216).

12. Schüklenk 2000, p. 973. Another contentious medical development was the research and development associated with the introduction of Norplant, approved by the U.S. Food and Drug Administration in 1990. Soheir Morsy's 1993 account of the development of the drug in Egypt and the use of Egyptian women as research subjects is illuminating for what it says about the ethics of medical

trials. See also Mintzes, Hardon, and Hanhart 1993, the edited volume in which Morsy's chapter appears.

13. World Medical Association 1983.

14. Gray, Quinn, Serwadda, et al. 2000.

15. Angell 1997a, p. 849.

16. The official title of the document, published simultaneously in several journals in early 1999, is "A Shared Statement of Ethical Principles for Those Who Shape and Give Health Care" (Benatar, Berwick, Bisognano, et al. 1999; Smith, Hiatt, and Berwick 1999a and 1999b). I had the good fortune to be involved in some of the follow-up discussions of the Tavistock Group, held in April 2000 at the American Academy of Arts and Sciences in Cambridge, Massachusetts. This meeting led to further clarification and expansion of the initial five principles into the following seven Tavistock principles:

Rights: People have a right to health and health care

Balance: Care of individual patients is central, but the health of populations is also our concern

Comprehensiveness: In addition to treating illness, we have an obligation to ease suffering, minimise disability, prevent disease, and promote health

Cooperation: Health care succeeds only if we cooperate with those we serve, each other, and those in other sectors

Improvement: Improving health care is a serious and continuing responsibility

Safety: Do no harm

Openness: Being open, honest, and trustworthy is vital in health care

(Berwick, Davidoff, Hiatt, et al. 2001, p. 616)

17. Benatar, Berwick, Bisognano, et al. 1999, p. 145; Smith, Hiatt, and Berwick 1999a, p. 250.

18. Sohl and Bassford 1986, p. 1175.

19. Sobrino 1988, p. 30.

20. Hippocrates' concise definition of medicine leaves little doubt what our mandate as healers should be: "I will define what I conceive medicine to be. In general terms, it is to do away with the suffering of the sick, to lessen the violence of their diseases, and to refuse to treat those who are over-ministered by their diseases, realizing that in such cases medicine is powerless" (from "The Art," cited in Sohl and Bassford 1986, p. 1176). Noting that this central concept of medicine—to heal the sick and do no harm—remains unchanged centuries later, Sohl and Bassford comment that "contemporary codes also emphasize the basic position of the patient-care norm" (ibid.).

21. For example, in a large study examining the relation between poverty and medical treatment of acute myocardial infarction in the United States, Rathore and colleagues found that black, female, and poor patients had inferior care during hospitalization and were not consistently offered even inexpensive therapies upon discharge (Rathore, Berger, Weinfurt, et al. 2000). Given the close association between race and class in the United States, it is also relevant to mention the growing body of evidence revealing significant racial and ethnic disparities in health outcomes, in type and quality of health care that African Americans and members of other minorities receive—even after certain access-related

factors such as education, income, and insurance status are controlled (Byrd and Clayton 2002; Fiscella, Franks, Gold, et al. 2000; Freeman and Payne 2000; Institute of Medicine 2002b; Schneider, Zaslavsky, and Epstein 2002). For an indepth discussion of the impact that lack of insurance has on both health status and health care outcomes, see Institute of Medicine 2002a.

22. The 2001 World Development Indicators say it all (World Bank 2001, pp. 98–100). Take Benin, for example, which has only one physician and two hospital beds for every 10,000 people; the same is true for Mali (data collected from 1990 to 1998). Eleven other African countries (Angola, Burkina Faso, Chad, Eritrea, The Gambia, Ethiopia, Malawi, Niger, Rwanda, Tanzania, and Uganda) and one Asian country (Nepal) have a physician-to-population ratio that is worse than 1:10,000, whereas the United States has 27 physicians for the same number of people. These ratios do not necessarily vary by a country's gross national product. Relatively poor Cuba, for example, has more physicians per capita population than any country in the world except Italy. As Chapter 2 noted, Cuba is also judged to have the most equitably financed health care system in Latin America.

23. Tomes 1998.

24. Thomas 1983.

25. A report by the World Bank in 2000, *The Burden of Disease Among the Global Poor,* details the striking differences between poor and nonpoor, noting that "disease patterns vary systematically across class" (Gwatkin and Guillot 2000, p. 3). Communicable diseases, which caused only 7.7 percent of deaths among the affluent, accounted for 58.6 percent of deaths among the globe's poor and 34.2 percent of deaths overall. The World Health Organization (1999c) presents similar figures for 1999, noting that infectious diseases caused approximately 25 percent of deaths worldwide—but accounted for at least 45 percent of deaths in low-income countries.

While the poor are dying of communicable diseases (tuberculosis and other respiratory infections, AIDS, diarrheal diseases, perinatal infections), the top five leading causes of death for the nonpoor are all noncommunicable diseases (ischemic heart disease, malignant neoplasms, cerebrovascular disease), according to the World Bank report. A striking example is pneumonia: 99 percent of deaths caused by pneumonia occur in developing countries (World Health Organization 1999c). Murray and Lopez (1996) also present telling statistics: while close to 0 percent of deaths in developed regions in 1990 were the result of poor water supply, sanitation, and personal and domestic hygiene (and therefore the pathogens that typically accompany such situations), 6.7 percent of deaths in developing regions—a total of 2,664,700 deaths—were the result of such conditions in that same year (p. 312). In terms of future epidemiological projections, the baseline scenario of the ten leading causes of death projected for 2020 differ for developed versus developing regions. While seven of the causes are the same on both lists, the remaining three listed for developing regions are preventable and treatable infectious diseases: tuberculosis, diarrheal disease, and HIV. Those for developed regions, on the other hand, include self-inflicted injuries, colon and rectal cancers, and diabetes mellitus (pp. 362–63). The World Bank terms the amount of excess death and disability experienced by the poor in comparison with the nonpoor the "Poor-Rich Gap," noting that communicable diseases account for 77 percent of this difference in deaths.

26. Of course, it may well be that my fellow clinicians are unaware of the country of origin of those who keep the hospital clean:

> No one asks
> where I am from,
> I must be
> From the country of janitors,
> I have always mopped this floor.
>> Martín Espada, "Jorge the
>> Church Janitor Finally Quits"

27. Churchill 1999, p. 255. The medical anthropologist Arthur Kleinman received no small amount of animus from medical ethicists when he suggested, in the *Encyclopedia of Bioethics,* that medical ethics was often quite divorced from any tangible social reality (Kleinman 1995).

28. For a discussion of the contributions anthropology could make to bioethics, see Marshall and Koenig 1996.

29. Churchill 1999, p. 259.

30. Benatar, Berwick, Bisognano, et al. 1999, p. 146.

31. Ibid., p. 145.

32. Wood, Braitstein, Montaner, et al. 2000, p. 2095.

33. Ibid.

34. This point was made in reference to the chief infectious causes of adult death (tuberculosis and HIV) in a series of publications seeking to cast treatment as a human right; see Farmer 2001a; Farmer 2001b; and Farmer, Léandre, Mukherjee, Claude, et al. 2001.

35. Perhaps one reason that France continues to refer to the "rights of the citizen" is because it expends no small amount of energy denying some within its borders those rights: "In France, the government has passed laws that not only limit migrants from their erstwhile colonies but even make it more difficult for migrants' children, themselves born in France, to become citizens" (Wallerstein 1995a, p. 160). Of course, other affluent European nations are almost as bad; Germany has a "racial" category for citizenship. The United States, a nation of immigrants, is also well known for widespread anti-immigrant views. See Bhabha 1998a and 1998b for an in-depth discussion of the legal and human rights implications of anti-immigrant sentiment.

36. For a classic account of class and color tension in pre-revolutionary Haiti, see James 1963.

37. Wallerstein 1995a, pp. 6–7. He continues: "But to be agencies of transformation, [groups] must be clear about their egalitarian objectives. Fighting for the rights of the group as one instance of the struggle for equality is quite different from fighting for the rights of the group to 'catch up' and move to the head of the line (which has in any case become for most groups an implausible objective)" (p. 7).

38. This liberal critique of physicians working in another country when they "should be" working in their own exposes another fundamental hypocrisy of

liberalism: that concerning immigration. It's worth quoting Wallerstein at some length:

> Let us take a simple, very important, and very immediately relevant issue: migra-
> tion. The political economy of the migration issue is extremely simple. The
> world-economy is more polarized than ever in two ways: socioeconomically and
> demographically. The gap is yawning between North and South and shows every
> sign of widening still further in the next several decades. The consequence is
> obvious. There is an enormous North-South migratory pressure.
>   Look at this from the perspective of liberal ideology. The concept of human
> rights obviously includes the right to move about. In the logic of liberalism, there
> should be no passports and no visas. Everyone should be allowed to work and
> settle everywhere, as is, for example, true within the United States and within
> most states today—certainly within any state that pretends to be a liberal state.
>   In practice, of course, most people in the North are literally aghast at the idea
> of open frontiers (1995a, p. 160).

39. Awareness and remediation of these structural patterns should be implicit in the doctor-patient contract: "It is clear today that the organization, adminis-tration and delivery of health care services are related to the socio-economic structure of each society.... If physicians do not investigate which economic sys-tems can best provide proper health care delivery and do not campaign for the introduction of those which do so, then they will fall into a cultural relativism, will no longer make the health of the patient the first consideration, but rather will allow political considerations to over-ride the physician's first duty" (Sohl and Bassford 1986, p. 1179).

40. In discussing U.S. journalists' critique of Cuba's AIDS programs, Aviva Chomsky notes: "United States media accounts have been fairly consistent in fo-cusing on the issue of freedom for those diagnosed HIV-positive and the ethical issues surrounding mandatory testing, rather than the health aspects of Cuba's AIDS programs. Ethical issues, however, have been narrowly defined by the U.S. media as individual independence from state interference. In this formulation, access or lack of access to medical treatment (much less to minimal standards of nutrition and shelter) is not an ethical issue" (2000, p. 339).

41. For considerations of the relationship between the Nuremberg code and American bioethics, see Faden, Lederer, and Moreno. 1996; Moreno 1997; Moreno and Lederer 1996; Pellegrino 1997; Pellegrino and Thomasma 2000; Sidel 1996. See also Aly, Chroust, and Pross 1994.

42. See, for example, White 2000. First, White argues that because syphilis in Macon County constituted a major public health problem, "a valid scientific, med-ical, and public health rationale was the basis for the initial design of the study" (p. 18). Second, he notes that a large percentage of the men followed were either over fifty years of age or had had syphilis infections for fifteen years or longer and that it was standard treatment in the 1930s and 1940s not to treat such men (p. 15). Third, he asserts that "the TSUS results were presented at medical meetings and published in mainstream peer-reviewed medical journals" (p. 18). Although White concedes that lying to study participants was problematic, he concludes with a nod to identity politics: "black professionals were experts on syphilis and seemingly valuable collaborators with white physicians in the TSUS" (p. 18).

43. Of course, this is a rhetorical point, too, since the U.S. Catholic Church should also of course excommunicate all Catholic physicians who are party to state-sponsored murder.

44. Virchow was committed to improving the health of the many, as opposed to just that of the few. "For if medicine is really to accomplish its great task," he wrote, "it must intervene in political and social life. It must point out the hindrances that impede the normal social functioning of vital processes, and effect their removal" (1849, p. 48). Navarro notes in a letter published in the *Lancet:* "Public-health institutions, including international ones, too often ignore the analysis by one of the founders of public health, Virchow, who noted that 'medicine is not only a biological, but also a social intervention and politics is public health in the most profound sense'" (1997, p. 1480). See also Eisenberg 1984.

45. Pellegrino makes a similar point: "One thing is certain: if health care is a commodity, it is for sale, and the physician is, indeed, a money-maker; if it is a human good, it cannot be for sale and the physician is a healer" (1999, p. 262).

46. An alternative strategy would be to depart from the individual and instead focus on the group, guided by an ethics of distributive justice, one involving a redistribution of resources. Iris Marion Young argues that an absence of justice implies complicity with the existing power structures: "An account of justice that sees the prevailing system not simply as 'benignly neglectful' of women, minorities, and the poor, but as positively hostile to them, must put its focus first on power rather than on how goods and services are handed out" (cited in Nelson and Nelson 1996, p. 355). Hilda Nelson and James Lindemann Nelson (1996) advocate a feminist approach to create a theory of justice in health care, one that focuses on the individual and considers patterns of power—and abuse of power—with the aim of empowering individuals. For a discussion of the role of feminism in bioethics, see the edited volume Wolf 1996. Nelson (1997) discusses the contributions of narratives to bioethics. See also Jos V. M. Welie's (1998) presentation of a philosophical-anthropological foundation for bioethics.

47. Clinton 2000.

48. Benatar, Berwick, Bisognano, et al. 1999, p. 146.

49. As the *Financial Times* reported in April 2000, *conservative* estimates are that between $130 and $140 billion of capital had left Russia since 1993. Meanwhile, during that same period, direct foreign investment was only $10 billion, and support from international financial institutions was also a mere fraction of the amount of capital lost, with the IMF and World Bank providing $25 billion (Peel 2000). Seven months earlier, the *Times* had reported that the Russian government was the world's most indebted country in 1998: public debt was a staggering 7.7 times the annual federal cash revenue. The second most indebted was Lebanon, with a public debt 6.3 times the government's revenue after more than twenty-five years of civil war (Thornhill and Ostrovsky 1999).

CHAPTER 9. RETHINKING HEALTH AND HUMAN RIGHTS

1. Universal Declaration of Human Rights 1948.

2. Telzak, Sepkowitz, Alpert, et al. 1995, p. 911. For papers reporting MDRTB cure rates greater than 80 percent, see reports of preliminary outcomes

in urban Peru (Farmer, Bayona, Shin, et al. 1998; Farmer, Kim, Mitnick, et al. 1999; Mitnick, Palacios, Shin, et al. 2001) and the more recent report of high cure rates in Turkey (Tahaoğlu, Törün, Sevim, et al. 2001). In an editorial accompanying this latter article in the *New England Journal of Medicine*, I argue that such efforts should be seen in a human rights framework (Farmer 2001b).

3. Amnesty International 1997, p. 31.

4. Interview by the author with Ivan Nikitovich Simonov, former Chief Inspector of Prisons and now with the Chief Board of Punishment Execution, Ministry of Internal Affairs, Russian Federation, Moscow, June 4, 1998.

5. Wedel 1998, p. 5. Another way of phrasing this, of course, is that structural violence has become more extreme in the post-Soviet era and that, as elsewhere, high levels of structural violence are associated with criminality. The examples cited in these pages—in Chapters 4 and 7, particularly—support this hypothesis. To the extent that Western advisers have been architects of many of these changes in Russia, they share responsibility for the prison-seated tuberculosis epidemic.

6. Interview by the author with Dr. Natalya Vezhina, Medical Director, TB Colony 33, Mariinsk, Kemerovo, Russian Federation, September 1998.

7. For example, see Dlugy 1999. As earlier chapters noted, anti-Russian prejudices are subtle but widespread in international TB circles.

8. See, for example, Alexander 1998. At about the same time, however, forces within the WHO Global Tuberculosis Programme began supporting the search for alternative forms of therapy for patients with MDRTB. For more on this process, see Farmer and Kim 1998; World Health Organization 1999a and 1999b.

9. This topic is discussed in Reyes and Coninx 1997. See also the exchange in Coker 2000 and Farmer and Kim 2000.

10. Farmer, Bayona, Shin, et al. 1998; Mitnick, Palacios, Shin, et al. 2001.

11. See Gupta, Kim, Espinal, et al. 2001.

12. For a rebuttal of these claims, see Farmer, Bayona, Becerra, et al. 1998. A WHO-led review (Espinal, Kim, Suarez, et al. 2000) more recently came to the same conclusion.

13. Michael Ignatieff points out that, despite the possible improvements brought about by human rights groups, their actions do not always fully coincide with the wishes of those for whom they purport to speak: "[Human rights activists] are not elected by the victim groups they represent, and in the nature of things they cannot be. But this leaves unresolved their right to speak for and on behalf of the people whose rights they defend.... Few mechanisms of genuine accountability connect NGOs and the communities in civil society whose interests they seek to advance" (2001, p. 10).

14. My translation from Haitian Creole. The original declaration—and also translations into French and Spanish and another English translation—may be found at the Partners In Health Web site, *http://www.pih.org.*

15. Cultural relativism as a "metaethical theory" has its role and, contrary to popular belief, is not incompatible with universal values. Although I cannot review the topic here, my thinking on these matters has been informed most by my fieldwork in Haiti, but also by others in and outside anthropology. See, for

example, Campbell 1972, Geertz 1984, Hatch 1983, Renteln 1988, and Schmidt 1955. Also see Talal Asad's discussion of torture: "Although the phrase 'torture or cruel, inhuman, or degrading treatment' serves today as a cross-cultural criterion for making moral and legal judgments about pain and suffering, it nevertheless derives much of its operative sense historically and culturally" (1997, p. 285). For an exploration of cultural relativism and bioethics, see Macklin 1999.

16. Steiner and Alston 1996, p. vi.

17. A notable precedent can be found in the multinational mobilization against King Leopold's brutal exploitation of the Congo; see Adam Hochschild's gripping account of "the first great international human rights movement of the twentieth century" (1998, p. 2). Ignatieff notes correctly that "all human rights activism in the modern world properly traces its origins back to the campaigns to abolish the slave trade and then slavery itself" (2001, p. 10).

18. For an examination of the search for justice in the aftermath of the genocides in Rwanda and Bosnia, both at the international level of the war crimes tribunals and at the personal level through the struggles of individual victims, see Neuffer 2001.

19. Neier 1998, p. 75. Binford makes a similar point: "The fact that human rights organizations key their analyses to international laws that provide substantial protection to civilians who live in the midst of civil war makes little difference, because the laws are not obeyed" (1996, p. 6). Why do states sign human rights accords that they do not intend to respect? In 1989, Louis Henkin wrote: "One can only speculate as to why States accepted these norms and agreements, but it may be reasonable to doubt whether those developments authentically reflected sensitivity to human rights generally. States attended to what occurred inside another State when such happenings impinged upon their political-economic interests" (quoted in Steiner and Alston 1996, p. 114).

20. Gutiérrez 1983, p. 87.

21. Sobrino 1988, p. 105.

22. Higgins is quoted in Steiner and Alston 1996, p. 141; emphasis in the original.

23. Keegan 1996. These disparities have only grown since the mid-1990s. By the end of the decade, the United Nations Development Programme estimated that the fifteen richest individuals on earth controlled more assets than the combined annual gross domestic product (GDP) of all of sub-Saharan Africa (United Nations Development Programme 1998). Furthermore, the wealth of the three richest people in the world exceeded the total annual GDP of the forty-eight least developed countries (United Nations Development Programme 1999).

24. Millen and Holtz 2000.

25. On the pathogenic effects of inequality, see Farmer 1999b; Wilkinson 1996; and Kawachi, Kennedy, Lochner, et al. 1997. See also the work of Didier Fassin (1996) and that of Dozon and Fassin (2001), as well as the volume edited by Leclerc, Fassin, Grandjean, et al. (2000). Although this literature is of recent vintage, the constitution of the World Health Organization (1946) underscores a similar point: "Unequal development in different countries in the

promotion of health and control of disease, especially communicable disease, is a common danger."

26. A growing number of public health practitioners and physicians have been pushing for a concerted effort to reduce inequalities in health; for a review, see Whitehead, Scott-Samuel, and Dahlgren 1998. One of the trends emerging from this literature is that, despite improvement in absolute health indicators for both rich and poor populations, the outcome gap is widening, and this rising inequity has its own pathogenic impact. For case studies from Brazil, see Victora, Vaughan, Barros, et al. 2000. One of the pioneers in U.S. efforts to set goals for reducing inequalities of health outcomes was Dr. Julius Richmond, who not coincidentally was the U.S. representative to the famous 1978 meeting in Almaty (formerly Alma-Ata), Kazakhstan, which issued the call for "health for all by the year 2000." Many were surprised that the U.S. delegation did not attempt to prevent the ratification of a document that claimed access to health care was a fundamental human right.

27. I am, of course, glossing a very complicated process in simple terms. The defeat of the social justice agenda of the Aristide government, which explicitly endorsed the "right to development," seemed almost complete by the time the Haitian government signed on to a structural adjustment project endorsed by the World Bank and the U.S. government; see Farmer 1995d for a more in-depth discussion of this process. But, as Chapter 2 suggests, the movement remains alive within Haiti. The concept of development as a new human right, most eloquently endorsed by Judge Mohammed Bedjaoui, president of the International Court of Justice, has been hotly contested by the United States, which Steiner and Alston (1996, p. 1113) describe as "an implacable opponent of the right to development." For a more detailed examination of the relationship between human rights and structural adjustment projects, see Skogly 1993.

28. For a consideration of obstacles to efforts to punish crimes against humanity in Haiti, see Chapter 2 of this book as well as Priscilla Hayner's work (2001). Brian Concannon (2000) is able to end his own overview on a positive note:

> After this Article's submission, the Raboteau Massacre trial reached its conclusion. The jury convicted sixteen of the twenty-two defendants in custody, most of whom received life sentences. The judge convicted all thirty-seven in absentia defendants, including the leaders of the dictatorship, all members of the military high command, and leaders of FRAPH, the main paramilitary organization. The court awarded $150 million in compensatory damages.
>
> The trial's principal lesson to the international community is that a poor country with an underdeveloped judiciary making a difficult democratic transition can still provide high-quality justice for its victims (pp. 248–49).

29. *Nunca Más*, the report of the Alfonsín-appointed Sábato commission (Comisión Nacional Sobre la Desaparición de Personas 1986), remains the best text on the subject. Its English translation is introduced by Ronald Dworkin, who writes of a "system of licensed sadism." See also Dussel, Finocchio, and Gojman 1997; Steadman 1997; Ciancaglini and Granovsky 1995. Andersen 1993 is close to a definitive treatment of the Argentine case. On El Salvador, the official report was published in *Estudios Centroamericanos;* see "De la locura a

la esperanza: La guerra de doce años en El Salvador" 1993. Hayner (2001) has recently reviewed the fate of some twenty truth commissions, including all those mentioned here.

30. Neier 1998, p. 33.

31. This view is compellingly defended by Neier, who wonders "why the Argentine prosecution of crimes against human rights started so promisingly and why it ended so badly" (1990, p. 34; see also Neier 1998). The later rearrest of General Massera may augur a resurgence of official interest in ending impunity in Argentina.

32. For overviews, see Guillermoprieto 1994, Chomsky 1985, and LaFeber 1984. For a case study from El Salvador, see the accounts of the El Mozote massacre by Binford (1996) and Danner (1993, 1994).

33. Bourdieu 1993, p. 944; my translation.

34. Ignatieff 2001, pp. 19–20, 22–23.

35. For an overview of critiques of anthropology as a colonial project, see Asad 1975. See also the classic essays by Hymes (1974) and Berreman (1974). As noted in the previous chapter, these debates resonate with recent critiques of U.S.-funded AIDS research in the developing world. For her comparison of placebo studies on HIV-infected mothers in Africa with the Tuskegee study, *New England Journal of Medicine* editor Marcia Angell was taken to task by prominent figures in the scientific community (e.g., Varmus and Satcher 1997), and two influential AIDS specialists resigned from the editorial board of the journal in protest (Saltus 1997). The debate continued with a *New York Times* front-page exploration of the ironies of U.S.-funded AIDS research in the Ivory Coast (French 1997). Angell justified her analogy by making a point-by-point comparison between the AIDS trials and the infamous syphilis study (1997b). See Chapter 8 of this book for more extensive discussion of these issues.

36. My translation, with the help of the songwriter Manno Charlemagne. From the album *Manno Charlemagne*, 1988, Mini Records.

37. See Farmer 1994 and Hancock 1989 for overviews of the type and extent of international aid to these regimes.

38. See Wallerstein 1995b.

39. Farmer 1992a.

40. Steiner and Alston 1996, p. 1110.

41. Harrison 1993, p. 102. For a discussion of this position, see Farmer 1994, p. 57. Lawrence Harrison subsequently became director of the entire agency.

42. Comandancia General del EZLN 1993; my translation.

43. Compare the situation in Chiapas to the impact of militarization in the Philippines, as described by Lynn Kwiatkowski (1998).

44. Physicians for Human Rights 1999, p. 4.

45. Neier 1998, p. 50.

46. I refer here to the case of Michael Fay, an eighteen-year-old U.S. citizen convicted of vandalizing cars and tearing down traffic signs in Singapore. According to the *Fort Worth Star-Telegram*, "Amnesty International sees the Fay case as one more reason to refocus international attention on the inhumaneness of flogging." But "many Americans," noted the article, "are surprisingly unsympathetic to the plight of the Ohio youth" (DeWitt 1994). The piece went on

to note that letters to the editor of the *Dayton Daily News,* Fay's hometown newspaper, were "running against the youth," and the Singapore embassy in Washington, D.C., asserted that the majority of mail it received supported Singapore's position.

47. This trend has already occasioned much commentary in the popular and scholarly literature. See, for example, Gitlin 1995, Glendon 1991, Hughes 1993, and Jacoby 1994. Gitlin noted trenchantly that "the politics of identity is silent on the deepest sources of social misery: the devastation of the cities, the draining of resources away from the public and into the private hands of the few. It does not organize to reduce the sickening inequality between rich and poor" (1995, p. 236).

48. See Steiner and Alston 1996, pp. 128–31, for an overview of the legal controversy over a hierarchy of rights. See also Alston's 1984 discussion of the proliferation of proposed rights, which have ranged from the "right to sleep" to the "right to tourism."

49. The passion of Chouchou Louis is recounted in Farmer 1994, chap. 7, and more briefly in Chapter 1 of this book. Precisely the same pattern has been well documented in El Salvador and Guatemala; see Farmer 1994, chap. 5, for a comparison between these two countries and Haiti. With the help of courageous colleagues in Haiti, it was possible for North Americans to work in solidarity on several levels. For example, an account of the murder of Chouchou Louis appeared under David Nyhan's name in the *Boston Globe* (Nyhan 1992); subsequent accounts appeared in a political magazine and in Farmer 1994. Pax Christi visited central Haiti in the spring of 1992 and interviewed torture victims and the families of the disappeared, including the widow of Chouchou Louis (see Pax Christi International 1992). The effects of the 1991 coup d'état on the health of the local population are explored in Farmer 1996a and Farmer and Bertrand 2000. For a penetrating view of "Operation Uphold Democracy," as the 1994 U.S.-led restoration of Aristide was termed, see Shacochis 1999. In the 2000 elections, the Haitian people again turned out in force (in contrast to the spurious reporting in the official press and the U.S. media) to hand an overwhelming majority to Aristide and other members of Fanmi Lavalas, the party he founded. To the majority of Haitians, Aristide is still associated with the primary goals of the Haitian popular movement—social and economic rights for the poor.

50. For more on these events and related topics, see Concannon 2000; see also the postscript to Chapter 2 of this book.

51. Even after indisputable evidence—eyewitness reports from sole survivor Rufina Amaya, forensic data, front-page stories in the *New York Times* and the *Washington Post*—of the Salvadoran army's murderous rampages against unarmed civilians, the Reagan administration had little trouble "recertifying" El Salvador as a country that respected human rights: "In the United States, the free press was not to be denied: El Mozote was reported; Rufina's story was told; the angry debate in Congress intensified. But then the Republican Administration, burdened as it was with the heavy duties of national security, denied that any credible evidence existed that a massacre had taken place; and the Democratic Congress, after denouncing, yet again, the murderous abuses of the Salvadoran

regime, in the end accepted the Administration's 'certification' that its ally was nonetheless making a 'significant effort to comply with internationally recognized human rights.' The flow of aid went on, and soon increased" (Danner 1993, p. 53). Meanwhile, the sole Latin American country that is not a U.S. client state has been the victim of repeated U.S. attempts to discredit it on human rights grounds. This is in large part because the United States has used human rights arguments as a means of advancing its own foreign policy but also because, as Schwab notes, "economic and social rights are fundamental in Cuba" (1999, p. 9).

52. Danner 1993, p. 132; Danner quotes from the Truth Commission's report, "De la locura a la esperanza: La guerra de doce años en El Salvador." See also Danner 1994.

53. As this book goes to press, Chiapas remains wracked by officially tolerated—perhaps sanctioned—paramilitary violence. See Chapter 3, postscript.

54. Physicians for Human Rights 1999, p. 4.

55. Virchow 1849, p. 48. See also Eisenberg 1984.

56. Mann and Tarantola 1998, p. 8. See also the collection of articles in Mann, Gruskin, Grodin, and Annas 1999. For a review of documents that provide the basis for an international human right to health, as established through international conventions and laws as well as in the constitutions of various nations (but not that of the United States), see Kinney 2001.

57. Interview by the author with Ivan Nikitovich Simonov, former Chief Inspector of Prisons and now with the Chief Board of Punishment Execution, Ministry of Internal Affairs, Russian Federation, Moscow, June 4, 1998.

58. Henkin 1990, p. 208.

59. Oscar Schachter has observed:

International law must also be seen as the product of historical experience in which power and the "relation of forces" are determinants. Those States with power (i.e., the ability to control the outcomes contested by others) will have a disproportionate and often decisive influence in determining the content of rules and their application in practice. Because this is the case, international law, in a broad sense, both reflects and sustains the existing political order and distribution of power (1991, p. 6).

Furthermore, legal commentary often reminds us of the power of normative, procedural thinking. During and after the Nuremberg trials, there was debate—again, cast in legal terms—as to whether the trials themselves were legal or merely reflected "victors' justice." The *American Journal of International Law* published some key trial documents in 1947: "It was urged on behalf of the defendants that a fundamental principle of all law—international and domestic—is that there can be no punishment of crime without a pre-existing law....It was submitted that ex post facto punishment is abhorrent to the law of all civilized nations" (see International Military Tribunal [Nuremberg] 1947, p. 19). In other words, some legalists seemed to argue that if there was no law against genocide or "aggressive war" on the books before the fact, it was therefore illegitimate to prosecute the Nazis for these actions. Those arguing the illegality of the Nuremberg trials were not fringe elements. Citing such concerns, Chief Justice Harlan

Fiske Stone referred to the "high-grade lynching party in Nuremberg" (quoted in Mason 1956, p. 746).

60. Farmer, Léandre, Mukherjee, Claude, et al. 2001.

61. I do not refer here to historical investigation, which is crucial to an understanding of the dynamics of structural violence. But the study of human rights abuses in the slave trade, for example, or in the silver mines of fifth-century B.C. Greece, is quite different from an investigation of ongoing, documentable suffering.

62. Neier 1998, p. xiii.

63. Steiner and Alston 1996, p. viii.

64. For more on this initiative, see *http://www.phrusa.org/campaigns/aids/links.html*.

65. For a review of widening outcome gaps and their relationship to economic policy, see Kim, Millen, Irwin, and Gershman 2000.

66. For an overview of this group and its "vitality of practice," see Farmer 1999b, chap. 1.

67. Ignatieff 2001, p. 35; paragraphing altered.

68. Krieger 1999, p. 295.

69. An example of this approach can be found in Asad's recent discussion of torture and modern human rights discourse. He notes: "If cruelty is increasingly represented in the language of rights (and especially of human rights), this is because *perpetual legal struggle* has now become the dominant mode of moral engagement in an interconnected, uncertain, and rapidly changing world" (1997, pp. 304–5).

70. Neugebauer 1999, p. 1474.

71. Mann 1998, pp. 145–46.

72. Neier 1998, pp. 23–24.

73. Physicians for Human Rights 1999, p. 12.

74. Gitlin 1995, p. 224.

75. Steiner and Alston 1996, p. 1140.

76. Ignatieff 2001, p. 172.

77. See, for example, the Web site titled Bill Gates's Personal Wealth Clock, available at *http://www.webho.com/WealthClock*.

AFTERWORD

1. Wilson 2000.

2. Despite the apathy of the developed world, the wounds in Latin America remain deep, as a recent letter from the Mothers of the Plaza de Mayo, a group of Argentinian women whose children were "disappeared," to Pope John Paul II suggests: "It took several days for us to assimilate your request to the House of Lords for clemency for the genocidal Pinochet. We address this letter to you as an ordinary person and ordinary citizen, because we find abhorrent the idea that a person like yourself, whose own body has not undergone the horrors of torture, rape, and all manner of violations of human rights, should ask as a pope, in Jesus' name, for clemency for the perpetrator of these acts" (Mothers of the Plaza de Mayo 1999, p. 895).

3. Banks 2000.

4. Of course others, including economist James K. Galbraith, have reached just the opposite conclusion. Writing of the debt crisis of the early 1980s, he notes that "matters were made worse by the concurrent triumph of neoliberalism in the United States and the United Kingdom in these same years. Following the debt crisis, the rich countries preached the 'magic of the marketplace' to the poor. No new financial architecture was created from the wreckage left by the commercial banks. Instead, the International Monetary Fund preached austerity, and then financial deregulation and privatization—sale of state assets at fire-sale prices to foreign investors" (2002, p. 24).

5. I refer to the $4.8 billion International Monetary Fund loan to Russia in 1998 that mysteriously vanished, perhaps finding its way to the Bank of New York and then to Swiss accounts, according to the FBI and Swiss officials (see N. Knox 2000, M. Walker 2000, and Whittell 2000).

6. A 1982 GAO audit stated that, since 1973, "the United States has provided Haiti about $218 million in food aid and economic assistance. After 8 years of operating in Haiti, AID is still having difficulty implementing its projects" (U.S. General Accounting Office 1982, p. i).

7. Hancock 1989.

8. Debt service is now one of the Peruvian government's largest expenses, as is the case for most indebted countries. In 2000, total debt service (calculated as the percentage of exports of goods and services) was 42.8 percent (World Bank 2002).

9. Fitch IBCA, the international rating agency, estimated that between 1993 and 1998 alone, capital flight out of Russia totaled a staggering $128.7 billion (Thornhill and Ostrovsky 1999).

10. Rey 1999.

11. For a recounting of this event, see Wilentz 1989.

12. This translation of "Weathervane" is by Catherine Brown (García Lorca 1995).

BIBLIOGRAPHY

Aalen, O.O., V.T. Farewell, D. De Angelis, et al. 1999. "New Therapy Explains the Fall in AIDS Incidence with a Substantial Rise in Number of Persons on Treatment Expected." *AIDS* 13 (1): 103–8.

Abbott, K. 1998. "Parolee with Tuberculosis Sues County Jail, State Prison." *Rocky Mountain News*, 2 April, p. A31.

Abdool-Karim, Q., and S.S. Abdool-Karim. 1999. "South Africa: Host to a New and Emerging HIV Epidemic." *Sexually Transmitted Infections* 75 (3): 139–40.

Abraham, L.K. 1993. *Mama Might Be Better Off Dead: The Failure of Health Care in Urban America.* Chicago: University of Chicago Press.

Abu-Lughod, J.L., ed. 1999. *Sociology for the Twenty-First Century: Continuities and Cutting Edges.* Chicago: University of Chicago Press.

Adams, R.N. 1970. *Crucifixion by Power.* Austin: University of Texas Press.

Adams, V. 1998. "Suffering the Winds of Lhasa: Politicized Bodies, Human Rights, Cultural Difference, and Humanism in Tibet." *Medical Anthropology Quarterly* 12 (1): 74–102.

Agosin, M. 1998. *An Absence of Shadows.* Fredonia, N.Y.: White Pine Press.

Albrecht, G.L., and J.W. Salmon. 1992. "Soviet Health Care in the Glasnost Era." In *Health Care Systems and Their Patients: An International Perspective,* edited by M.M. Rosenthal and M. Frenkel, pp. 247–66. Boulder: Westview Press.

Alexander, A. 1998. "Money Isn't the Issue; It's (Still) Political Will." *TB Monitor* 5 (5): 53.

Alston, P. 1984. "Conjuring Up New Human Rights: A Proposal for Quality Control." *American Journal of International Law* 78 (3): 607–21.

Aly, G., P. Chroust, and C. Pross. 1994. *Cleansing the Fatherland: Nazi Medicine and Racial Hygiene.* Baltimore: Johns Hopkins University Press.

American Medical Association Council on Ethical and Judicial Affairs. 1995. "Ethical Issues in Managed Care." *Journal of the American Medical Association* 273 (4): 330–35.

American Association for the Advancement of Science. 2002a. "Forensic Anthropologists Threatened in Guatemala." 21 March. Available at *http://shr .aaas.org/aaashran/alert.php?a_id=213*.

———. 2002b. "Further Violence Directed at Forensic Science Teams." 16 May. Available at *http://shr.aaas.org/aaashran/alert.php?a_id=219*.

American College of Physicians. 1997. "Inner-City Health Care." *Annals of Internal Medicine* 126 (6): 485–90.

American Hospital Association. 1992. A Patient's Bill of Rights. Available at *http://www.aha.org/resource/pbillofrights.asp*.

Americas Watch and the National Coalition for Haitian Refugees. 1993. *Silencing a People: The Destruction of Civil Society in Haiti*. New York: Human Rights Watch.

Americas Watch, National Coalition for Haitian Refugees, and Physicians for Human Rights. 1991. *Return to the Darkest Days: Human Rights in Haiti Since the Coup*. New York and Boston: Americas Watch.

Amnesty International. 1997. *Torture in Russia: "This Man-Made Hell."* London: Amnesty International.

———. 1998. *Amnesty International Report 1998*. London: Amnesty International Publications.

———. 2002. *United States of America: A Safe Haven for Torturers*. New York: Amnesty International USA Publications.

Anders, G. 1994. "Money Machines: HMOs Pile Up Billions in Cash, Try to Decide What to Do with It." *Wall Street Journal,* 21 December, p. A1.

———. 1996. *Health Against Wealth: HMOs and the Breakdown of Medical Trust*. Boston: Houghton Mifflin.

Andersen, M. 1993. *Dossier Secreto*. Boulder: Westview Press.

Andrulis, D.P., and B. Carrier. 1999. *Managed Care in the Inner City: The Uncertain Promise for Providers, Plans, and Communities*. San Francisco: Jossey-Bass.

Angell, M. 1997a. "The Ethics of Clinical Research in the Third World." *New England Journal of Medicine* 337 (12): 847–49.

———. 1997b. "Tuskegee Revisited." *Wall Street Journal,* 28 October, p. A22.

———. 2000a. "The Ethics of Research in Developing Countries." *New England Journal of Medicine* 343 (5): 363.

———. 2000b. "Investigators' Responsibilities for Human Subjects in Developing Countries." *New England Journal of Medicine* 342 (13): 967–69.

———. 2000c. "The Pharmaceutical Industry: To Whom Is It Accountable?" *New England Journal of Medicine* 342 (25): 1902–4.

Annas, G.J. 1993. "Detention of HIV-Positive Haitians at Guantánamo: Human Rights and Medical Care." *New England Journal of Medicine* 329 (8): 589–92.

Annas, G.J., and M.A. Grodin. 1996. "Medicine and Human Rights: Reflections on the Fiftieth Anniversary of the Doctors' Trial." *Health and Human Rights* 2 (1): 7–21.

Arboleda-Flórez, J., H. Stuart, P. Freeman, and M. A. González-Block. 1999. *Acceso a los servicios de salud en el marco del TLC.* Washington, D.C.: Organización Panamericana de la Salud.

Aristide, J. B. 1990. *In the Parish of the Poor: Writings from Haiti.* Maryknoll, N.Y.: Orbis Books.

———. 1992. *Théologie et politique.* Montreal: Les Éditions du CIDIHCA.

———. 2000. *Eyes of the Heart: Seeking a Path for the Poor in the Age of Globalization.* Monroe, Maine: Common Courage Press.

Armada, F., C. Muntaner, and V. Navarro. 2001. "Health and Social Security Reforms in Latin America: The Convergence of the World Health Organization, the World Bank, and Transnational Corporations." *International Journal of Health Services* 31 (4): 729–68.

Arnesen, I. 1993. "HIV Prisoners." *The Nation,* 4 January, pp. 4–5.

Asad, T. 1997. "On Torture, or Cruel, Inhuman, and Degrading Treatment." In *Social Suffering,* edited by A. Kleinman, V. Das, and M. Lock, pp. 285–308. Berkeley: University of California Press.

———, ed. 1975. *Anthropology and the Colonial Encounter.* London: Ithaca Press and Humanities.

Ashbury, C. H. 1991. "The Orphan Drug Act: The First 7 Years." *Journal of the American Medical Association* 265 (7): 893–97.

Babcock, B. A., S. Deller, A. E. Ross, et al. 1996. *Sex Discrimination and the Law: History, Practice, and Theory.* Boston: Little, Brown.

Bachman, R., and L. Saltzman. 1995. *Violence Against Women: Estimates from the Redesigned Survey.* Washington, D.C.: U.S. Department of Justice, Office of Justice Programs, Bureau of Statistics.

Baer, H., and M. Singer. 1997. *Medical Anthropology and the World System.* Westport, Conn.: Bergin and Garvey.

Ball, P. 1999. AAAS/CIIDH Database of Human Rights Violations in Guatemala (ATV20.1). Available at *http://hrdata.aaas.org/ciidh/data.html.*

Ball, P., P. Kobrak, and H. F. Spirer. 1999. "State Violence in Guatemala, 1960–1996: A Quantitative Reflection." Available at *http://hrdata.aaas.org/ciidh/data.html.*

Banks, G. 2000. "Stuffy Boston Smartens Up." *International Herald Tribune,* 3 March, p. 18.

Baptiste, J. E., and B. Maguire. 2001. "Intransigence Is a Nonstarter." *South Florida Sun-Sentinel,* 11 June, p. A25.

Barbacci, M., J. T. Repke, and R. E. Chaisson. 1991. "Routine Prenatal Screening for HIV Infection." *Lancet* 337 (8743): 709–11.

Barnum, H. N. 1986. "Cost Savings from Alternative Treatments for Tuberculosis." *Social Science and Medicine* 23 (9): 847–50.

Barraza-Lloréns, M., S. Bertozzi, E. González-Pier, et al. 2002. "Addressing Inequality in Health and Health Care in Mexico." *Health Affairs* 21 (3): 47–56.

Barreiro, A. 1982. *Basic Ecclesial Communities: The Evangelization of the Poor.* Maryknoll, N.Y.: Orbis Books.

Bartley, M., D. Blane, and G. D. Smith. 1998. "Introduction: Beyond the Black Report." *Sociology of Health and Illness* 20 (5): 563–77.

Bastian, I., L. Rigouts, A. Van Deun, et al. 2000. "Directly Observed Treatment, Short-Course Strategy, and Multidrug-Resistant Tuberculosis: Are Any Modifications Required?" *Bulletin of the World Health Organization* 78 (2): 238–51.

Becerra, M. C., P. E. Farmer, and J. Y. Kim. 1999. "The Problem of Drug-Resistant Tuberculosis: An Overview." In *The Global Impact of Drug-Resistant Tuberculosis,* edited by Program in Infectious Disease and Social Change, pp. 1–38. Boston: Harvard Medical School and the Open Society Institute.

Becerra, M. C., J. Freeman, J. Bayona, et al. 2000. "Using Treatment Failure Under Effective Directly Observed Short-Course Chemotherapy Programs to Identify Patients with Multidrug-Resistant Tuberculosis." *International Journal of Tuberculosis and Lung Disease* 4 (2): 108–14.

Beck, A. J., J. C. Karberg, and P. M. Harrison. 2002. "Prison and Jail Inmates at Midyear 2001." *Bureau of Justice Statistics Bulletin,* April.

Bedjaoui, M. 1991. "The Right to Development." In *International Law: Achievements and Prospects,* edited by M. Bedjaoui, pp. 1177–92. Paris: United Nations Educational, Scientific, and Cultural Organization.

Bell, B. 2001. *Walking on Fire: Haitian Women's Stories of Survival and Resistance.* Ithaca, N.Y.: Cornell University Press.

Benatar, S. R. 2001. "Commentary: Justice and Medical Research: A Global Perspective," *Bioethics* 15(4): 333–40.

Benatar, S. R., D. M. Berwick, M. Bisognano, et al. 1999. "A Shared Statement of Ethical Principles for Those Who Shape and Give Health Care." *Annals of Internal Medicine* 130 (2): 144–47.

Bennett, L. R., L. Manderson, and Global Forum for Health Research. 2000. *Eliminating Sexual Violence Against Women: Towards a Global Initiative. Report of the Consultation on Sexual Violence Against Women.* Melbourne: Key Centre for Women's Health in Society, University of Melbourne.

Bereano, P. 1995. "Patent Pending: The Race to Own DNA; Guaymi Tribe Was Surprised to Discover They Were Invented." *Seattle Times,* 27 August, p. B5.

Bergquist, C., R. Penaranda, and G. Sánchez, eds. 1992. *Violence in Colombia: The Contemporary Crisis in Historical Perspective.* Wilmington, Del.: Scholarly Resources.

Berlinguer, G. 1999. "Globalization and Global Health." *International Journal of Health Services* 29 (3): 579–95.

Berreman, G. D. 1974. "Bringing It All Back Home: Malaise in Anthropology." In *Reinventing Anthropology,* edited by D. Hymes, pp. 83–98. New York: Random House.

Berryman, P. 1987. *Liberation Theology: Essential Facts About the Revolutionary Movement in Latin America and Beyond.* New York: Pantheon Books.

Berwick, D. 2002. " 'We All Have AIDS': Case for Reducing the Cost of HIV Drugs to Zero." *British Medical Journal* 324 (7331): 214–16.

Berwick, D., F. Davidoff, H. Hiatt, et al. 2001. "Refining and Implementing the Tavistock Principles for Everybody in Health Care." *British Medical Journal* 323 (7313): 616–20.

Betancourt, E.F. 1988. "Cuba's Callous War on AIDS." *New York Times,* 11 February.

Bhabha, J. 1998a. "Enforcing the Human Rights of Citizens and Non-Citizens in the Era of Maastricht: Some Reflections on the Importance of States." *Development and Change* 29: 697–724.

———. 1998b. " 'Get Back to Where You Once Belonged': Identity, Citizenship, and Exclusion in Europe." *Human Rights Quarterly* 20: 592–627.

Bifani, P., B. Pjikaytis, V. Kapur, et al. 1996. "Origin and Interstate Spread of a New York City Multidrug-Resistant *Mycobacterium tuberculosis* Clone Family." *Journal of the American Medical Association* 275 (6): 452–57.

Bill Gates Personal Wealth Clock. Available at *http://www.webho.com/Wealth Clock.*

Binford, L. 1996. *The El Mozote Massacre.* Tucson: University of Arizona Press.

Birns, L., and M.M. McCarthy. 2001. "Haiti Needs U.S. Aid, Not Ineffective Manipulation." *Miami Herald,* 21 December, p. 7B.

Black, G. 1988. *The Good Neighbor: How the United States Wrote the History of Central America and the Caribbean.* New York: Pantheon Books.

Blagov, S. 2002. "Health Sector Struggles with Drug Abuse, AIDS." Inter Press News Service, 7 March.

Boff, L. 1989. *Faith on the Edge: Religion and Marginalized Existence.* 1st ed. San Francisco: Harper and Row.

Boff, L., and C. Boff. 1987. *Introducing Liberation Theology.* Maryknoll, N.Y.: Orbis Books.

Boletín de la Organización Panamericana de la Salud-Cuba. 2002. 1 April. 7 (1): 4.

Bonhoeffer, D. 1972. *Letters and Papers from Prison.* New York: Macmillan.

Borge, T. 1987. *Christianity and Revolution.* Maryknoll, N.Y.: Orbis Books.

Bosk, C.L. 1999. "Professional Ethicist Available: Logical, Secular, Friendly." *Daedalus* 128 (4): 47–68.

Boston Public Health Commission, Research and Technology Services. 2001. *The Health of Boston 2001.* Boston: Boston Public Health Commission.

Bourdieu, P. 1990. *In Other Words: Essays Towards a Reflexive Sociology.* Cambridge: Polity.

———. 1996. *Sur la télévision.* Paris: Raisons d'Agir.

———. 1998. *La domination masculine.* Paris: Éditions du Seuil.

———. 2000a. *Propos sur le champ politique.* Lyon: Presses Universitaires de Lyon.

———. 2000b. *Les structures sociales de l'économie.* Paris: Éditions du Seuil.

———, ed. 1993. *La misère du monde.* Paris: Éditions du Seuil.

Bourgois, P. 1990. "Confronting Anthropological Ethics: Ethnographic Lessons from Central America." *Journal of Peace Research* 27 (1): 43–54.

———. 1995. *In Search of Respect: Selling Crack in El Barrio.* Cambridge: Cambridge University Press.

Brandt, A.M. 1978. "Racism and Research: The Case of the Tuskegee Syphilis Study." *Hastings Center Report* 8 (6): 21–29.

———. 1987. *No Magic Bullet: A Social History of Venereal Disease in the United States Since 1880.* New York: Oxford University Press.

Braun, M.M., B.I. Truman, B. Maguire, et al. 1989. "Increasing Incidence of Tuberculosis in a Prison Inmate Population: Association with HIV Infection." *Journal of the American Medical Association* 261 (3): 393–97.

Briceño-León, R., and V. Zubillaga. 2002. "Violence and Globalization in Latin America." *Current Sociology* 50 (1): 19–37.

British Medical Association. 2001. *The Medical Profession and Human Rights: Handbook for a Changing Agenda.* London: Zed Books.

Brown, R.M. 1993. *Liberation Theology: An Introductory Guide.* Louisville: Westminster/John Knox Press.

Burdick, J. 1993. *Looking for God in Brazil: The Progressive Catholic Church in Urban Brazil's Religious Arena.* Berkeley: University of California Press.

Burns, J.F. 2001. "U.S. Envoy Sees Her Role Reverse." *International Herald Tribune,* 26 November.

Bush, J. 2001. "For Nicaragua: A Proven Democratic Leader." *Miami Herald,* 1 November, p. 7B.

Butler, K. 2000. "Grand Marnier Workers Toil for 2 Pounds a Day on Haiti Plantation." *Independent* (London), 16 July, p. 3.

"Buying into the Orphan Drug Market." 1995. *Lancet* 346 (8980): 917.

Byrd, W.M., and L.A. Clayton. 2002. *An American Health Dilemma.* Vol. 2, *Race, Medicine, and Health Care in the United States, 1900–2000.* New York: Routledge.

Caldwell, J.C., S. Findley, P. Caldwell, et al., eds. 1990. *What We Know About Health Transition: The Cultural, Social, and Behavioural Determinants of Health. The Proceedings of an International Workshop, Canberra, May 1989.* Canberra: Health Transition Centre, Australian National University.

Callahan, D. 1999. "The Social Sciences and the Task of Bioethics." *Daedalus* 128 (4): 275–94.

Campbell, D. 1972. "Herskovits, Cultural Relativism, and Metascience." In *Cultural Relativism: Perspectives in Cultural Pluralism,* edited by M. Herskovits, pp. 289–315. New York: Random House.

Campbell, D. 2001. "Getting the Right Result: Nicaragua's Election Showed the U.S. Still Won't Allow a Free Vote." *Guardian,* 7 November, p. 17.

Capron, A.M. 1999. "What Contributions Have Social Science and the Law Made to the Development of Policy on Bioethics?" *Daedalus* 128 (4): 295–325.

Caputo, J.D. 1993. *Against Ethics: Contributions to a Poetics of Obligation with Constant Reference to Deconstruction.* Bloomington: Indiana University Press.

Carmack, R., ed. 1988. *Harvest of Violence: The Mayan Indians and the Guatemalan Crisis.* Norman: University of Oklahoma Press.

Carney, J.G. 1987. *To Be a Revolutionary.* San Francisco: Harper and Row.

Castaneda, J. 1998. "In Mexico, the Good, the Bad, and the Difference." *Washington Post,* 25 January, p. C2.

Castillo, O. 1993. "Apolitical Intellectuals." Translated by M. Randall. In *Against Forgetting: Twentieth Century Poetry of Witness,* edited by C. Forché, pp. 607–8. New York: Norton.

Castro, A., P. Farmer, and L. Barberia. 2002. "Control of HIV/AIDS in Cuba: A Briefing Memo for President Carter's Visit to Cuba." Carter Center, Atlanta.

Castro, F. 1987. *Fidel and Religion: Castro Talks on Revolution and Religion with Frei Betto*. Translated by Cuban Center for Translation and Interpretation. New York: Simon and Schuster.

Cates, W., and T. J. Coates. 2000. "The Ethics of Research in Developing Countries." *New England Journal of Medicine* 343 (5): 362.

Centers for Disease Control and Prevention. 1989. "Prevention and Control of Tuberculosis in Correctional Institutions: Recommendations of the Advisory Committee for the Elimination of Tuberculosis." *Morbidity and Mortality Weekly Report* 38 (18): 313–25.

———. 1991. "Tuberculosis Mortality in the United States: Final Data, 1990." *Morbidity and Mortality Weekly Report* 40: SS23–SS27.

———. 1992a. "Famine-Affected, Refugee, and Displaced Populations: Recommendations for Public Health Issues." *Morbidity and Mortality Weekly Report* 41 (RR–13): 1–76.

———. 1992b. "Tuberculosis Transmission in a State Correctional Institution: California, 1990–1991." *Morbidity and Mortality Weekly Report* 41 (49): 927–29.

———. 2001. "Public Health Dispatch: Update: Outbreak of Poliomyelitis—Dominican Republic and Haiti, 2000–2001." *Morbidity and Mortality Weekly Report* 50 (39): 855–56.

Chapman, A., and L. Rubenstein, eds. 1998. *Human Rights and Health: The Legacy of Apartheid*. Washington, D.C.: American Association for the Advancement of Science.

Charlemagne, M. 1988. *Manno Charlemagne*. Recording. Mini Records.

Chelala, C. 2000. "Bolivian Soldiers Double Up as Health Workers." *Lancet* 355 (9220): 2057.

Chen, M.-S. 1998. "Howard Waitzkin: Intellectual for the Disadvantaged?" *Journal of Health and Social Behavior* 39: 4–6.

Chien, A., M. Connors, and K. Fox. 2000. "The Drug War in Perspective." In *Dying for Growth: Global Inequality and the Health of the Poor*, edited by J. Y. Kim, J. V. Millen, A. Irwin, and J. Gershman, pp. 293–327. Monroe, Maine: Common Courage Press.

Chirac, P., T. von Schoen-Angerer, T. Kasper, et al. 2000. "AIDS: Patent Rights Versus Patient Rights." *Lancet* 356 (9228): 502.

Chokr, N. N. 1999. "Human Rights: Beyond Universalism and Cultural Relativism—Toward a Dynamic, Contextual, and Cross-Cultural Approach." *Applied Philosophy* (online journal). Available at *http://www.rd-inc.com/HumanRights.doc*.

Chomsky, A. 2000. " 'The Threat of a Good Example': Health and Revolution in Cuba." In *Dying for Growth: Global Inequality and the Health of the Poor*, edited by J. Y. Kim, J. V. Millen, A. Irwin, and J. Gershman, pp. 331–57. Monroe, Maine: Common Courage Press.

Chomsky, N. 1985. *Turning the Tide: U.S. Intervention in Central America and the Struggle for Peace*. Boston: South End Press.

———. 1993. *Year 501: The Conquest Continues*. Boston: South End Press.

———. 1994. *World Orders Old and New.* New York: Columbia University Press.

———. 1998. "The United States and the Challenge of Relativity." In *Human Rights Fifty Years On: A Reappraisal,* edited by T. Evans, pp. 24–56. Manchester, England: Manchester University Press.

———. 1999. *The Umbrella of U.S. Power: The Universal Declaration of Human Rights and the Contradictions of U.S. Policy.* New York: Seven Cities Press.

———. 2000. *Rogue States.* Cambridge, Mass.: South End Press.

Chomsky, N., and E. Herman. 1979a. *After the Cataclysm.* Boston: South End Press.

———. 1979b. *The Political Economy of Human Rights.* Boston: South End Press.

———. 1979c. *The Washington Connection and Third World Fascism.* Boston: South End Press.

Chopp, R. S. 1986. *The Praxis of Suffering: An Interpretation of Liberation and Political Theologies.* Maryknoll, N.Y.: Orbis Books.

Christakis, N. A. 1999. "Prognostication and Bioethics." *Daedalus* 128 (4): 197–214.

Churchill, L. R. 1997. "Bioethics in Social Context." In *The Social Medicine Reader,* edited by G. E. Henderson, N. M. P. King, R. P. Strauss, et al., pp. 310–20. Durham: Duke University Press.

———. 1999. "Are We Professionals? A Critical Look at the Social Role of Bioethicists." *Daedalus* 128 (4): 253–74.

Ciancaglini, S., and M. Granovsky. 1995. *Más que la verdad: El Juicio a las Juntas.* Buenos Aires: Planeta.

"Cientos de miles de chinos han contraído el sida por vender su sangre al gobierno." 2001. *El País,* 1 June, p. 1.

CID/Gallup. 2000. Haiti Public Opinion Poll, October.

CIIDH (International Center for Human Rights Research). 1999. "Draining the Sea: An Analysis of Terror in Three Rural Communities in Guatemala (1980–1984)." Available at *http://hrdata.aaas.org/ciidh/dts/dataproj.html.*

Clinton, W. J. 1997. Remarks by the President in Apology for Study Done in Tuskegee. 16 May. Available at *http://www.cdc.gov/nchstp/od/tuskegee/clintonp.htm.*

———. 2000. State of the Union Address. 27 January. Available at *http://www.pbs.org/newshour/bb/white_house/jan-june00/sotu4.html.*

Clinton, W. J., and A. Gore. 1992. *Putting People First.* New York: Times Books.

Coatsworth, J. H. 2000. "Conflict with Cuba Is Finally Coming to an End." *Boston Globe,* 22 May, p. A11.

Coburn, D. 2000. "Income Inequality, Social Cohesion, and the Health Status of Populations: The Role of Neo-Liberalism." *Social Science and Medicine* 51 (1): 135–46.

Cohen, L. 1999. "Where It Hurts: Indian Material for an Ethics of Organ Transplantation." *Daedalus* 128 (4): 135–65.

Cohen, M. S. 2000. "Preventing Sexual Transmission of HIV—New Ideas from Sub-Saharan Africa." *New England Journal of Medicine* 342 (13): 970–72.

Coker, R. 2000. "'Extrapolitis' a Disease More Threatening Than TB in Russia?" *European Journal of Public Health* 10 (2): 148–50.

Cole, D. 1999. *No Equal Justice: Race and Class in the American Criminal Justice System.* New York: The New Press.

Collier, G. A. 1994. *Basta! Land and the Zapatista Rebellion in Chiapas.* Oakland, Calif.: Institute for Food and Development Policy.

———. 1997. "Reaction and Retrenchment in the Highlands of Chiapas in the Wake of the Zapatista Rebellion." *Journal of Latin American Anthropology* 3 (1): 14–31.

Collier, G. A., P. J. Farías Campero, J. E. Pérez, and V. P. White. 2000. "Socio-Economic Change and Emotional Illness Among the Highland Maya of Chiapas, Mexico." *Ethos* 28 (1): 20–53.

Colson, E. 1971. *The Social Consequences of Resettlement: The Impact of the Kariba Resettlement upon the Gwembe Tonga.* Manchester, England: Manchester University Press.

Colwell, R. R., P. R. Epstein, D. Gubler, et al. 1999. "Climate Change and Human Health." *Science* 279 (5353): 968–69.

Comandancia General del EZLN. 1993. *Declaración de la Selva Lacandona.* Selva Lacandona, Chiapas, Mexico. Available at *http://www.ezln.org /documentos/1994/199312xx.es.htm.*

Comaroff, J., and J. L. Comaroff, eds. 1993. *Modernity and Its Malcontents: Ritual and Power in Postcolonial Africa.* Chicago: University of Chicago Press.

———, eds. 2001. *Millennial Capitalism and the Culture of Neoliberalism.* Durham, N.C.: Duke University Press.

Comisión Económica para América Latina y el Caribe. 1997. *La economía Cubana: Reformas estructurales y desempeño en los noventa.* Mexico: Fondo de Cultura Económica.

Comisión Nacional Sobre la Desaparición de Personas. 1986. *Nunca Más: The Report of the Argentine National Commission on the Disappeared.* New York: Farrar, Straus and Giroux.

Concannon, B. 2000. "Beyond Complementarity: The International Criminal Court and National Prosecutions, a View from Haiti." *Columbia Human Rights Law Review* 32 (1): 201–50.

———. 2001a. "Justice for Haiti: The Raboteau Trial." *International Lawyer* 35 (2): 641–47.

———. 2001b. "No Reconciliation Without Justice." *Criminal Justice Matters* 44: 21–24.

———. n.d. Untitled essay available at *http://www.uchastings.edu/boswell_01 /Brian%20on%20Dec%2017.htm.*

Coninx, R., B. Eshaya-Chauvin, and H. Reyes. 1995. "Tuberculosis in Prisons." *Lancet* 346 (8984): 1238–39.

Constable, P. 1991. "After Coup, Haiti Remains in Grip of 'Low Key' Repression by Military." *Boston Globe,* 12 December, p. 2.

Contreras, J. 2002. "Is the United States a Haven for Torturers?" *Newsweek,* Web exclusive, 12 April.

Cortright, D., and G. A. Lopez. 1999. "Are Sanctions Just? The Problematic Case of Iraq." *Journal of International Affairs* 52: 735–55.

Council on Hemispheric Affairs. 2001. "Upcoming Nicaraguan Elections." Press release, 30 October. Available at *http://www.coha.org/Press_Releases/01–21-Nicaragua(extended).htm.*

Court, J., and F. Smith. 1999. *Making a Killing: HMOs and the Threat to Your Health.* Monroe, Maine: Common Courage Press.

"Criticized Research Quantifies the Risk of AIDS Infection." 2000. *New York Times,* 30 March, p. A16.

Csordas, T. 1990. "Embodiment as a Paradigm for Anthropology." *Ethos* 18 (1): 5–47.

———, ed. 1994. *Embodiment and Experience: The Existential Ground of Culture and Self.* New York: Cambridge University Press.

Cunningham, H. 1998. "Patenting the Primitive: Colonial Encounters in Post-Colonial Contexts." *Critique of Anthropology* 18 (2): 205–33.

Cunningham, H., and S. Scharper. 1996. Human Genome Project Patenting Indigenous People. Third World Network Features, 23 February. Available at *http://www.dartmouth.edu/~cbbc/courses/bio4/bio4–1996/Human Genome3rdWorld.html.*

Cunningham, R.M. 1983. "Entrepreneurialism in Medicine." *New England Journal of Medicine* 309 (21): 1313–14.

Dale, R. 2000. "Now More Than Ever, Rich Nations Need the Cooperation of the Poorer States." *International Herald Tribune,* 3 March, p. 15.

Dalton, H.L., S. Burris, and Yale AIDS Law Project, eds. 1987. *AIDS and the Law: A Guide for the Public.* New Haven: Yale University Press.

Daniels, N., B.P. Kennedy, and I. Kawachi. 1999. "Why Justice Is Good for Our Health: The Social Determinants of Health Inequalities." *Daedalus* 128 (4): 215–51.

Danner, M. 1993. "The Truth of El Mozote." *New Yorker,* 6 December, pp. 50–133.

———. 1994. *The Massacre at El Mozote.* New York: Vintage Books.

Das, V. 1999. "Public Good, Ethics, and Everyday Life: Beyond the Boundaries of Bioethics." *Daedalus* 128 (4): 99–133.

Davis, M. 2001. *Late Victorian Holocausts.* London: Verso.

"De la locura a la esperanza: La guerra de doce años en El Salvador. Informe de la Comisión de la Verdad." 1993. *Estudios Centroamericanos* 533: 161–326.

"Death in Chiapas." 1997. *New York Times,* 25 December, p. A26.

Deaton, A. 1999. "Inequalities in Income and Inequalities in Health: Increasing Inequality in America." Paper prepared for conference on Increasing Inequality in America, 12–13 March, Bush School of Public Policy, Texas A&M University, College Station, Texas.

"A Decade of Global Wealth." 1999. *Forbes,* 5 July, pp. 154–55.

"Declaration of Helsinki IV, 41st World Medical Assembly, Hong Kong, September 1989." 1992. In *The Nazi Doctors and the Nuremberg Code: Human Rights in Human Experimentation,* edited by G.J. Annas and M.A. Grodin, pp. 339–42. New York: Oxford University Press.

Declaration of Indigenous People of the Western Hemisphere Regarding the Human Genome Diversity Project. 1995. Alaska Native Knowledge Network. Available at *http://www.ankn.uaf.edu/declaration.html.*

Department of Health, Republic of South Africa. 1995. *Health Trends in South Africa 1994.* Pretoria: Department of Health.

Desjarlais, R., L. Eisenberg, B. Good, et al. 1995. *World Mental Health: Problems and Priorities in Low-Income Countries.* New York: Oxford University Press.

Desormeaux, J., M.P. Johnson, J.S. Coberly, et al. 1996. "Widespread HIV Counseling and Testing Linked to a Community-Based Tuberculosis Control Program in a High-Risk Population." *Bulletin of the Pan American Health Organization* 30 (1): 1–8.

DeWitt, K. 1994. "Many Americans Back Singapore's Decision to Flog Teen." *Fort Worth Star-Telegram,* 10 April, p. 4.

Dirección Nacional de Estadísticas del Ministerio de Salud Pública, de la República de Cuba. 1998. Portal de salud de Cuba: Sistema de salud. Available at *http://www.sld.cu/sistema_de_salud/estrategias.html.*

Dlugy, Y. 1999. "The Prisoners' Plague." *Newsweek,* 5 July, pp. 18–20.

Doner, K.S. 1995. "Managed Care: Ethical Issues." *Journal of the American Medical Association* 274 (8): 609.

Donnelly, J. 1985. *The Concept of Human Rights.* New York: St. Martin's Press.

dos Anjos, M.F. 1996. "Medical Ethics in the Developing World: A Liberation Theology Perspective." *Journal of Medicine and Philosophy* 21 (6): 629–37.

Dostoyevsky, F. 1985. *The House of the Dead.* Translated by D. McDuff. London: Penguin Books.

Dowd, M. 2002. "Office of Strategic Mendacity." *New York Times,* 20 February, p. A21.

Downing, T.E., and G. Kushner. 1988. Introduction to *Human Rights and Anthropology,* edited by T.E. Downing and G. Kushner, pp. 1–8. Cambridge, Mass.: Cultural Survival.

———. 1992. "Human Rights and Anthropology: The Challenge for Anthropologists." *Man and Life* 18 (1–2): 21–30.

Dozon, J.-P., and D. Fassin. 2001. *Critique de la santé publique.* Paris: Belland.

Dubos, R., and J. Dubos. 1952. *The White Plague: Tuberculosis, Man, and Society.* Boston: Little, Brown.

Dussel, I., S. Finocchio, and S. Gojman. 1997. *Haciendo memoria en el país de nunca más.* Buenos Aires: Eudeba.

Dye, C., S. Scheele, P. Dolin, et al. 1999. "Global Burden of Tuberculosis: Estimated Incidence, Prevalence, and Mortality by Country." *Journal of the American Medical Association* 282 (7): 677–86.

Dyer, O. 2002. "Prisoners' Treatment Is 'Bordering on Torture,' Charity Says." *British Medical Journal* 324 (7331): 187.

Eagleson, J., and P. Sharper, eds. 1979. *Puebla and Beyond: Documentation and Commentary.* Maryknoll, N.Y.: Orbis Books.

Eindhoven, A.C. 1994. "Commentary: Setting the Record Straight—A Reply to Howard Waitzkin." *American Journal of Public Health* 84 (3): 490–94.

Eisenberg, L. 1984. "Rudolf Ludwig Karl Virchow, Where Are You Now That We Need You?" *American Journal of Medicine* 77: 524–32.

———. 1999. "Whatever Happened to the Faculty on the Way to the Agora?" *Archives of Internal Medicine* 159 (19): 2251–56.

Elton, C. 2002. "Despite Threats, Guatemalan Scientists Dig for the Truth." *Christian Science Monitor,* 27 March, p. 8.

Emanuel, E. J. 2000. "Justice and Managed Care: Four Principles for the Just Allocation of Health Care Resources." *Hastings Center Report* 30 (3): 8–16.

Emanuel, E. J., and N. N. Dubler. 1995. "Preserving the Physician-Patient Relationship in the Era of Managed Care." *Journal of the American Medical Association* 273 (4): 323–29.

"The Embodiment of Violence." 1998. *Medical Anthropology Quarterly* 12 (1).

Engelhardt, H. T. 1998. "Critical Care: Why There Is No Global Bioethics." *Journal of Medicine and Philosophy* 23 (6): 643–51.

Engelhardt, H. T., Jr., and M. A. Rie. 1988. "Morality for the Medical-Industrial Complex: A Code of Ethics for the Mass Marketing of Health Care." *New England Journal of Medicine* 319 (16): 1086–89.

Engleman, E. 2002. "Experts Warn Russia's Fight Against TB Is Far from Over." Associated Press, 22 March.

Equipo Argentino de Antropología Forense (Argentine Forensic Anthropology Team). 1996. *Biannual Report 1994–1995.* Buenos Aires: EAAF.

Equipo de Antropología Forense de Guatemala (Guatemalan Forensic Anthropology Team). 1997. *Las masacres en Rabinal: Estudio histórico antropológico de las masacres de Plan de Sánchez, Chichupac y Río Negro 1997.* Editorial Serviprensa, C.A., Guatemala: Fundación de Antropología Forense de Guatemala.

Espada, M. 1994. *Poetry Like Bread.* Willimantic, Conn.: Curbstone Press.

Espinal, M. A., S. J. Kim, P. G. Suarez, et al. 2000. "Standard Short-Course Chemotherapy for Drug Resistant Tuberculosis: Treatment Outcomes in Six Countries." *Journal of the American Medical Association* 283 (19): 2537–45.

Fabian, J. 1983. *Time and the Other: How Anthropology Makes Its Object.* New York: Columbia University Press.

Faden, R. R., S. E. Lederer, and J. D. Moreno. 1996. "U.S. Medical Researchers, the Nuremberg Doctors Trial, and the Nuremberg Code: A Review of Findings of the Advisory Committee on Human Radiation Experiments." *Journal of the American Medical Association* 276 (20): 1667–71.

Fainaru, S. 1999. "U.S. Is a Haven for Suspected War Criminals." *Boston Globe,* 2 May, p. A1.

Falla, R. 1992. *Masacres de la Selva, Ixcan, Guatemala, 1975–1982.* Guatemala City: Universidad de San Carlos de Guatemala.

Farmer, P. E. 1988. "Bad Blood, Spoiled Milk: Bodily Fluids as Moral Barometers in Rural Haiti." *American Ethnologist* 15 (1): 62–83.

———. 1990. "Sending Sickness: Sorcery, Politics, and Changing Concepts of AIDS in Rural Haiti." *Medical Anthropology Quarterly* 4 (1): 6–27.

———. 1992a. *AIDS and Accusation: Haiti and the Geography of Blame.* Berkeley: University of California Press.

———. 1992b. "Birth of the Klinik: The Making of Haitian Professional Psychiatry." In *Ethnopsychiatry,* edited by A. Gaines, pp. 251–72. Albany: SUNY Press.

———. 1992c. "New Disorder, Old Dilemmas: AIDS and Anthropology in Haiti." In *The Time of AIDS*, edited by G. Herdt and S. Lindenbaum, pp. 287–318. Los Angeles: Sage.

———. 1994. *The Uses of Haiti.* Monroe, Maine: Common Courage Press.

———. 1995a. "Culture, Poverty, and the Dynamics of HIV Transmission in Rural Haiti." In *Culture and Sexual Risk: Anthropological Perspectives on AIDS*, edited by H. T. Brummelhuis and G. Herdt, pp. 3–28. Newark, N.J.: Gordon and Breach.

———. 1995b. "Medicine and Social Justice." *America* 173 (2): 13–17.

———. 1995c. "Pestilence and Restraint: Haitians, Guantánamo, and the Logic of Quarantine." In *AIDS and the Public Debate: Historical and Contemporary Perspectives*, edited by C. Hannaway, V. A. Harden, and J. Parascandola, pp. 139–52. Burke, Va.: IOS Press.

———. 1995d. "The Significance of Haiti." In *Haiti: Dangerous Crossroads*, edited by North American Congress on Latin America, pp. 217–30. Boston: South End Press.

———. 1996a. "Haiti's Lost Years: Lessons for the Americas." *Current Issues in Public Health* 2: 143–51.

———. 1996b. "On Suffering and Structural Violence: A View from Below." *Daedalus* 125 (1): 261–83.

———. 1996c. "Social Inequalities and Emerging Infectious Diseases." *Emerging Infectious Diseases* 2 (4): 259–69.

———. 1997a. "AIDS and Anthropologists: Ten Years Later." *Medical Anthropology Quarterly* 11 (4): 516–25.

———. 1997b. "Ethnography, Social Analysis, and the Prevention of Sexually Transmitted HIV Infection." In *The Anthropology of Infectious Disease*, edited by M. Inhorn and P. Brown, pp. 413–38. Amsterdam: Gordon and Breach.

———. 1997c. "Letter from Haiti." *AIDS Clinical Care* 9 (11): 83–85.

———. 1997d. "Social Scientists and the New Tuberculosis." *Social Science and Medicine* 44 (3): 347–58.

———. 1998a. "Inequalities and Antivirals." *Pharos* 61 (2): 34–38.

———. 1998b. "A Visit to Chiapas." *America* 178 (10): 14–18.

———. 1999a. "Cruel and Unusual: Drug-Resistant Tuberculosis as Punishment." In *Sentenced to Die? The Problem of TB in Prisons in East and Central Europe and Central Asia*, edited by V. Stern and R. Jones, pp. 70–88. London: International Centre for Prison Studies, King's College.

———. 1999b. *Infections and Inequalities: The Modern Plagues.* Berkeley: University of California Press.

———. 1999c. "Managerial Successes, Clinical Failures." *International Journal of Tuberculosis and Lung Disease* 3 (5): 365–67.

———. 1999d. "Pathologies of Power: Rethinking Health and Human Rights." *American Journal of Public Health* 89 (10): 1486–96.

———. 1999e. "TB Superbugs: The Coming Plague on All Our Houses." *Natural History* 108 (3): 46–53.

———. 2000. "Prevention Without Treatment Is Not Sustainable." *National AIDS Bulletin* 13 (6): 6–9, 40.

————. 2001a. *Infections and Inequalities: The Modern Plagues.* 2d ed., with a new preface. Berkeley: University of California Press.

————. 2001b. "The Major Infectious Diseases in the World—To Treat or Not to Treat?" *New England Journal of Medicine* 345 (3): 208–10.

Farmer, P. E., J. Bayona, M. Becerra, et al. 1997. "Poverty, Inequality, and Drug Resistance: Meeting Community Needs in the Global Era." In *Proceedings of the International Union Against Tuberculosis and Lung Disease, North American Region Conference,* 27 February–2 March, Chicago, Ill., pp. 88–101.

————. 1998. "The Dilemma of MDRTB in the Global Era." *International Journal of Tuberculosis and Lung Disease* 2 (11): 869–76.

Farmer, P. E., J. Bayona, S. Shin, et al. 1998. "Preliminary Results of Community-Based MDRTB Treatment in Lima, Peru." *International Journal of Tuberculosis and Lung Disease* 2 (11 Suppl. 2): S371.

Farmer, P. E., and D. Bertrand. 2000. "Hypocrisies of Development and the Health of the Haitian Poor." In *Dying for Growth: Global Inequality and the Health of the Poor,* edited by J. Y. Kim, J. V. Millen, A. Irwin, and J. Gershman, pp. 65–89. Monroe, Maine: Common Courage Press.

Farmer, P. E., and C. L. Briggs. 1999. "Hidden Epidemics of Tuberculosis. Infectious Disease and Social Inequalities: From Hemispheric Insecurity to Global Cooperation." Working paper 239, Latin American Program, Woodrow Wilson Center for Scholars, Washington, D.C.

Farmer, P. E., M. Connors, and J. Simmons, eds. 1996. *Women, Poverty, and AIDS: Sex, Drugs, and Structural Violence.* Monroe, Maine: Common Courage Press.

Farmer, P. E., and J. Y. Kim. 1998. "Community-Based Approaches to the Control of Multidrug-Resistant Tuberculosis: Introducing 'DOTS-Plus.' " *British Medical Journal* 317 (7159): 671–74.

————. 2000. "Resurgent TB in Russia: Do We Know Enough to Act?" *European Journal of Public Health* 10 (2): 150–52.

Farmer, P. E., J. Y. Kim, C. Mitnick, et al. 1999. "Responding to Outbreaks of MDRTB: Introducing 'DOTS-Plus.' " In *Tuberculosis: A Comprehensive International Approach,* 2d ed., edited by L. B. Reichman and E. S. Hershfield, pp. 447–69. New York: Marcel Dekker.

Farmer, P. E., A. S. Kononets, S. E. Borisov, et al. 1999. "Recrudescent Tuberculosis in the Russian Federation." In *The Global Impact of Drug-Resistant Tuberculosis,* edited by Program in Infectious Disease and Social Change, pp. 39–84. Boston: Harvard Medical School and the Open Society Institute.

Farmer, P. E., F. Léandre, J. S. Mukherjee, M. S. Claude, et al. 2001. "Community-Based Approaches to HIV Treatment in Resource-Poor Settings." *Lancet* 358 (9279): 404–9.

Farmer, P. E., F. Léandre, J. S. Mukherjee, R. Gupta, et al. 2001. "Community-Based Treatment of Advanced HIV Disease: Introducing DOT-HAART (Directly Observed Therapy with Highly Active Antiretroviral Therapy)." *Bulletin of the World Health Organization* 79 (12): 1145–51.

Farmer, P. E., and E. Nardell. 1998. "Nihilism and Pragmatism in Tuberculosis Control." *American Journal of Public Health* 88 (7): 4–5.

Farmer, P. E., S. Robin, S. L. Ramilus, et al. 1991. "Tuberculosis, Poverty, and 'Compliance': Lessons from Rural Haiti." *Seminars in Respiratory Infections* 6 (4): 254–60.

Farmer, P. E., and B. Rylko-Bauer. 2001. "L' 'exceptionnel' système de santé américain: Critique d'une médecine à vocation commerciale" (The "exceptional" American health care system: Critique of the for-profit approach). *Actes de la Recherche en Sciences Sociales* 139: 13–30.

Farmer, P. E., D. A. Walton, and M. C. Becerra. 2000. "International Tuberculosis Control in the 21st Century." In *Tuberculosis: Current Concepts and Treatment,* 2d ed., edited by L. N. Friedman, pp. 475–96. Boca Raton: CRC Press.

Farmer, P. E., D. A. Walton, and J. J. Furin. 2000. "The Changing Face of AIDS: Implications for Policy and Practice." In *The Emergency of AIDS: The Impact on Immunology, Microbiology, and Public Health,* edited by K. Mayer and H. Pizer, pp. 139–61. Washington, D.C.: American Public Health Association.

Fassin, D. 1996. *L'Espace politique de la santé: Essai de généalogie.* Paris: Presses Universitaires de France.

Feinsilver, J. 1993. *Healing the Masses: Cuban Health Politics at Home and Abroad.* Berkeley: University of California Press.

Feldberg, G. 1995. *Disease and Class: Tuberculosis and the Shaping of Modern North American Society.* New Brunswick, N.J.: Rutgers University Press.

Feldman, E., and R. Bayer, eds. 1999. *Blood Feuds: AIDS, Blood, and the Politics of Medical Disaster.* New York: Oxford University Press.

Ferm, D. M. 1986. *Third World Liberation Theologies: An Introductory Survey.* Maryknoll, N.Y.: Orbis Books.

Feshbach, M. 1995. *Environmental and Health Atlas of Russia.* Moscow: PAIMS; Bethseda, Md.: Foundation for International Arts and Education.

Field, M., and J. Twigg, eds. 2000. *Russia's Torn Safety Nets: Health and Social Welfare During the Transition.* New York: St. Martin's Press.

Fiscella, K., P. Franks, M. R. Gold, et al. 2000. "Inequality in Quality: Addressing Socioeconomic, Racial, and Ethnic Disparities in Health Care." *Journal of the American Medical Association* 283 (19): 2579–84.

Fisk, M. 2000. *Toward a Healthy Society: The Morality and Politics of Health Care Reform.* Lawrence: University Press of Kansas.

Forster, E. M. 1971. *Maurice.* New York: Norton.

Foucault, M. 1975. *Surveiller et punir: Naissance de la prison.* Paris: Gallimard.

Fox, R. C. 1999. "Is Medical Education Asking Too Much of Bioethics?" *Daedalus* 128 (4): 1–25.

Freeden, M. 1991. *Rights.* Minneapolis: University of Minnesota Press.

Freeman, H. P., and R. Payne. 2000. "Racial Injustice in Health Care." *New England Journal of Medicine* 342 (14): 1045–47.

Freire, P. 1986. *Pedagogy of the Oppressed.* New York: Continuum.

French, H. 1997. "AIDS Research in Africa: Juggling Risks and Hope." *New York Times,* 9 October, pp. A1, A14.

Freudenheim, M. 1995. "Penny-Pinching HMOs Showed Their Generosity in Executive Paychecks." *New York Times,* 11 April, p. D1.

———. 2000. "Aetna to Shed Customers and Jobs in Effort to Cut Health Care Costs." *New York Times,* 19 December, p. A1.

Freudenheim, M., and C. Krauss. 1999. "Dancing to a New Health Care Beat; Latin America Becomes Ripe for U.S. Companies' Picking." *New York Times,* 16 June, p. C1.

Frieden, T. R., E. Fujiwara, R. Washko, et al. 1995. "Tuberculosis in New York City: Turning the Tide." *New England Journal of Medicine* 333 (4): 229–33.

Friedman, T. L. 1993. "U.S. to Release 158 Haitian Detainees." *New York Times,* 10 June, p. A12.

Fundación de Antropología Forense de Guatemala. 2000. *Cuatro casos para-digmáticos solicitados por la Comisión para el Esclarecimiento Histórico de Guatemala: Informe de las investigaciones antropológico-forenses e históri-cas realizadas en las comunidades de Panzós, Belén, Acul y Chel.* Editorial Serviprensa, C.A., Guatemala: Fundación de Antropología Forense de Guatemala.

Galbraith, J. K. 2002. "A Perfect Crime: Global Inequality." *Daedalus* 131 (1): 11–25.

Galeano, E. 1973. *Open Veins of Latin America: Five Centuries of the Pillage of a Continent.* New York: Monthly Review Press.

———. 1983. *Days and Nights of Love and War.* New York: Monthly Review Press.

———. 1988. *Memory of Fire.* New York: Pantheon Books.

———. 1991. *The Book of Embraces.* New York: Norton.

Gall, O. 1998. "The Historical Structure of Racism in Chiapas." *Social Identi-ties* 4 (2): 235–61.

Galtung, J. 1969. "Violence, Peace, and Peace Research." *Journal of Peace Re-search* 6 (3): 167–91.

Garcia, P. M., L. A. Kalish, J. Pitt, et al. 1999. "Maternal Levels of Plasma Human Immunodeficiency Virus Type 1 RNA and the Risk of Perinatal Transmis-sion." *New England Journal of Medicine* 341 (6): 394–402.

García Lorca, F. 1995. *Federico García Lorca: Selected Verse.* Edited by C. Mau-rer. New York: Farrar, Straus and Giroux.

Garrett, L. 1994. *The Coming Plague: Newly Emerging Diseases in a World Out of Balance.* New York: Farrar, Straus and Giroux.

———. 1997. "Crumbled Empire, Shattered Health." *Newsday* series, 26 Oc-tober–18 November.

———. 1998. "TB Surge in Former East Bloc." *Newsday,* 25 March, p. A21.

———. 2000. *Betrayal of Trust: The Collapse of Global Public Health.* New York: Hyperion.

Gates, H. L., Jr., and C. West. 1996. *The Future of the Race.* New York: Knopf.

Geertz, C. 1984. "Anti-Anti-Relativism." *American Anthropologist* 86 (2): 263–78.

———. 1988. *Works and Lives: The Anthropologist as Author.* Stanford: Stan-ford University Press.

Gellner, E. 1985. *Relativism and the Social Sciences.* Cambridge: Cambridge Uni-versity Press.

Gerth, J., and S. G. Stolberg. 2000. "Medicine Merchants: Birth of a Blockbuster; Drug Makers Reap Profits on Tax-Backed Research." *New York Times*, 23 April, p. 1.

Gewirth, A. 1978. *Reason and Morality*. Chicago: University of Chicago Press.

———. 1982. *Human Rights: Essays on Justification and Applications*. Chicago: University of Chicago Press.

Gibbons, E. D. 1999. *Sanctions in Haiti: Human Rights and Democracy Under Assault*. Westport, Conn.: Praeger.

Gibbons, E. D., and R. Garfield. 1999. "The Impact of Economic Sanctions on Health and Human Rights in Haiti, 1991 to 1994." *American Journal of Public Health* 89 (10): 1499–504.

Ginzberg, E. 1999. "The Uncertain Future of Managed Care." *New England Journal of Medicine* 340 (2): 144–46.

Gitlin, T. 1995. *The Twilight of Common Dreams*. New York: Metropolitan Books.

Glasser, I., and R. Bridgman. 1999. *Braving the Street: The Anthropology of Homelessness*. New York: Berghahn Books.

Glendon, M. A. 1991. *Rights Talk: The Impoverishment of Political Discourse*. New York: Free Press.

Global Exchange. 1998. *On the Offensive: Intensified Military Occupation in Chiapas Six Months Since the Massacre at Acteal*. San Francisco: Global Exchange.

———. 2000. Global Exchange Chiapas Timeline—2000. Available at *http://www.globalexchange.org/campaigns/mexico/chiapas/2000.html*.

Goldberg, C. 2000. "Emergency Crews Worry as Hospitals Say, 'No Vacancy.' " *New York Times*, 17 December, p. 39.

Goldberg, C., and S. Kishkovsky. 2000. "Russia's Doctors Are Beggars at Work, Paupers at Home." *New York Times*, 16 December, p. A1.

Golden, T. 1995. "Patients Pay High Price in Cuba's War on AIDS." *New York Times*, 16 October, pp. A1, A10.

Good, M. D. 1999. "Clinical Realities and Moral Dilemmas: Contrasting Perspectives from Academic Medicine in Kenya, Tanzania, and America." *Daedalus* 128 (4): 167–96.

Gordimer, N. 1999. *Living in Hope and History: Notes from Our Century*. New York: Farrar, Straus and Giroux.

Gore, C. 1922. *Property, Its Duties and Rights, Historically, Philosophically, and Religiously Regarded; Essays by Various Writers, with an Introduction by the Bishop of Oxford*. New York: Macmillan.

Gossen, G. H. 1974. *Chamulas in the World of the Sun: Time and Space in a Maya Oral Tradition*. Cambridge, Mass.: Harvard University Press.

———. 1999. *Telling Maya Tales: Tzotzil Identities in Modern Mexico*. New York: Routledge.

Gould, C. 1988. *Rethinking Democracy: Freedom and Social Cooperation in Politics, Economy, and Society*. Cambridge: Cambridge University Press.

———. 1996. "Group Rights and Social Ontology." *Philosophical Forum* 28 (1–2): 73–86.

———. 2001. "Two Concepts of Universality and the Problem of Cultural Relativism." In *Cultural Identity and the Nation State,* edited by C. Gould and P. Pasquino, pp. 67–84. Boulder: Rowman and Littlefield.

Gould, J. 1990. *To Lead as Equals: Rural Protest and Political Consciousness in Chinandega, Nicaragua, 1912–1979.* Chapel Hill: University of North Carolina Press.

Gould, P. 1996. *The Slow Plague: A Geography of the AIDS Pandemic.* Cambridge, Mass.: Blackwell.

Gourevitch, P. 1998. *We Wish to Inform You That Tomorrow We Will Be Killed with Our Families.* New York: Farrar, Straus and Giroux.

Govier, T. 1997. "The Right to Eat and the Duty to Work." In *Contemporary Moral Issues,* 4th ed., edited by W. Cragg and C.M. Koggel, pp. 433–43. Toronto: McGraw-Hill Ryerson.

Granich, R., B. Jacobs, J. Mermin, et al. 1995. "Cuba's National AIDS Program: The First Decade." *Western Journal of Medicine* 163 (2): 139–44.

Grann, D. 2001. "Giving 'the Devil' His Due." *Atlantic Monthly* 287 (6): 54–75.

Gray, R.H., T.C. Quinn, D. Serwadda, et al. 2000. "The Ethics of Research in Developing Countries." *New England Journal of Medicine* 343 (5): 361–62.

Greco, D.B. 2000. "The Ethics of Research in Developing Countries." *New England Journal of Medicine* 343 (5): 362.

Green, L. 1998. "Lived Lives and Social Suffering: Problems and Concerns in Medical Anthropology." *Medical Anthropology Quarterly* 12 (1): 3–7.

———. 1999. *Fear as a Way of Life: Mayan Widows in Rural Guatemala.* New York: Columbia University Press.

Greene, G. 1939. *Another Mexico / The Lawless Roads.* New York: Viking Press.

———. 1940. *The Power and the Glory.* New York: Viking Press.

———. 1973. *The Honorary Consul.* New York: Washington Square Press.

Greifinger, R., N. Heywood, and J. Glaser. 1993. "Tuberculosis in Prison: Balancing Justice and Public Health." *Journal of Law, Medicine, and Ethics* 21 (3–4): 332–41.

Grodin, M.A., and G.J. Annas. 1996. "Legacies of Nuremberg: Medical Ethics and Human Rights." *Journal of the American Medical Association* 276 (20): 1682–83.

Grodin, M.A., C.J. Annas, and L.H. Glantz. 1993. "Medicine and Human Rights: A Proposal for International Action." *Hastings Center Report* 23 (4): 8–12.

Gruening, E. 1928. *Mexico and Its Heritage.* New York: Century.

"Guatemalan Peace Vows Unfulfilled." 2000. *St. Louis Post-Dispatch,* 29 December, p. B6.

Guay, L.A., P. Musoke, T. Fleming, et al. 1999. "Intrapartum and Neonatal Single-Dose Nevirapine Compared with Zidovudine for Prevention of Mother-to-Child Transmission of HIV-1 in Kampala, Uganda: HIVNET 012 Randomised Trial." *Lancet* 354 (9181): 795–802.

"La guerra en los Andes." 1992. *Allpanchis,* no. 39 (special issue).

Guillermoprieto, A. 1994. *The Heart That Bleeds: Latin America Now.* New York: Knopf.

Gulden, T. 2002. "Spatial and Temporal Patterns in Civil Violence: Guatemala 1988–1986." Working paper 29, Brookings Center on Social and Economic

Dynamics. Available at *http://www.brook.edu/dybdocroot/es/dynamics/papers/guatemala/guatemala.pdf*.

Gunderman, R. 1998. "Medicine and the Pursuit of Wealth." *Hastings Center Report* 28 (1): 9–13.

Gupta, R., J. Y. Kim, M. A. Espinal, et al. 2001. "Responding to Market Failures in Tuberculosis Control." *Science* 293 (5532): 1049–51.

Gutiérrez, E. D., C. Zielinski, and C. Kendall. 2000. "The Globalization of Health and Disease: The Health Transition and Global Change." In *The Handbook of Social Studies in Health and Medicine,* edited by G. Albrecht, R. Fitzpatrick, and S. Scrimshaw, pp. 84–99. London: Sage.

Gutiérrez, G. 1973. *A Theology of Liberation: History, Politics, and Salvation.* Maryknoll, N.Y.: Orbis Books.

———. 1983. *The Power of the Poor in History.* Maryknoll, N.Y.: Orbis Books.

———. 1987. *On Job: God-Talk and the Suffering of the Innocent.* Maryknoll, N.Y.: Orbis Books.

———. 1993. *Las Casas: In Search of the Poor of Jesus Christ.* Maryknoll, N.Y.: Orbis Books.

Gwatkin, D. R., and M. Guillot. 2000. *The Burden of Disease Among the Global Poor: Current Situation, Future Trends, and Implications for Strategy.* Washington, D.C.: World Bank.

"Haitians Abused and Abandoned." 1992. *Boston Globe,* 28 April, p. 18.

Hallinan, J. T. 2001. *Going Up the River: Travels in a Prison Nation.* New York: Random House.

Hancock, G. 1989. *The Lords of Poverty: The Power, Prestige, and Corruption of the International Aid Business.* New York: Atlantic Monthly Press.

Handwerker, W. P. 1997. "Universal Human Rights and the Problem of Unbounded Cultural Meanings." *American Anthropologist* 99 (4): 799–809.

Hanks, T. D. 1983. *God So Loved the Third World.* Maryknoll, N.Y.: Orbis Books.

Hansen, H., and N. E. Groce. 2001. "From Quarantine to Condoms: Shifting Policies and Problems of HIV Control in Cuba." *Medical Anthropology* 19: 259–92.

Harbury, J. 1994. *Bridge of Courage: Life Stories of the Guatemalan Compañeros and Compañeras.* Monroe, Maine: Common Courage Press.

Harrison, L. 1993. "Voodoo Politics." *Atlantic Monthly* 271 (6): 101–8.

Harry, D. 2000. "Indigenous People Should Control Research That Could Affect Them." *St. Louis Post-Dispatch,* 24 September, p. F3.

Hartigan, K. 1992. "Matching Humanitarian Norms with Cold, Hard Interests: The Making of Refugee Policies in Mexico and Honduras, 1980–89." *International Organization* 46 (3): 709–30.

Harvard Study Team. 1991. "The Effect of the Gulf Crisis on the Children of Iraq." *New England Journal of Medicine* 325 (13): 977–80.

Harvey, N. 1998. *The Chiapas Rebellion: The Struggle for Land and Democracy.* Durham: Duke University Press.

Hasan, M. M. 1996. "Let's End the Non-Profit Charade." *New England Journal of Medicine* 334 (16): 1055–57.

Hatch, E. 1983. *Culture and Morality: The Relativity of Values in Anthropology.* New York: Columbia University Press.

Hayner, P. B. 2001. *Unspeakable Truths: Confronting State Terror and Atrocity.* New York and London: Routledge.

Health Action AIDS. A Physicians for Human Rights project in coordination with Partners In Health. Available at *http://www.phrusa.org/campaigns/aids/phr_pih.html.*

Heaney, S. 1998. *Opened Ground: Selected Poems, 1966–1996.* New York: Farrar, Straus and Giroux.

Heggenhougen, H. K. 1995. "The Epidemiology of Functional Apartheid and Human Rights Abuses." *Social Science and Medicine* 40 (3): 281–84.

———. 1999. "Are the Marginalized the Slag-Heap of Globalization? Disparity, Health, and Human Rights." *Health and Human Rights* 4 (1): 205–13.

———. 2000. "More Than Just 'Interesting!' Anthropology, Health, and Human Rights." *Social Science and Medicine* 50 (9): 1171–75.

Hellman, J. A. 2000. "Real and Virtual Chiapas: Magic Realism and the Left." *Socialist Register,* July, pp. 161–86.

Henkin, L. 1983. *Right v. Might: International Law and the Use of Force.* New York: Columbia University Press.

———. 1990. *International Law: Politics, Values, and Functions. General Course on Public International Law.* Boston: M. Nijhoff.

Henry, C., and P. E. Farmer. 1999a. "Risk Analysis: Infections and Inequalities in a Globalizing Era." *Development* 42 (4): 31–34. Available at *http://www.sagepub.co.uk/journals/Details/issue/sample/a010917.pdf.*

———. 1999b. "Risk Analysis: Infections and Inequalities in a Globalizing Era." Abstract. Conference on "Responses to Globalization: Rethinking Equity and Health," Society for International Development, 13 July, Geneva.

Héritier, F., ed. 1996. *De la violence.* Paris: Éditions Odile Jacob.

———. 1999. *De la violence II.* Paris: Éditions Odile Jacob.

Hernández Castillo, R. A. 1998a. "Reflexiones en torno a la masacre de Acteal: ¿Antropología para qué?" *Gaceta del Tecolote Maya* 3 (1): 1–2.

———, ed. 1998b. *La otra palabra: Mujeres y violencia en Chiapas, antes y después de Acteal.* Mexico City: Centro de Investigaciones y Estudios Superiores en Antropología Social (CIESAS), Grupo de Mujeres de San Cristóbal A.C. Colectivo de Encuentro entre Mujeres (COLEM), Centro de Investigación y Acción para la Mujer (CIAM).

Hewitt de Alcántara, C. 1984. *Anthropological Perspectives on Rural Mexico.* London: Routledge and Kegan Paul.

Hilts, P. 1993. "Haitians Held at Guantánamo Unconscious in a Hunger Strike." *New York Times,* 15 February, p. A7.

Himmelstein, D., S. Woolhandler, and I. Hellander. 2001. *Bleeding the Patient: The Consequences of Corporate Health Care.* Monroe, Maine: Common Courage Press.

Hindley, J. 1996. "Towards a Pluralcultural Nation: The Limits of Indigenismo and Article 4." In *Dismantling the Mexican State?* edited by R. Aitken, N. Craske, G. A. Jones, and D. E. Stansfield, pp. 225–43. New York: St. Martin's Press.

Hinton, A. L. 2002a. "Introduction: Genocide and Anthropology." In *Genocide: An Anthropological Reader*, edited by Alexander Laban Hinton, pp. 1–23. Oxford: Blackwell Publishers.

———, ed. 2002b. *Annihilating Difference: The Anthropology of Genocide*. Berkeley: University of California Press.

———, ed. 2002c. *Genocide: An Anthropological Reader*. Oxford: Blackwell Publishers.

"History Repeating by Haitian Return." 1992. *St. Louis Post-Dispatch*, 9 February, p. B2.

Hochschild, A. 1998. *King Leopold's Ghost: A Story of Greed, Terror, and Heroism in Colonial Africa*. Boston: Houghton-Mifflin.

Hoffman, S. 1981. *Duties Beyond Borders: On the Limits and Possibilities of Ethical International Politics*. Syracuse: Syracuse University Press.

Holman, E. A., R. C. Silver, and H. Waitzkin. 2000. "Traumatic Life Events in Primary Care Patients: A Study in an Ethnically Diverse Sample." *Archives of Family Medicine* 9 (9): 802–10.

"How the Industries Stack Up." 2000. *Fortune*, 17 April, pp. F25–29.

———. 2001. *Fortune*, 16 April, pp. F24–28.

———. 2002. *Fortune*, 15 April, pp. F24–27.

Howe, E. G. 1986. "Ethical Issues Regarding Mixed Agency of Military Physicians." *Social Science and Medicine* 23 (8): 803–15.

Hughes, R. 1993. *Culture of Complaint: The Fraying of America*. New York: Oxford University Press.

Human Rights Office of the Archdiocese of Guatemala. 1999. *Guatemala: Never Again!* Maryknoll, N.Y.: Orbis Books.

Human Rights Watch. 2000. *Punishment and Prejudice: Racial Disparities in the War on Drugs*. New York: Human Rights Watch.

Human Rights Watch/Americas. 1997. *Implausible Deniability: State Responsibility for Rural Violence in Mexico*. New York: Human Rights Watch.

Human Rights Watch/Americas, Jesuit Refugee Service/USA, and National Coalition for Haitian Refugees. 1994. "Fugitives from Injustice: The Crisis of Internal Displacement in Haiti." Report 6 (10).

Human Rights Watch/Americas and National Coalition for Haitian Refugees. 1994. "Terror Prevails in Haiti: Human Rights Violations and Failed Diplomacy." *Haiti Insight* 6 (5): 1–47.

Hymes, D. 1974. "The Uses of Anthropology: Critical, Political, Personal." In *Reinventing Anthropology*, edited by D. Hymes, pp. 3–79. New York: Random House.

Ignatieff, M. 2001. *Human Rights as Politics and Idolatry*. Princeton: Princeton University Press.

Iguíñiz, J. 1995. *Deuda externa en América Latina: Exigencias éticas desde la doctrina social de la Iglesia, Lima*. Lima: Instituto Bartolomé de Las Casas.

Indigenous Peoples Council on Biocolonialism. Web site at *http://www.ipcb.org*.

Institute of Medicine. 2001. *Coverage Matters: Insurance and Health Care*. Washington, D.C.: National Academy Press.

————. 2002a. *Care Without Coverage: Too Little, Too Late.* Washington, D.C.: National Academy Press.

————. 2002b. *Unequal Treatment: Confronting Racial and Ethnic Disparities in Health Care.* Washington, D.C.: National Academy Press.

Inter-American Commission on Human Rights. 1994. *Report on the Situation of Human Rights in Haiti.* Washington, D.C.: Inter-American Commission on Human Rights.

International Military Tribunal (Nuremberg). 1947. "Judgment and Sentences." *American Journal of International Law* 41 (1): 172–333.

Iriart, C., E. E. Merhy, and H. Waitzkin. 2000. "La atención gerenciada en América Latina: Transnacionalización del sector salud en el contexto de la reforma." *Caderños de Saúde Pública* 16 (1): 95–105.

————. 2001. "Managed Care in Latin America: The New Common Sense in Health Policy Reform." *Social Science and Medicine* 52(8): 1243–53.

Ito, M., Y. Nishibe, and Y. K. Inoue. 1998. "Isolation of Inoue-Melnick Virus from Cerebrospinal Fluid of Patients with Epidemic Neuropathy in Cuba." *Archives of Pathology and Laboratory Medicine* 122 (6): 520–22.

Jacoby, R. 1994. *Dogmatic Wisdom: How the Culture Wars Divert Education and Distract America.* New York: Doubleday.

James, C. L. R. 1963. *The Black Jacobins: Toussaint L'Ouverture and the San Domingo Revolution.* New York: Vintage Books.

————. 1980. *The Black Jacobins.* London: Allison and Busby.

Janzen, J. M., and R. K. Janzen. 2000. *Do I Still Have a Life? Voices from the Aftermath of War in Rwanda and Burundi.* Publications in Anthropology, no. 20. Lawrence: University of Kansas.

Jean-Louis, R. 1989. "Diagnostic de l'état de santé en Haïti." *Forum Libre* 1 (*Médecine, Santé et Démocratie en Haïti*): 11–20.

Jencks, C. 2002. "Does Inequality Matter?" *Daedalus* 131 (1): 49–65.

Jenkins, J. H. 1998. "The Medical Anthropology of Political Violence: A Cultural and Feminist Agenda." *Medical Anthropology Quarterly* 12 (1): 122–31.

Johnson, K. 1993. "Judicial Acquiescence to the Executive Branch's Pursuit of Foreign Policy and Domestic Agendas in Immigration Matters: The Case of the Haitian Asylum Seekers." *Georgetown Immigration Law Journal* 7 (1): 1–37.

Johnston, B. R. 1994a. "The Abuse of Human Environmental Rights: Experience and Response." In *Who Pays the Price? The Sociocultural Context of Environmental Crisis,* edited by B. R. Johnston, pp. 219–32. Washington, D.C.: Island Press.

————. 1994b. "Environmental Degradation and Human Rights Abuse." In *Who Pays the Price? The Sociocultural Context of Environmental Crisis,* edited by B. R. Johnston, pp. 7–15. Washington, D.C.: Island Press.

————. 1994c. "Experimenting on Human Subjects: Nuclear Weapons Testing and Human Rights Abuse." In *Who Pays the Price? The Sociocultural Context of Environmental Crisis,* edited by B. R. Johnston, pp. 131–41. Washington, D.C.: Island Press.

Joint United Nations Programme on HIV/AIDS. 2000. *Report on the Global HIV/AIDS Epidemic, June 2000.* Geneva: Joint United Nations Programme on HIV/AIDS.

Jonas, S. 1991. *The Battle for Guatemala: Rebels, Death Squads, and U.S. Power.* Boulder: Westview Press.

———. 1997. "The Peace Accords: An End and a Beginning." *Report on the Americas, New York: North American Congress on Latin America (NACLA)* 30 (6): 6–10.

Jones, J. H. 1993. *Bad Blood: The Tuskegee Syphilis Experiment.* New York: Free Press.

Junod, S. W. 2000. "Diethylene Glycol Deaths in Haiti." *Public Health Reports* 115 (1): 78–86.

Juviler, P. 2000. "Political Community and Human Rights in Postcommunist Russia." In *Human Rights: New Perspectives, New Realities,* edited by A. Pollis and P. Schwab, pp. 115–37. Boulder: Lynne Rienner.

Kahn, J. 2001. "Rich Nations Consider Fund of Billions to Fight AIDS." *New York Times,* 29 April, p. A10.

Kaiser Family Foundation. 1999. "United States: Infant Death Rate per 1,000 Live Births, by Race/Ethnicity, 1999." Available at *http://www.statehealthfacts.kff.org/cgi-bin/healthfacts.cgi?action=profile&area=United+States&category=Health+Status&subcategory=Infants&topic=Infant+Deaths+by+Race%2fEthnicity.*

Karshan, M. 2000. "The Haitian People Achieve Environmental Justice for Earth Day." Haitian Government Press Release on Ash Removal. 22 April. Available at *http://www.essentialaction.org/return/government.txt.*

Kassirer, J. P. 1998. "Managing Care: Should We Adopt a New Ethic?" *New England Journal of Medicine* 339 (6): 397–98.

Katz, C. 1992. "All the World Is Staged: Intellectuals and the Projects of Ethnography." *Society and Space* 10: 495–510.

Kauffman, L. A. 1993. "The Diversity Game." *Village Voice,* 31 August, pp. 29, 32.

Kaufman, C. 1998. "Contraceptive Use in South Africa Under Apartheid." *Demography* 35 (4): 421–34.

Kaveny, C. 1999. "Commodifying the Polyvalent Good of Health Care." *Journal of Medicine and Philosophy* 24 (3): 207–23.

Kawachi, I., B. P. Kennedy, K. Lochner, et al. 1997. "Social Capital, Income Inequality, and Mortality." *American Journal of Public Health* 87 (9): 1491–98.

Kazionny, B., C. Wells, H. Kluge, et al. 2001. "Implications of the Growing HIV-1 Epidemic for Tuberculosis Control in Russia." *Lancet* 358 (9292): 1513–14.

Kearney, M. 1995. "The Local and the Global: The Anthropology of Globalization and Transnationalism." *Annual Review of Anthropology* 24: 547–65.

Keegan, V. 1996. "Highway Robbery by the Super-Rich." *Guardian,* 22 July, p. 16.

Kernaghan, C. 1993. *Haiti After the Coup: Sweatshop or Real Development.* New York: U.S. National Labor Committee.

Keshavjee, S., S. Weiser, and A. Kleinman. 2001. "Medicine Betrayed: Hemophilia Patients and HIV in the U.S." *Social Science and Medicine* 53 (8): 1081–94.

Kilborn, P. T., and L. Clemetson. 2002. "Gains of 90's Did Not Lift All, Census Shows." *New York Times,* 5 June, pp. A1, A20.

Kim, J. Y., J. V. Millen, A. Irwin, and J. Gershman, eds. 2000. *Dying for Growth: Global Inequality and the Health of the Poor.* Monroe, Maine: Common Courage Press.

Kimerling, M. E., H. Kluge, N. Vezhnina, et al. 1999. "Inadequacy of the Current WHO Re-Treatment Regimen in a Central Siberian Prison: Treatment Failure and MDRTB." *International Journal of Tuberculosis and Lung Disease* 3 (5): 451–53.

Kinney, E. D. 2001. "The International Human Right to Health: What Does This Mean for Our Nation and World?" *Indiana Law Review* 34: 1457–75.

Kipnis, K., and D. T. Meyers, eds. 1985. *Economic Justice: Private Rights and Public Responsibilities.* Totowa, N.J.: Rowman and Littlefield.

Kirkpatrick, J. 1981. "Establishing a Viable Human Rights Policy." Speech delivered at Human Rights Conference, 4 April, Kenyon College, Gambier, Ohio. Available at *http://www.thirdworldtraveler.com/HumanRightsDocuments /Kirkpatrick_HRPolicy.html.*

Kirsch, J. D., and M. Arana Cedeño. 1999. "Informed Consent for Family Planning for Poor Women in Chiapas, Mexico." *Lancet* 354 (9176): 419–20.

Klein, D. E., G. Sullivan, D. L. Wolcott, et al. 1987. "Changes in AIDS Risk Behaviors Among Homosexual Male Physicians and University Students." *American Journal of Psychiatry* 144 (6): 742–47.

Klein, N. 2000. *No Logo! Taking Aim at the Brand Bullies.* Toronto: Knopf Canada.

Kleinman, A. 1995. "Anthropology of Medicine." In *Encyclopedia of Bioethics,* edited by W. T. Reich, pp. 1667–72. New York: Simon and Schuster.

———. 1999. "Moral Experience and Ethical Reflection: Can Ethnography Reconcile Them? A Quandary for the 'New Bioethics.'" *Daedalus* 128 (4): 69–97.

Kleinman, A., L. Eisenberg, and B. Good. 1978. "Culture, Illness, and Care: Clinical Lessons from Anthropologic and Cross-Cultural Research." *Annals of Internal Medicine* 88 (2): 251–58.

Kleist, T. 1997. "Mexican Gunmen Slay 42; Chiapas Village Targeted." *Chicago Sun-Times,* 23 December, p. 1.

Knowlton, B. 2000. "U.S. Appeals Court Hands Victory to Elian's Father." *International Herald Tribune,* 2 June, pp. 1, 8.

Knox, N. 2000. "Swiss Judge Traces Trail of Laundered Russian Funds." *USA Today,* 24 August, p. B1.

Knox, R. A. 2000. "Health Officials Track New TB Strain." *Boston Globe,* 21 April, p. B4.

Koggel, C. 1998. *Perspectives on Equality: Constructing a Relational Theory.* Totowa, N.J.: Rowman and Littlefield.

Kolata, G., and K. Eichenwald. 1999. "For the Uninsured, Experiments May Provide the Only Treatment." *New York Times,* 22 June, p. A1.

Koss, M., P. Koss, and J. Woodruff. 1991. "Deleterious Effects of Criminal Victimization on Women's Health and Medical Utilization." *Archives of Internal Medicine* 151 (2): 342–47.

Krieger, N. 1999. "Embodying Inequality: A Review of Concepts, Measures, and Methods for Studying Health Consequences of Discrimination." *International Journal of Health Services* 29 (2): 295–352.

Kwiatkowski, L. M. 1998. *Struggling with Development: The Politics of Hunger and Gender in the Philippines.* Boulder: Westview Press.

LaFeber, W. 1984. *Inevitable Revolutions: The United States in Central America*. New York: Norton.

Lambert, P., M. Tauber, and A. Tresinowski. 2002. "After the Jackpot." *People* 57 (22): 82–88.

Lancaster, R. 1988. *Thanks to God and the Revolution*. New York: Columbia University Press.

Lanchin, M. 2000. "Secret Haunts El Salvador." *San Francisco Chronicle,* 23 March, pp. A1, A10.

Laqueur, W., and B. Rubin, eds. 1990. *The Human Rights Reader*. Rev. ed. New York: New American Library.

Laurell, A. C. 2001. "Health Reform in Mexico: The Promotion of Inequality." *International Journal of Health Services* 31 (2): 291–321.

Lawless, R. 1992. *Haiti's Bad Press*. Rochester, Vt.: Schenkman.

Lawyers Committee for Human Rights. 1990. *Paper Laws, Steel Bayonets: Breakdown of the Rule of Law in Haiti*. New York: Lawyers Committee for Human Rights.

Le Caisne, L. 2000. *Prison: Une ethnologue en centrale*. Paris: Éditions Odile Jacob.

Leacock, E. B. 1981. *Myths of Male Dominance*. New York: Monthly Review Press.

Leaning, J., S. Briggs, and L. Chen, eds. 1999. *Humanitarian Crises: The Medical and Public Health Response*. Cambridge, Mass.: Harvard University Press.

Leatherman, T. L. 1998. "Illness, Social Relations, and Household Production and Reproduction in the Andes of Southern Peru." In *Building a New Bio-cultural Synthesis: Political-Economic Perspectives on Human Biology,* edited by A. L. Goodman and T. L. Leatherman, pp. 245–67. Ann Arbor: University of Michigan Press.

Leclerc, A., D. Fassin, H. Grandjean, et al., eds. 2000. *Les inégalités sociales de santé*. Paris: Éditions la Découverte et Syros.

Lee, B. 2002. "Statement of Congresswoman Barbara Lee: New Partnership for Haiti Resolution." Statement introducing H. Cong. Res. 382, on behalf of the Congressional Black Caucus Haiti Task Force. 18 April, Washington, D.C.

Leiner, M. 1994. *Sexual Politics in Cuba: Machismo, Sexuality, and AIDS*. Boulder: Westview Press.

Lemarchand, R. 1997. "The Rwanda Genocide." In *Century of Genocides: Eyewitness Accounts and Critical Views,* edited by S. Totten, W. S. Parsons, and I. W. Charny, pp. 408–23. New York: Garland.

Levins, R. 2000. "Is Capitalism a Disease? The Crisis in U.S. Public Health." *Monthly Review* 52 (4): 8–33.

Lewin, M. E., and S. Altman, eds. 2000. *America's Health Care Safety Net: Intact But Endangered*. Washington, D.C.: National Academy Press.

Li, J. T. C. 1996. "The Patient-Physician Relationship: Covenant or Contract." *Mayo Clinic Proceedings* 71: 917–18.

———. 1998. "The Physician as Advocate." *Mayo Clinic Proceedings* 73: 1022–24.

———. 1999. "Humility and the Practice of Medicine." *Mayo Clinic Proceedings* 74: 529–30.

Liebow, E. 1993. *Tell Them Who I Am: The Lives of Homeless Women.* New York: Free Press.

Liguori, A.L. 1995. "Health, Human Rights, and Dignity: Reflections from the Mexican Experience." *Health and Human Rights* 1 (3): 298–305.

Lindsay, M.K., J. Grant, H.B. Peterson, et al. 1993. "Human Immunodeficiency Virus Infection Among Patients in a Gynecology Emergency Department." *Obstetrics and Gynecology* 81 (6): 1012–15.

Loescher, G. 1988. "Humanitarianism and Politics in Central America." *Political Science Quarterly* 103 (2): 295–320.

Löytönen, M., and P. Maasilta. 1998. "Multi-Drug Resistant Tuberculosis in Finland: A Forecast." *Social Science and Medicine* 46 (6): 695–702.

Lurie, M., A. Harrison, D. Wilkinson, et al. 1997. "Circular Migration and Sexual Networking in Rural Kwazulu/Natal: Implications for the Spread of HIV and Other Sexually Transmitted Diseases." *Health Transition Review* 7 (Supplement 3): 17–27.

Lurie, P., and S.M. Wolfe. 1997. "Unethical Trials of Interventions to Reduce Perinatal Transmission of the Human Immunodeficiency Virus in Developing Countries." *New England Journal of Medicine* 337 (12): 853–56.

Lush, T. 2002. "Pastor Arrested as War Criminal." *St. Petersburg Times,* 1 May, p. A1.

MacDonald, T.H. 1999. *A Developmental Analysis of Cuba's Health Care System Since 1959.* Lewiston, N.Y.: Edwin Mellen Press.

Macklin, R. 1999. *Against Relativism: Cultural Diversity and the Search for Ethical Universals in Medicine.* New York: Oxford University Press.

Madrick, J. 2002. "A Rise in Child Poverty Rates Is at Risk in U.S." *New York Times,* 13 June, p. C2.

Magnarella, P.J. 1994. "Anthropology, Human Rights, and Justice." *International Journal of Anthropology* 9 (1): 3–7.

Mann, J. 1998. "AIDS and Human Rights: Where Do We Go from Here?" *Health and Human Rights* 3 (1): 143–49.

Mann, J.M., S. Gruskin, M.A. Grodin, and G.J. Annas. 1999. *Health and Human Rights.* New York and London: Routledge.

Mann, J., and D. Tarantola. 1998. "Responding to HIV/AIDS: A Historical Perspective." *Health and Human Rights* 2 (4): 5–8.

Marcos, S. 2001. *Our Word Is Our Weapon: Selected Writings.* Edited by J. Ponce de León. New York: Seven Stories Press.

Marcos, S., and the Zapatista Army of National Liberation. 1995. *Shadows of Tender Fury: The Letters and Communiqués of Subcomandante Marcos and the Zapatista Army of National Liberation.* New York: Monthly Review Press.

Marks, S.P. 1999. "Economic Sanctions as Human Rights Violations: Reconciling Political and Public Health Imperatives." *American Journal of Public Health* 89 (10): 1509–13.

Marmot, M. 1994. "Social Differentials in Health Within and Between Populations." *Daedalus* 123 (4): 197–216.

Marmot, M., M. Bobak, and G.D. Smith. 1995. "Explanations for Social Inequalities in Health." In *Societies and Health,* edited by B.C. Amick, S. Levine, A.R. Tarlov, and D.C. Walsh, pp. 172–210. New York: Oxford University Press.

Marmot, M. G., G. D. Smith, and S. A. Stansfeld. 1991. "Health Inequalities Among British Civil Servants: The Whitehall II Study." *Lancet* 337 (8754): 1387–93.

Marshall, P. A., and B. A. Koenig. 1996. "Bioethics in Anthropology: Perspectives on Culture, Medicine, and Morality." In *Medical Anthropology: Contemporary Theory and Method,* edited by C. F. Sargent and T. M. Johnson, pp. 349–73. Westport, Conn.: Praeger.

Martín-Baró, I. 1994. *Writings for a Liberation Theology.* Cambridge, Mass.: Harvard University Press.

Martínez, S. 1996. "Indifference Within Indignation: Anthropology, Human Rights, and the Haitian Bracero." *American Anthropologist* 98 (1): 17–25.

Maruschak, L. M. 1999. "HIV in Prisons 1997." *Bureau of Justice Statistics Bulletin,* November, pp. 1–12.

Mas, P., J. L. Pelegrino, M. G. Guzman, et al. 1997. "Viral Isolation from Cases of Epidemic Neuropathy in Cuba." *Archives of Pathology and Laboratory Medicine* 121 (8): 825–33.

Maskovsky, J. 1999. " 'Fighting for Our Lives': Poverty and AIDS Activism in Neoliberal Philadelphia." Ph.D. diss., Temple University.

———. 2000. " 'Managing' the Poor: Neoliberalism, Medicaid HMOs, and the Triumph of Consumerism Among the Poor." *Medical Anthropology* 19: 121–46.

Mason, T. A. 1956. *Harlan Fiske Stone: Pillar of the Law.* New York: Viking Press.

Mauer, M. 1999. *Race to Incarcerate: The Sentencing Project.* New York: The New Press.

Mayer, E. 1992. "Peru in Deep Trouble: Mario Vargas Llosa's 'Inquest in the Andes' Reexamined." In *Rereading Cultural Anthropology,* edited by G. E. Marcus, pp. 181–219. Durham: Duke University Press.

McCord, C., and H. Freeman. 1990. "Excess Mortality in Harlem." *New England Journal of Medicine* 322 (3): 173–77.

McCormick, E. 1993. "HIV-Infected Haitian Refugees: An Argument Against Exclusion." *Georgetown Immigration Law Journal* 7 (1): 149–71.

McCully, P. 1996. *Silenced Rivers: The Ecology and Politics of Large Dams.* London: Zed Books.

McNeil, D. G., Jr. 2000a. "Medical Merchants: A Special Report; Drug Makers and 3rd World: Study in Neglect." *New York Times,* 21 May, p. 1.

———. 2000b. "Medicine Merchants: Patients and Patents; As Devastating Epidemics Increase, Nations Take On Drug Companies." *New York Times,* 9 July, p. A8.

———. 2000c. "No Limit: Writing the Bill for Global AIDS." *New York Times,* 2 July, p. 4.

———. 2000d. "Selling Cheap 'Generic' Drugs, India's Copycats Irk Industry." *New York Times,* 1 December, pp. A1, A14.

Médecins Sans Frontières. 2001. "Fatal Imbalance: The Crisis in Research and Development for Drugs for Neglected Diseases." Available at *http://www .msf.org/content/page.cfm?articleid=032387D3–7D09–49E3–99FC231DB E03F7B7.*

Merleau-Ponty, M. 1945. *Phénoménologie de la perception.* Paris: Gallimard.

Messer, E. 1993. "Anthropology and Human Rights." *Annual Review of Anthropology* 22: 221–49.

———. 1997. "Pluralist Approaches to Human Rights." *Journal of Anthropological Research* 53: 293–317.

Mexico Solidarity Network. 2000. News and Analysis Archive. News Summary, 1–7 August.

Millen, J. V., and T. H. Holtz. 2000. "Dying for Growth, Part I: Transnational Corporations and the Health of the Poor." In *Dying for Growth: Global Inequality and the Health of the Poor,* edited by J. Y. Kim, J. V. Millen, A. Irwin, and J. Gershman, pp. 177–223. Monroe, Maine: Common Courage Press.

Miłosz, C. 1973. *Selected Poems.* Hopewell, N.J.: Ecco Press.

———. 1978. *Bells in Winter.* Hopewell, N.J.: Ecco Press.

———, ed. 1983. *Postwar Polish Poetry.* 3d ed. Berkeley: University of California Press.

Ministry of Public Health of Cuba. 2000. *Health Care Situation in Cuba: Basic Indicators 1999.* Havana: National Health Statistics Bureau, Ministry of Public Health.

Ministry of Social Development, Mexico. 2000. "Chiapas: State-Level Indigenous Profile." Available at *http://www.sedesol.gob.mx/perfiles/estatal/chiapas/00_summary.html.*

Mintz, S. 1974. *Caribbean Transformations.* Baltimore: Johns Hopkins University Press.

———. 1977. "The So-Called World System: Local Initiative and Local Response." *Dialectical Anthropology* 2 (4): 253–70.

———. 1997. "The Localization of Anthropological Practice: From Area Studies to Transnationalism." *Critique of Anthropology* 18 (2): 117–33.

Mintzes, B., A. Hardon, and J. Hanhart, eds. 1993. *Norplant: Under Her Skin.* Amsterdam: Wemos and Women's Health Action Foundation.

Misión de Verificación de las Naciones Unidas en Guatemala (MINUGUA). 1999. *Noveno informe sobre derechos humanos de MINUGUA.* Guatemala City: MINUGUA.

Mitchell, J. 1943. *McSorley's Wonderful Saloon.* New York: Duell, Sloan and Pearce.

Mitnick, C., E. Palacios, S. Shin, et al. 2001. "Treatment Outcomes in 75 Patients with Chronic Multidrug-Resistant Tuberculosis Enrolled in Aggressive Community-Based Therapy in Urban Peru." *International Journal of Tuberculosis and Lung Disease* 5 (11) Supplement 1: S156–57.

Mittal, A., and P. Rosset, eds. 1999. *America Needs Human Rights.* Oakland, Calif.: Food First Books.

Monmaney, T. 1997. "Gene Sleuths Seek Asthma's Secrets on Remote Island; Residents, Who Apparently Inherited Susceptibility, Have Come Under the Microscope of a Booming Biotech Industry." *Los Angeles Times,* 30 April, p. A1.

Moore, M., and J. W. Anderson. 1997. "45 Villagers Slaughtered in Restive Mexican State; Human Rights Workers Blame Ruling Party." *Washington Post,* 24 December, p. A8.

Moreno, J.D. 1997. "Reassessing the Influence of the Nuremberg Code on American Medical Ethics." *Journal of Contemporary Health Law and Policy* 13 (2): 347–60.

Moreno, J.D., and S.E. Lederer. 1996. "Revising the History of the Cold War Research Ethics." *Kennedy Institute of Ethics Journal* 6 (3): 223–37.

Morsy, S.A. 1993. "Bodies of Choice: Norplant Experimental Trials on Egyptian Women." In *Norplant: Under Her Skin,* edited by B. Mintzes, A. Hardon, and J. Hanhart, pp. 89–114. Amsterdam: Wemos and Women's Health Action Foundation.

Mosley, W.H., J.L. Bobadilla, and D.T. Jamison. 1993. "The Health Transition: Implications for Health Policy in Developing Countries." In *Disease Control Priorities in Developing Countries,* edited by D.T. Jamison, W.H. Mosley, A.R. Measham, and J.L. Bobadilla, pp. 673–99. New York: Oxford Medical Publications.

Mothers of the Plaza de Mayo. 1999. "Letter to Pope John Paul II." *International Journal of Health Services* 29 (4): 895–96.

Mullings, A.M.A. 2000. "The Ethics of Research in Developing Countries." *New England Journal of Medicine* 343 (5): 362.

Murphy, A. 2000. *The Triumph of Evil: The Reality of the U.S.A.'s Cold War Victory.* Fucecchio: European Press Academic Publishing.

Murray, J.L., and A.D. Lopez. 1996. *The Global Burden of Disease: A Comprehensive Assessment of Mortality and Disability from Diseases, Injuries, and Risk Factors in 1990 and Projected to 2020.* Boston: Harvard School of Public Health on behalf of the World Health Organization and the World Bank.

Mushlin, A.I., and F.A. Appel. 1977. "Diagnosing Potential Noncompliance: Physicians' Ability in a Behavioral Dimension of Medical Care." *Archives of Internal Medicine* 137 (3): 318–21.

Nader, L. 1972. "Up the Anthropologist—Perspectives Gained from Studying Up." In *Reinventing Anthropology,* edited by D. Hymes, pp. 284–311. New York: Pantheon Books.

Nagengast, C. 1994. "Violence, Terror, and the Crisis of the State." *Annual Review of Anthropology* 23: 109–36.

———. 1997. "Women, Minorities, and Indigenous Peoples: Universalism and Cultural Relativity." *Journal of Anthropological Research* 53: 349–69.

Nagengast, C., and T. Turner. 1997. "Introduction: Universal Human Rights Versus Cultural Relativity." *Journal of Anthropological Research* 53: 269–72.

Nash, J. 1995. "The Reassertion of Indigenous Identity: Mayan Responses to State Intervention in Chiapas." *Latin American Research Review* 30 (5): 7–42.

National Center for Health Statistics. 1998. *Health, United States, 1998, with Socioeconomic Status and Health Chartbook.* Hyattsville, Md.: National Center for Health Statistics.

———. 2000. *Health, United States, 2000, with Adolescent Health Chartbook.* Hyattsville, Md.: National Center for Health Statistics.

National Endowment for Democracy. Web site at *http://www.ned.org/about/about.html.*

National Institute for Health Care Management. 2001. "Prescription Drugs and Mass Media Advertising, 2000." Available at *http://www.nihcm.org /DTCbrief2001.pdf.*

———. 2002a. "Changing Patterns of Pharmaceutical Innovation." Available at *http://nihcm.org/innovations.pdf.*

———. 2002b. "Prescription Drug Expenditures in 2001: Another Year of Escalating Costs." Available at *http://www.nihcm.org/spending2001.pdf.*

Navarro, V. 1981a. "The Economic and Political Determinants of Human (Including Health) Rights." In *Imperialism, Health, and Medicine,* edited by V. Navarro, pp. 53–76. Farmingdale, N.Y.: Baywood.

———. 1981b. "The Underdevelopment of Health or the Health of Underdevelopment: An Analysis of the Distribution of Human Health Resources in Latin America." In *Imperialism, Health, and Medicine,* edited by V. Navarro, pp. 15–36. Farmingdale, N.Y.: Baywood.

———. 1990. "Race or Class Versus Race and Class: Mortality Differentials in the United States." *Lancet* 336 (8725): 1238–40.

———. 1997. "WHO: Where There Is No Vision, the People Perish." *Lancet* 350 (9089): 1480–81.

———. 1998. "Whose Globalization?" *American Journal of Public Health* 88 (5): 742–43.

"Nearly 1,000,000 Locked Up in Russian Prisons." 2002. Interfax, 5 January. Available at *http://www.cdi.org/russia/johnson/6006-3.cfm.*

Neier, A. 1990. "What Should Be Done About the Guilty?" *New York Review of Books,* 1 February, pp. 32–35.

———. 1998. *War Crimes: Brutality, Genocide, Terror, and the Struggle for Justice.* New York: Times Books.

Neill, K. G. 2001. "Dancing with the Devil: Health, Human Rights, and the Export of U.S. Models of Managed Care to Developing Countries." *Cultural Survival Quarterly* 24 (4): 61–63.

Nelson, H. L., ed. 1997. *Stories and Their Limits: Narrative Approaches to Bioethics.* New York: Routledge.

Nelson, H. L., and J. L. Nelson. 1996. "Justice in the Allocation of Health Care Resources: A Feminist Account." In *Feminism and Bioethics: Beyond Reproduction,* edited by S. M. Wolf, pp. 351–70. New York: Oxford University Press.

Nelson-Pallmeyer, J. 1992. *Brave New World Order: Must We Pledge Allegiance?* Maryknoll, N.Y.: Orbis Books.

Neptune-Anglade, M. 1986. *L'autre moitié du développement: À propos du travail des femmes en Haiti.* Pétion-Ville, Haiti: Éditions des Alizés.

Neruda, P. 1974. *Five Decades: A Selection (Poems 1925–1970).* New York: Grove Press.

Neuffer, E. 2001. *The Key to My Neighbor's House: Seeking Justice in Bosnia and Rwanda.* New York: Picador.

Neugebauer, R. 1999. "Research on Violence in Developing Countries: Benefits and Perils." *American Journal of Public Health* 89 (10): 1473–74.

Newbury, C. 1988. *The Cohesion of Oppression: Clientship and Ethnicity in Rwanda, 1860–1960.* New York: Columbia University Press.

Nguyen, V. K. 2000. "The Shape of Things to Come?" *Globe and Mail,* 11 July, p. A15.

Nickel, J. 1987. *Making Sense of Human Rights: Philosophical Reflections on the Universal Declaration of Human Rights.* Berkeley: University of California Press.

Nightingale, E., K. Hannibal, J. Geiger, et al. 1990. "Apartheid Medicine: Health and Human Rights in South Africa." *Journal of the American Medical Association* 264 (16): 2097–102.

Nordstrom, C. 1998. "Terror Warfare and the Medicine of Peace." *Medical Anthropology Quarterly* 12 (1): 103–21.

Norris, C. 1990. *What's Wrong with Postmodernism: Critical Theory and the Ends of Philosophy.* Baltimore: Johns Hopkins University Press.

———. 1992. *Uncritical Theory: Postmodernism, Intellectuals, and the Gulf War.* Amherst: University of Massachusetts Press.

Norton, M. 2002. "Haiti Clamors for Release of Blocked Loans That Might Take Years to Disburse." Associated Press, 11 March.

"The Nuremberg Code." 1949–1953. In *Trials of War Criminals Before the Nuremberg Military Tribunals Under Control Council Law No. 10,* Nuremberg, October 1946–April 1949, pp. 181–82. Washington, D.C.: U.S. Government Printing Office.

Nussbaum, M., and A. Sen. 1993. *The Quality of Life.* Oxford: Oxford University Press.

Nutter, D. O. 1984. "Access to Care and the Evolution of Corporate, For-Profit Medicine." *New England Journal of Medicine* 311 (14): 917–19.

Nyhan, D. 1992. "Murder in Haiti." *Boston Globe,* 19 March, p. A17.

Obiora, L. A. 1997. "Bridges and Barricades: Rethinking Polemics and Intransigence in the Campaign Against Female Circumcision." *Case Western Reserve Law Review* 47 (2): 275–379.

Oficina los Derechos Humanos del Arzobispado de Guatemala (ODHAG). 1998. *Guatemala: Nunca Más.* Guatemala City: Informe Proyecto Interdiocesano de Recuperación de la Memoria Histórica.

Okin, S. 1981. "Liberty and Welfare: Some Basic Issues in Human Rights Theory." In *Human Rights,* edited by J. R. Pennock and J. W. Chapman, pp. 232–56. New York: New York University Press.

Olujic, M. B. 1998. "Embodiment of Terror: Gendered Violence in Peacetime and Wartime in Croatia and Bosnia-Herzegovina." *Medical Anthropology Quarterly* 12 (1): 31–50.

O'Neill, W. 1993. "The Roots of Human Rights Violations in Haiti." *Georgetown Immigration Law Journal* 7 (1): 87–117.

Organs Watch. University of California, Berkeley. Web site at *http://sunsite .berkeley.edu/biotech/organswatch/.*

Orwell, G. 1933. *Down and Out in Paris and London.* New York: Harcourt Brace.

———. 1968. *The Collected Essays, Journalism, and Letters of George Orwell.* Vol. 4, *In Front of Your Nose, 1945–1950.* New York: Penguin Books.

Ott, K. 1996. *Fevered Lives: Tuberculosis in American Culture Since 1870.* Cambridge, Mass.: Harvard University Press.

Packard, R. 1989. *White Plague, Black Labor: Tuberculosis and the Political Economy of Health and Disease in South Africa.* Berkeley: University of California Press.

Pan American Health Organization. 2001. Haiti: Country Health Profiles. Available at *http://www.paho.org/English/SHA/prflHAI.htm.*

Partners In Health. Web site at *www.pih.org.*

Patterson, O. 1979. "On Slavery and Slave Formations." *New Left Review* 117: 31–67.

Paul VI. 1967. Populorum Progresio. Available at *http://www.osjspm.org /cst/pp.htm.*

Pax Christi International. 1992. *Pax Christi Newsletter.* April, vol. 13. Brussels: Pax Christi International.

Pear, R. 2001. "HMOs Plan to Drop Medicare, Calling Fees Too Low." *New York Times,* 22 September, p. A8.

Peel, Q. 2000. "Russia's Invitation to Reform: To Revive His Country's Economy, Vladimir Putin Must Be Able to Attract Foreign Investment and Technology." *Financial Times,* 17 April, p. 23.

Pellegrino, E. 1997. "The Nazi Doctors and Nuremberg: Some Moral Lessons Revisited." *Annals of Internal Medicine* 127 (4): 307–8.

———. 1999. "The Commodification of Medical and Health Care: The Moral Consequences of a Paradigm Shift from a Professional to a Market Ethic." *Journal of Medicine and Philosophy* 24 (3): 243–66.

Pellegrino, E. D., and D. C. Thomasma. 2000. "Dubious Premises—Evil Conclusions: Moral Reasoning at the Nuremberg Trials." *Cambridge Quarterly of Health Care Ethics* 9 (2): 261–74.

Pereira, W. 1981. *Inhuman Rights: The Western System and Global Human Rights Abuse.* New York: Apex.

Pérez-Stable, E. J. 1999. "Managed Care Arrives in Latin America." *New England Journal of Medicine* 340 (14): 1110–12.

Perry, M. 1998. *The Idea of Human Rights: Four Inquiries.* Oxford: Oxford University Press.

Peterson, M. A., ed. 1999. "Managed Care Backlash." *Journal of Health Politics, Policy, and Law* 24 (5): 873–1218 (theme issue).

Pharmaceutical Research and Manufacturers of America. 2001. "Global Partnerships: Humanitarian Programs of the Pharmaceutical Industry in Developing Nations." Available at *http://world.phrma.org/Phrma_2001Booklet.pdf.*

———. 2002. "New Medicines in Development for Infectious Diseases." Available at *http://www.phrma.org/searchcures/newmeds/resources/2002–04–03 .56.pdf.*

Physicians for Human Rights. 1999. *Health Care Held Hostage: Human Rights Violations and Violations of Medical Neutrality in Chiapas, Mexico.* Boston: Physicians for Human Rights.

Pierre-Antoine, L. 2002. "Aux origines des événements du décembre 2001." *Haïti-Progrès,* 27 February–5 March, 19 (50): 11–14.

Pitcher, L. 1998. " 'The Divine Impatience:' Ritual, Narrative, and Symbolization in the Practice of Martyrdom in Palestine." *Medical Anthropology Quarterly* 12 (1): 8–30.

Pixley, G. V., and C. Boff. 1989. *The Bible, the Church, and the Poor*. Maryknoll, N.Y.: Orbis Books.

Polier, N., and W. Roseberry. 1989. "Tristes Tropes: Post-Modern Anthropologists Encounter the Other and Discover Themselves." *Economy and Society* 18 (2): 245–64.

Pollack, A. 2001. "News Analysis: Defensive Drug Industry Fuels Fight over Patents." *New York Times*, 20 April, p. A6.

Pollack, R., and L. O'Rourke. 2001. *Off the Charts: Pay, Profits, and Spending by Drug Companies*. June. Washington, D.C.: Families USA.

Pollack, R., J. Woods, and L. O'Rourke. 2001. *Healthy Pay for Health Plan Executives*. June. Washington, D.C.: Families USA.

Pollak, M. 1988. *Les homosexuels et le SIDA: Sociologie d'une epidémie*. Paris: A. M. Matailie.

Poppendieck, J. 1998. *Sweet Charity? Emergency Food and the End of Entitlement*. New York: Viking Press.

Portaels, F., L. Rigouts, and I. Bastian. 1999. "Addressing Multidrug-Resistant Tuberculosis in Penitentiary Hospitals and in the General Population of the Former Soviet Union." *International Journal of Tuberculosis and Lung Disease* 3 (7): 582–88.

Powell, C. 1993. " 'Life' at Guantánamo: The Wrongful Detention of Haitian Refugees." *Reconstruction* 2 (2): 58–68.

Power, S. 2002 *"A Problem from Hell": America and the Age of Genocide*. New York: Basic Books.

Powles, J. W., and N. E. Day. 1997. "Consumption of Alcohol and Mortality in Russia." *Lancet* 350 (9082): 956.

Program in Infectious Disease and Social Change, ed. 1999. *The Global Impact of Drug-Resistant Tuberculosis*. Boston: Harvard Medical School and the Open Society Institute.

Pruchnicki, A. 1997. "First, Do No Harm (Pending Prior Approval)." *New England Journal of Medicine* 337 (22): 1627–28.

Puleo, M. 1994. *The Struggle Is One: Voices and Visions of Liberation*. Albany: SUNY Press.

Quesada, J. 1998. "Suffering Child: An Embodiment of War and Its Aftermath in Post-Sandinista Nicaragua." *Medical Anthropology Quarterly* 12 (1): 51–73.

Quinn, T. C., M. J. Wawer, N. Sewankambo, et al. 2000. "Viral Load and Heterosexual Transmission of Human Immunodeficiency Virus Type 1." *New England Journal of Medicine* 342 (13): 921–29.

Racine, M. M. B. 1999. *Like the Dew That Waters the Grass: Words from Haitian Women*. Washington, D.C.: EPICA.

Rathore, S. S., A. K. Berger, K. P. Weinfurt, et al. 2000. "Race, Sex, Poverty, and the Medical Treatment of Acute Myocardial Infarction in the Elderly." *Circulation: Journal of the American Heart Association* 102 (6): 642–48.

Rawls, J. 1999. *The Law of Peoples*. Cambridge, Mass.: Harvard University Press.

Reichman, L. B. 1997. "Tuberculosis Elimination—What's to Stop Us?" *International Journal of Tuberculosis and Lung Disease* 1 (1): 3–11.

Relman, A. 1991. "Shattuck Lecture—The Health Care Industry: Where Is It Taking Us?" *New England Journal of Medicine* 325 (12): 854–59.

———. 1998. "Education to Defend Professional Values in the New Corporate Age." *Academic Medicine* 73 (12): 1229–33.

Renteln, A.D. 1988. "Relativism and the Search for Human Rights." *American Anthropologist* 90 (1): 56–72.

Reverby, S.M., ed. 2000. *Tuskegee Truths: Rethinking the Tuskegee Syphilis Study.* Chapel Hill: University of North Carolina Press.

Rey, T. 1999. "Junta, Rape, and Religion in Haiti, 1993–1994." *Journal of Feminist Studies in Religion* 15 (2): 73–100.

Reyes, H., and R. Coninx. 1997. "Pitfalls of Tuberculosis Programmes in Prisons." *British Medical Journal* 315 (7120): 1447–50.

Reyes-Frausto, S., M.A. Lezana-Fernández, M.C. Garcia Peña, et al. 1998. "Maternal Mortality Regionalization and Trend in Mexico (1937–1995)." *Archives of Medical Research* 29 (2): 165–72.

Ridgeway, J., ed. 1994. *The Haiti Files: Decoding the Crisis.* Washington, D.C.: Essential Books.

"Rifampicin or Ethambutol in the Routine Treatment of Tuberculosis." 1973. *British Medical Journal* 4 (892): 568.

Rifkin, J. 2000. "The Price of Life: A Call for Radical Reform, As the Guardian Launches Its Special Inquiry into the Onrush of Gene Patenting." *Guardian* (London), 15 November, p. 22.

Rimsha, N., H. Waitzkin, I. Pena, et al. 1996. "Local Research and Legal Advocacy for the Medically Indigent." *American Journal of Public Health* 86 (6): 883–85.

Rivera, L.N. 1992. *A Violent Evangelism: The Political and Religious Conquest of the Americas.* Louisville: Westminster/John Knox Press.

Robbins, I.P. 1999. "Managed Care in Prisons as Cruel and Unusual Punishment." *Journal of Criminal Law and Criminology* 90 (1): 195–237.

Robert, D., and R. Machado. 2001. "Haiti: Economic Situation and Prospects." Inter-American Development Bank, Country Economic Assessment. Available at *http://www.iadb.org/regions/re2/sep/ha-sep.htm.*

Roemer, M.I. 1998. "The Globalization of Public Health." *American Journal of Public Health* 88 (5): 744.

Rosaldo, M., and L. Lamphere, eds. 1974. *Women, Culture, and Society.* Stanford: Stanford University Press.

Roseberry, W. 1996. "The Unbearable Lightness of Anthropology." *Radical History Review* (65): 5–25.

Rosenberg, C.E. 1999. "Meanings, Politics, and Medicine: On the Bioethical Enterprise and History." *Daedalus* 128 (4): 27–46.

Ross, J. 1995. *Rebellion from the Roots: Indian Uprising in Chiapas.* Monroe, Maine: Common Courage Press.

———. 2000. *The War Against Oblivion: Zapatista Chronicles, 1994–2000.* Monroe, Maine: Common Courage Press.

Ross-Robinson, H. "Dame Eugenia: 'Nobody Is Listening to the Haitian People!'" *Haiti Confidential,* August 2001.

Rothman, D.J. 1984. "Were Tuskegee and Willowbrook 'Studies in Nature'?" *Hastings Center Report* 12 (1): 5–7.

Rouillon, A., S. Perdrizet, and R. Parrot. 1976. "Transmission of Tubercle Bacilli: The Effects of Chemotherapy." *Tubercle* 57: 275–99.

Rout, L. 1976. *The African Experience in Spanish America.* Cambridge: Cambridge University Press.

Rowley, S. H. 1989. "Cuba's AIDS Center Resembles Prison." *Chicago Tribune,* 17 April, p. C22.

Roy, A. 1999. *Cost of Living.* London: Flamingo.

Rühl, C., V. Pokrovsky, and V. Vinogradov. 2002. "The Economic Consequences of HIV in Russia." World Bank report. Available at *http://www.worldbank.org.ru/eng/group/hiv/.*

Rus, J. 1994. "The 'Comunidad Revolucionaria Institucional': The Subversion of Native Government in Highland Chiapas, 1936–1968." In *Everyday Forms of State Formation: Revolution and the Negotiation of Rule in Modern Mexico,* edited by G. Joseph and D. Nugent, pp. 265–300. Durham: Duke University Press.

"Russia's Population to Continue to Decline." 2000. *New York Times,* 6 December, p. A10.

Rylko-Bauer, B., and P. Farmer. 2002. "Managed Care or Managed Inequality? A Call for Critiques of Market-Based Medicine." *Medical Anthropology Quarterly* 16 (4): 476–502.

Saltus, R. 1997. "Journal Departures Reflect AIDS Dispute." *Boston Globe,* 16 October, p. A11.

Santana, S., L. Faas, and K. Wald. 1991. "Human Immunodeficiency Virus in Cuba: The Public Health Response of a Third World Country." *International Journal of Health Services* 21 (3): 511–37.

Sawyer, J. 1999. "The Dirt May Hold Their Only Hope." *St. Louis Post-Dispatch,* 1 August, p. A10.

Schachter, O. 1991. *International Law in Theory and Practice.* Boston: M. Nijhoff.

Scheffler, S. 1981. "Natural Rights, Equality, and the Minimal State." In *Reading Nozick: Essays on Anarchy, State, and Utopia,* edited by J. Paul, pp. 148–68. Totowa, N.J.: Rowman and Littlefield.

Scheper-Hughes, N. 1993. "AIDS, Public Health, and Human Rights in Cuba." *Lancet* 342 (8877): 965–67.

———. 1994. "An Essay: 'AIDS and the Social Body.'" *Social Science and Medicine* 39 (7): 991–1003.

———. 1996a. "Small Wars and Invisible Genocides." *Social Science and Medicine* 43 (5): 889–900.

———. 1996b. "Theft of Life: The Globalization of Organ Stealing Rumors." *Anthropology Today* 12 (3): 3–11.

———. 1998. "Organ Trade: The New Cannibalism." *The New Internationalist,* April, no. 300, pp. 14–17.

———. 2000a. "The Global Traffic of Human Organs." *Current Anthropology* 41 (2): 191–224.

———. 2000b. "Sacred Wounds: Writing with the Body." Introduction to *The Soft Vengeance of a Freedom Fighter,* by Albie Sachs, 2d ed., pp. xi–xxiv. Berkeley: University of California Press.

———. n.d. "AIDS and Human Rights in Cuba—A Second Look." Department of Anthropology, University of California, Berkeley. Photocopy.

Schiff, H., ed. 1995. *Holocaust Poetry*. New York: St. Martin's Press.

Schirmer, J. 1991. "The Guatemalan Military Project: An Interview with Gen. Héctor Gramajo." *Harvard International Review* 13 (3): 1–13.

Schlesinger, S., and S. Kinzer. 1999. *Bitter Fruit: The Story of the American Coup in Guatemala*. Cambridge, Mass.: Harvard University, David Rockefeller Center for Latin American Studies.

Schmidt, H. 1971. *The United States Occupation of Haiti, 1915–1934*. New Brunswick, N.J.: Rutgers University Press.

Schmidt, P. F. 1955. "Some Criticisms of Cultural Relativism." *Journal of Philosophy* 52 (25): 780–91.

Schmitt, E. 1991. "U.S. Base Is an Oasis to Haitians." *New York Times,* 28 November, p. A6.

Schneider, E. C., A. M. Zaslavsky, and A. M. Epstein. 2002. "Racial Disparities in the Quality of Care for Enrollees in Medicare Managed Care." *Journal of the American Medical Association* 287 (10): 1288–94.

Schoenholtz, A. 1993. "Aiding and Abetting Persecutors: The Seizure and Return of Haitian Refugees in Violation of the U.N. Refugee Convention and Protocol." *Georgetown Immigration Law Journal* 7 (1): 67–85.

Schoofs, M. 2000. "Glaxo Enters Fight in Ghana on AIDS Drug." *Wall Street Journal,* 1 December, p. A3.

Schoultz, L. 1979. "U.S. Policy Toward Human Rights in Latin America: A Comparative Analysis of Two Administrations." *Denver Journal of International Law and Policy* 8 (special issue): 591–605.

Schüklenk, U. 2000. "Protecting the Vulnerable: Testing Times for Clinical Research Ethics." *Social Science and Medicine* 51 (6): 969–77.

Schwab, P. 1999. *Cuba: Confronting the U.S. Embargo*. New York: St. Martin's Press.

Segundo, J. L. 1976. *The Liberation of Theology*. Maryknoll, N.Y.: Orbis Books.

———. 1980. *Our Idea of God*. Dublin: Gill and Macmillan.

Sen, A. 1981. *Poverty and Famines: An Essay on Entitlement and Deprivation*. Oxford: Clarendon Press.

———. 1985a. *Commodities and Capabilities*. Amsterdam: North-Holland.

———. 1985b. "Well-Being, Agency, and Freedom: The Dewey Lectures, 1984." *Journal of Philosophy* 82 (4): 169–221.

———. 1987. *On Ethics and Economics*. Oxford: Blackwell.

———. 1992a. *Inequality Reexamined*. New York: Russell Sage Foundation.

———. 1992b. "Missing Women." *British Medical Journal* 304 (6827): 587–88.

———. 1993. "The Economics of Life and Death." *Scientific American* 268 (5): 40–47.

———. 1998. "Mortality as an Indicator of Economic Success and Failure." (Text of the Innocenti Lecture of UNICEF, delivered in Florence, March 1995.) *Economic Journal* 108 (446): 1–25.

———. 1999. *Development as Freedom*. New York: Knopf.

———. 2000. "Will There Be Any Hope for the Poor?" *Time,* 22 May, pp. 94–95.

Sentencing Project. 2001. "U.S. Continues to Be World Leader in Rate of Incarceration." Available at *http://www.sentencingproject.org/news/usn01.pdf*.

———. 2002a. "New Inmate Population Figures Show Continued Growth, Prospects for Change in Policy Unclear." Available at *http://www.sentencingproject.org/news/inmatepop-apr02.pdf.*

———. 2002b. "Prison Privatization and the Use of Incarceration." Available at *http://www.sentencingproject.org/news/pub1053.pdf.*

Serrill, M. S. 1996. "Mexico's Black Mood." *Time International Magazine,* 7 October, vol. 148, no. 15. Available at *http://www.time.com/time/international/1996/961007/mexico.html.*

Shacochis, B. 1999. *The Immaculate Invasion.* New York: Penguin Books.

Shearer, W. T., T. C. Quinn, P. LaRussa, et al. 1997. "Viral Load and Disease Progression in Infants Infected with Human Immunodeficiency Virus Type 1." *New England Journal of Medicine* 336 (19): 1337–42.

Sheldon, G. F. 1998. "Professionalism, Managed Care, and the Human Rights Movement." *Bulletin of the American College of Surgeons* 83 (12): 13–33.

Sher, G. 1983. "Health Care and the 'Deserving Poor.'" *Hastings Center Report* 13 (2): 9–12.

Shue, H. 1996. *Basic Rights: Subsistence, Affluence, and U.S. Foreign Policy.* 2d ed. Princeton: Princeton University Press.

Shuger, S. 2000. "Supreme Court Cover-Up." Today's Papers, *Slate,* 30 March. Available at *http://slate.msn.com/?id=1004976.*

Shute, S., and S. Hurley, eds. 1993. *On Human Rights: The Oxford Amnesty Lectures.* New York: Basic Books.

Sidel, V. W. 1996. "The Social Responsibilities of Health Professionals: Lessons from Their Role in Nazi Germany." *Journal of the American Medical Association* 276 (20): 1679–81.

Sidel, V. W., and R. Sidel. 1977. *A Healthy State: An International Perspective on the Crisis in United States Medical Care.* New York: Pantheon Books.

Simpson, C. 1993. *The Splendid Blond Beast: Money, Law, and Genocide in the Twentieth Century.* New York: Grove Press.

Singer, M. 1994. "AIDS and the Health Crisis of the U.S. Urban Poor: The Perspective of Critical Medical Anthropology." *Social Science and Medicine* 39 (7): 931–48.

———. 1998. "The Development of Critical Medical Anthropology: Implications for Biological Anthropology." In *Building a New Biocultural Synthesis: Political-Economic Perspectives on Human Biology,* edited by A. L. Goodman and T. L. Leatherman, pp. 93–123. Ann Arbor: University of Michigan Press.

Singer, M., and H. Baer. 1995. *Critical Medical Anthropology.* Amityville, N.Y.: Baywood.

"Sixteen Charged in Chiapas Massacre." 1997. *Los Angeles Times,* 27 December, p. A4.

Skogly, S. 1993. "Structural Adjustment and Development: Human Rights—An Agenda for Change." *Human Rights Quarterly* 15: 751–78.

Skolnick, A. 1992. "Some Experts Suggest the Nation's 'War on Drugs' Is Helping Tuberculosis Stage a Deadly Comeback." *Journal of the American Medical Association* 268 (22): 3177–78.

Smeeding, T., L. Rainwater, and G. Burtless. 2001. "United States Poverty in a Cross-National Context." Working paper prepared for the IRP Conference

"Understanding Poverty in America: Progress and Problems," 22–24 May 2000, Madison, Wisconsin.

Smith, C. 1990. "The Militarization of Civil Society in Guatemala: Economic Reorganization as a Continuation of War." *Latin American Perspectives* 67 (4): 8–41.

Smith, J. F. 1997. "Christmas Lights Still Burn in Chiapas Massacre Chapel; Mexico: Investigators Seek Evidence at Site Where 45 Worshippers Were Gunned Down; Government Is Assailed." *Los Angeles Times,* 25 December, p. A1.

Smith, R., H. Hiatt, and D. Berwick. 1999a. "Shared Ethical Principles for Everybody in Health Care: A Working Draft from the Tavistock Group." *British Medical Journal* 318 (7178): 248–51.

———. 1999b. "A Shared Statement of Ethical Principles for Those Who Shape and Give Health Care: A Working Draft from the Tavistock Group." *Annals of Internal Medicine* 130 (2): 143–47.

Snider, D. E., Jr., L. Salinas, and G. D. Kelly. 1989. "Tuberculosis: An Increasing Problem Among Minorities in the United States." *Public Health Reports* 104 (6): 646–53.

Sobrino, J. 1988. *Spirituality of Liberation: Toward Political Holiness.* Maryknoll, N.Y.: Orbis Books.

"Social Suffering." 1996. *Daedalus* 125 (1).

Sohl, P., and H. A. Bassford. 1986. "Codes of Medical Ethics: Traditional Foundations and Contemporary Practice." *Social Science and Medicine* 22 (11): 1175–79.

Sontag, D., and L. Richardson. 1997. "Doctors Withhold H.I.V. Pill Regimen from Some." *New York Times,* 2 March, pp. 1, 31.

"South Florida Braces for Haitian Time Bomb." 1993. *Orlando Sentinel,* 11 January, p. A1.

Specter, M. 1994. "Climb in Russia's Death Rate Sets Off Population Implosion." *New York Times,* 6 March, p. 1.

———. 1997. "AIDS Onrush Sends Russia to the Edge of an Epidemic." *New York Times,* 18 May, p. A1.

———. 1998. "Citadel of Russia's Wasteful Health System." *New York Times,* 4 February, p. A1.

———. 2000. "At a Western Outpost of Russia, AIDS Spreads 'Like a Forest Fire.'" *New York Times,* 4 December, p. A1.

Stanley, A. 1998. "Russians Lament the Crime of Punishment." *New York Times,* 8 January, p. A1.

Starn, O. 1992. "Missing the Revolution: Anthropologists and the War in Peru." In *Rereading Cultural Anthropology,* edited by G. E. Marcus, pp. 152–80. Durham: Duke University Press.

Stavenhagen, R. 1996a. *Ethnic Conflicts and the Nation-State.* Houndmills, Basingstoke, Hampshire: Macmillan, in association with United Nations Research Institute for Social Development; New York: St. Martin's Press.

———. 1996b. "Indigenous Rights: Some Conceptual Problems." In *Constructing Democracy: Human Rights, Citizenship, and Society in Latin America,* edited by E. Jelin and E. Hershberg, pp. 141–60. Boulder: Westview Press.

Stea, D., S. Elguea, and C. Pérez Bustillo. 1997. "Environment, Development, and Indigenous Revolution in Chiapas." In *Life and Death Matters: Human Rights and the Environment at the End of the Millennium,* edited by B.R. Johnston, pp. 213–37. Walnut Creek, Calif.: Altamira Press.

Steadman, K.J. 1997. "Struggling for a 'Never Again': A Comparison of the Human Rights Reports in Post-Authoritarian Argentina and Chile." Bachelor's thesis, Harvard University.

Stein, D. 1992. "Making Sense of America's Refugee Policy." *USA Today,* September, 121 (2568): 13–15.

Steinbock, B. 1996. "The Concept of Coercion and Long-Term Contraceptives." In *Coerced Contraception? Moral and Policy Challenges of Long-Acting Birth Control,* edited by E.H. Moskowitz and B. Jennings, pp. 53–78. Washington, D.C.: Georgetown University Press.

Steiner, H., and P. Alston. 1996. *International Human Rights in Context: Law, Politics, Morals.* New York: Oxford University Press.

Stephen, L., and G.A. Collier. 1997. "Reconfiguring Ethnicity, Identity, and Citizenship in the Wake of the Zapatista Rebellion." *Journal of Latin American Anthropology* 3 (1): 2–13.

Stephens, J. 2000. "Where Profits and Lives Hang in the Balance: Finding an Abundance of Subjects and Lack of Oversight Abroad, Big Drug Companies Test Offshore to Speed Products to Market." *Washington Post,* 17 December, p. A1.

Stern, H.F. 1995. "When Money and Biomedicine Mix: A Tale of Two Colliding Discourses." *Mind and Human Interaction* 6 (2): 84–97.

Stern, V. 1998. *A Sin Against the Future: Imprisonment in the World.* London: Penguin Books.

Stern, V., and R. Jones. 1999. *Sentenced to Die? The Problem of TB in Prisons in East and Central Europe and Central Asia.* London: International Centre for Prison Studies, King's College.

Stocker, K., H. Waitzkin, and C. Iriart. 1999. "The Exportation of Managed Care to Latin America." *New England Journal of Medicine* 340 (14): 1131–36.

Stokes Newbold [Richard Newbold Adams and Manning Stokes Nash]. 1957. "Receptivity to Communist Fomented Agitation in Rural Guatemala." *Economic Development and Cultural Change* 5: 338–61.

Stolberg, S.G., and J. Gerth. 2000. "Keeping Down the Competition; How Companies Stall Generics and Keep Themselves Healthy." *New York Times,* 23 July, p. 1.

Styblo, K. 1984. *Epidemiology of Tuberculosis.* The Hague: Royal Netherlands Tuberculosis Association.

Sumartojo, E. 1993. "When Tuberculosis Treatment Fails: A Social Behavioral Account of Patient Adherence." *American Review of Respiratory Disease* 147 (5): 1311–20.

Sutherland, I., and P.M. Fayers. 1975. "The Association of the Risk of Tuberculosis Infection with Age." *Bulletin of the International Union Against Tuberculosis* 50: 70–81.

Swarns, R.L. 2000. "Loans to Buy AIDS Drugs Are Rejected by Africans." *New York Times,* 22 August, p. A6.

Syfers, J. 2000. "Human Rights Versus Classical Liberalism: A Study in the Theory of Value." In *Not for Sale: In Defense of Public Goods,* edited by A. Anton, M. Fisk, and N. Holmstrom, pp. 145–70. Boulder: Westview Press.

"Symposium: The Haitian Refugee Crisis: A Closer Look." 1993. *Georgetown Immigration Law Journal* 7 (1): 1–147.

Szulc, T. 1986. *Fidel: A Critical Portrait.* New York: Avon Books.

Szymborska, W. 1981. *Sounds, Feelings, Thoughts.* Translated by M. J. Krynski and R. A. Maguire. Princeton: Princeton University Press.

———. 1995. *View with a Grain of Sand: Selected Poems.* Translated by S. Baranczak and C. Cavanagh. New York: Harcourt, Brace.

Tahaoğlu, K., T. Törün, T. Sevim, et al. 2001. "The Treatment of Multidrug-Resistant Tuberculosis in Turkey." *New England Journal of Medicine* 345 (3): 170–74.

Tang, D. 2000. "Disease Called Threat to Security." *Washington Times,* 30 June, p. A17.

Tangeman, M. 1995. *Mexico at the Crossroads: Politics, the Church, and the Poor.* Maryknoll, N.Y.: Orbis Books.

Taubes, G. 1997. "Resurgent Mosquitoes, Dengue in Cuba." *Science* 277 (5323): 174.

Tauer, C. 1989. "AIDS: Human Rights and Public Health." *Medical Anthropology* 10 (2–3): 177–92.

Taylor, E., C. Besse, and T. Healing. 1994. "Tuberculosis in Siberia." *Lancet* 343: 968.

Tedlock, B. 1982. *Time and the Highland Maya.* Albuquerque: University of New Mexico Press.

Tedlock, D. 1993. *Breath on the Mirror: Mythic Voices and Visions of the Living.* San Francisco: HarperCollins.

Telzak, E. E., K. Sepkowitz, P. Alpert, et al. 1995. "Multidrug-Resistant Tuberculosis in Patients Without HIV Infection." *New England Journal of Medicine* 333 (14): 907–11.

t'Hoen, E. 2000. Statement from Médecins Sans Frontières, Campaign for Access to Essential Medicines. Health Issues Group DG Trade, 26 June, Brussels. Available at *http://trade-info.cec.eu.int/civil_soc/documents/meeting/me-25-msf.pdf.*

Thomas, C. W. 2000. "Correctional Privatization in the United States: An Examination of Its Modern History and Future Potential." Paper presented at the Mental Health in Corrections Symposium, 22 June, Kansas City, Missouri.

Thomas, L. 1983. *The Youngest Science: Notes of a Medicine-Watcher.* New York: Viking Press.

Thornhill, J., and A. Ostrovsky. 1999. "IMF Agrees Russia Is Keeping to Conditions of Loan." *Financial Times,* 24 September, p. 3.

Thornton, S. 1996. "Cultural Rights, Multiculturalism, and Cultural Relativism." In *Teaching for Citizenship in Europe,* edited by A. Osler, H. F. Rathenaw, and H. Starkey, pp. 23–34. Stoke-on-Trent: Trentham Books.

Tjaden, P., and N. Thoennes. 1998. *Prevalence, Incidence, and Consequences of Violence Against Women: Findings from the National Violence Against Women Survey.* Washington, D.C.: U.S. Department of Justice, National Institute of Justice/CDC Research in Brief.

Tomes, N. 1998. *The Gospel of Germs: Men, Women, and the Microbe in American Life.* Cambridge, Mass.: Harvard University Press.

Tomkins, A., and C.J. Henry. 1992. "Comparison of Nutrient Composition of Refugee Rations and Pet Foods." *Lancet* 340 (8815): 367–68.

Trouiller, P., and P. Olliaro. 1999. "Drug Development Output: What Proportion for Tropical Diseases?" *Lancet* 354 (9173): 164.

Trouillot, M-R. 1990. *Haiti, State Against Nation: The Origins and Legacy of Duvalierism.* New York: Monthly Review Press.

Turett, G.S., E.E. Telzak, L.V. Torian, et al. 1995. "Improved Outcomes for Patients with Multidrug-Resistant Tuberculosis." *Clinical Infectious Diseases* 21: 1238–44.

Turner, T. 1997. "Human Rights, Human Difference: Anthropology's Contribution to an Emancipatory Cultural Politics." *Journal of Anthropological Research* 53: 273–92.

Turque, B., S. Reiss, M. Liu, et al. 1993. "Why Our Borders Are Out of Control." *Newsweek,* 9 August, p. 25.

Turshen, M. 1986. "Health and Human Rights in a South African Bantustan." *Social Science and Medicine* 22 (9): 887–92.

———. 1989. *The Politics of Public Health.* New Brunswick, N.J.: Rutgers University Press.

———. 1999. *Privatizing Health Services in Africa.* New Brunswick, N.J.: Rutgers University Press.

Tuskegee Syphilis Ad Hoc Advisory Panel. 1973. *Final Report.* Washington, D.C.: U.S. Public Health Service.

Tutu, D.M. 1999. *No Future Without Forgiveness.* London: Rider.

UNAIDS/World Health Organization. 2000. Haiti: Epidemiological Fact Sheets on HIV/AIDS and Sexually Transmitted Infections, 2000 Update. Available at *http://www.who.int/emc-hiv/fact_sheets/pdfs/haiti_en.pdf.*

United Nations. 2000. "Raboteau Verdict in Haiti a 'Landmark in Fight Against Impunity,' But Case Not Yet Finished, Says UN Independent Expert." Press release, 20 November. Available at *http://www.unhchr.ch/huricane/huricane.nsf/view01/720D87DC442C8259C125699D005C63B6?opendocument.*

United Nations Development Programme. 1990. *Human Development Report, 1990.* New York: Oxford University Press for UNDP.

———. 1998. *Human Development Report, 1998.* New York: Oxford University Press for UNDP.

———. 1999. *Human Development Report, 1999.* New York : Oxford University Press for UNDP.

———. 2001. *Human Development Report, 2001.* New York: Oxford University Press for UNDP.

United Nations Human Rights Commission. 1995. *Situation of Human Rights in Haiti.* Geneva: United Nations Economic and Social Council.

Universal Declaration of Human Rights. 1948. Adopted and proclaimed by General Assembly resolution 217 A (III), 10 December. Available at *http://www.un.org/Overview/rights.html.*

U.S. Central Intelligence Agency. 2000a. "The Global Infectious Disease Threat and Its Implications for the United States." NIE 99–17D, January. Available at *www.cia.gov/cia/publications/nie/report/nie99–17d.html.*

———. 2000b. *The World Factbook 2000*. Available at *http://www.umsl .edu/services/govdocs/wofact2000/*.

———. 2001. *The World Factbook 2001*; entry for "Haiti." Available at *http:// www.cia.gov/cia/publications/factbook/*.

U.S. Department of Justice and Federal Bureau of Investigation. 1999. *Crime in the United States, 1998*. Washington, D.C.: U.S. Government Printing Office.

———. 2000. *Crime in the United States, 2000*. Washington, D.C.: U.S. Government Printing Office.

U.S. General Accounting Office. 1982. *Assistance to Haiti: Barriers, Recent Program Changes, and Future Options*. Washington, D.C.: U.S. General Accounting Office.

U.S. House. 2002. H. Cong. Res. 382, "Urging the President to end any embargo against Haiti and to no longer require, as a condition of providing humanitarian and development assistance to Haiti, the resolution of the political impasse in Haiti, and for other purposes." 107th Cong., 2d sess. 18 April.

Uvin, P. 1998. *Aiding Violence: The Development Enterprise in Rwanda*. West Hartford, Conn.: Kumarian Press.

Varmus, H., and D. Satcher. 1997. "Ethical Complexities of Conducting Research in Developing Countries." *New England Journal of Medicine* 337 (14): 1003–5.

Vasseur, V. 2000. *Médecin-chef à la prison de la santé*. Paris: Le Cherche Midi Éditeur.

Verdier, R. I., D. W. Fitzgerald, W. D. Johnson, et al. 2000. "Trimethoprim-Sulfamethoxazole Compared with Ciprofloxacin for Treatment and Prophylaxis of *Isospora belli* and *Cyclospora cayetanensis* Infection in HIV-Infected Patients." *Annals of Internal Medicine* 132 (11): 885–88.

Victora, C. G., J. P. Vaughan, F. C. Barros, et al. 2000. "Explaining Trends in Inequities: Evidence from Brazilian Child Health Studies." *Lancet* 356 (9235): 1093–98.

Vidal, C. 1996. "Le génocide des Rwandais tutsi: Cruauté délibérée et logiques de haine." In *De la violence*, edited by F. Héritier, pp. 327–66. Paris: Éditions Odile Jacob.

Virchow, R. L. K. 1849. *Die einheitsrebungen in der wissenschaftlichen medicin*. Berlin: Druck und Verlag von G. Reimer.

Wacquant, L. 1999. *Les prisons de la misère*. Paris: Raisons d'Agir.

———. 2002. *Prisons of Poverty*. Expanded ed. Minneapolis: University of Minnesota Press.

Wagner, R. 1975. *The Invention of Culture*. Englewood Cliffs, N.J.: Prentice-Hall.

Waitzkin, H. 1984. "The Strange Career of Managed Competition: From Military Failure to Medical Success?" *American Journal of Public Health* 84 (3): 482–89.

———. 1991. *The Politics of Medical Encounters: How Patients and Doctors Deal with Social Problems*. New Haven: Yale University Press.

———. 1998. "Is Our Work Dangerous? Should It Be?" *Journal of Health and Social Behavior* 39: 7–17.

———. 2000. *The Second Sickness: Contradictions of Capitalist Health Care.* Lanham, Md.: Rowman and Littlefield.

Waitzkin, H., and C. Iriart. 2000. "How the United States Exports Managed Care to Third-World Countries." *Monthly Review* 52 (1): 21–35.

———. 2001. "How the United States Exports Managed Care to Developing Countries." *International Journal of Health Services* 31 (3): 495–505.

Waitzkin, H., and H. Magaña. 1997. "The Black Box in Somatization: Unexplained Physical Symptoms, Culture, and Narratives of Trauma." *Social Science and Medicine* 45 (6): 811–25.

Waitzkin, H., K. Wald, R. Kee, R. Danielson, et al. 1997. "Primary Care in Cuba: Low- and High-Technology Developments Pertinent to Family Medicine." *Journal of Family Practice* 45 (3): 250–58.

Walberg, P., M. McKee, V. Shkolnikov, et al. 1998. "Economic Change, Crime, and Mortality Crisis in Russia: A Regional Analysis." *British Medical Journal* 317 (7154): 312–18.

Waldholz, M. 1996. "New AIDS Treatment Raises Tough Question of Who Will Get It." *Wall Street Journal,* 3 July, p. A1.

Wali, A. 1989. *Kilowatts and Crisis: Hydroelectric Power and Social Dislocation in Eastern Panama.* Boulder: Westview Press.

Walker, A. 2000. "Haitian Orphan's Story Draws No Crowds." *Boston Globe,* 18 April, p. A4.

Walker, M. 2000. "Money Laundering? 'It's Capital Flight.'" *Straits Times* (Singapore), 14 January, p. 69.

Walker, S. L. 1997. "Rebels Call for Army Pullout from Chiapas; Zapatistas Come to Mexico City to Press Demands." *San Diego Union-Tribune,* 13 September, p. A2.

Wallerstein, I. 1974. *The Modern World-System: Capitalist Agriculture and the Origins of the European World-Economy in the Sixteenth Century.* San Diego: Academic Press.

———. 1987. "World-Systems Analysis." In *Social Theory Today,* edited by A. Giddens and J. Turner, pp. 309–24. Stanford: Stanford University Press.

———. 1994. "Response to Eric Wolf." *Current Anthropology* 35 (1): 9–12.

———. 1995a. *After Liberalism.* New York: The New Press.

———. 1995b. "The Insurmountable Contradictions of Liberalism: Human Rights and the Rights of Peoples in the Geoculture of the Modern World-System." *South Atlantic Quarterly* 46: 1161–78.

Ward, J., S. Kleinman, D. Douglas, et al. 1988. "Epidemiologic Characteristics of Blood Donors with Antibody to Human Immunodeficiency Virus." *Transfusion* 28: 198–301.

Ward, M. 1993. "A Different Disease: HIV/AIDS and Health Care for Women in Poverty." *Culture, Medicine, and Psychiatry* 17 (4): 413–30.

Wardman, A. G., A. J. Knox, M. F. Muers, and R. L. Page. 1988. "Profiles of Noncompliance with Antituberculosis Therapy." *British Journal of Diseases of the Chest* 82: 285–89.

Wasserstrom, R. 1983. *Class and Society in Central Chiapas.* Berkeley: University of California Press.

Watanabe, J.M. 2002. "Silence and Solidarity Across a Watershed of War: The Heritage of U.S. Complicity in Guatemala." *American Anthropologist* 104 (1): 330–34.

Waterston, A. 1993. *Street Addicts in the Political Economy.* Philadelphia: Temple University Press.

———. 1999. *Love, Sorrow, and Rage: Destitute Women in a Manhattan Residence.* Philadelphia: Temple University Press.

Wedel, J.R. 1998. *Collision and Collusion: The Strange Case of Western Aid to Eastern Europe, 1989–1998.* New York: St. Martin's Press.

Weise, J. 1971. "The Interaction of Western and Indigenous Medicine in Haiti in Regard to Tuberculosis." Ph.D. diss., Department of Anthropology, University of North Carolina at Chapel Hill.

Welie, J.V.M. 1998. *In the Face of Suffering: The Philosophical-Anthropological Foundations of Clinical Ethics.* Omaha: Creighton University Press.

West, C. 1989. *The American Evasion of Philosophy: A Genealogy of Pragmatism.* Madison: University of Wisconsin Press.

———. 1993. *Prophetic Thought in Postmodern Times.* Monroe, Maine: Common Courage Press.

———. 1999. *The Cornel West Reader.* New York: Basic Civitas Books.

White, R.M. 2000. "Unraveling the Tuskegee Study of Untreated Syphilis." *Archives of Internal Medicine* 160 (5): 585–98.

Whitehead, M., A. Scott-Samuel, and G. Dahlgren. 1998. "Setting Targets to Address Inequalities in Health." *Lancet* 351 (9111): 1279–82.

Whittell, G. 2000. "Russian Leader Faces Pounds 3bn Questions." *Times* (London), 25 July, p. 15.

Widmer, S.R. 1999. "Essentializing Malnutrition: Foreign Attempts to Improve Nutrition in Tanzania, 1921–1975." Bachelor's thesis, Harvard University.

Wilentz, A. 1989. *The Rainy Season: Haiti After Duvalier.* New York: Simon and Schuster.

Wilkinson, R.G. 1996. *Unhealthy Societies: The Afflictions of Inequality.* London: Routledge.

Williams, E. 1970. *From Columbus to Castro: The History of the Caribbean, 1492–1969.* London: Andre Deutsch.

Williams, P.J. 1991. *The Alchemy of Race and Rights.* Cambridge, Mass.: Harvard University Press.

Wilson, J. 2000. "Human Rights Groups Criticise Straw Decision to Release Ex-Dictator But Hail Precedent That No One Is Above the Law." *Guardian,* 3 March, p. 1.

Wilson, W.J. 1980. *The Declining Significance of Race: Blacks and Changing American Institutions.* Chicago: University of Chicago Press.

Wines, M. 2000a. "Capitalism Comes to Russian Health Care." *New York Times,* 22 December, p. A1.

———. 2000b. "Heroin Carries AIDS to a Region in Siberia." *New York Times,* 24 April, pp. A1, A8.

Wines, M., and A. Zuger. 2000. "In Russia, the Ill and Infirm Include Health Care Itself." *New York Times,* 4 December, p. A1.

Wittgenstein, L. 1958. *Philosophical Investigations.* Translated by G.E.M. Anscombe. Oxford: Basil Blackwell.

Wolf, S.M., ed. 1996. *Feminism and Bioethics: Beyond Reproduction.* New York: Oxford University Press.

Womack, J. 1968. *Zapata and the Mexican Revolution.* New York: Vintage Books.

———. 1999. *Rebellion in Chiapas: An Historical Reader.* New York: The New Press.

Wood, E., P. Braitstein, J.S. Schechter, et al. 2000. "Extent to Which Low-Level Use of Antiretroviral Treatment Could Curb the AIDS Epidemic in Sub-Saharan Africa." *Lancet* 355 (9221): 2095–100.

World Bank. 1993. *World Development Report 1993.* Oxford: Oxford University Press.

———. 1994a. *Social Indicators of Development.* Baltimore: Johns Hopkins University Press.

———. 1994b. *World Development Report 1994.* Oxford: Oxford University Press.

———. 1999. *Confronting AIDS: Public Priorities in a Global Epidemic.* New York: Oxford University Press.

———. 2000a. *The Burden of Disease Among the Global Poor: Current Situation, Future Trends, and Implications for Strategy.* Washington, D.C.: World Bank.

———. 2000b. World Development Indicators 2000. Available at *http://www. worldbank.org/data/wdi2000/index.htm.*

———. 2001. *World Development Indicators.* Table 2.15. Washington, D.C.: International Bank.

———. 2002. Development Indicators Database. Available at *http://devdata .worldbank.org/external/CPProfile.asp?SelectedCountry=PER&CCODE= PER&CNAME=Peru&PTYPE=CP.*

"World Bank Forecasts 5.4 Million HIV Cases in Russia by 2020." 2002. Dow Jones Business News. Available at *http://story.news.yahoo.com/news? tmpl=story&u=/dowjones/20020515/bs_dowjones/world_bank_ forecasts _5_4_million_hiv_cases_in_russia_by_2020.*

World Health Organization. 1946. Constitution of the World Health Organization. Adopted by the International Health Conference, 22 July, New York. Available at *http://www.yale.edu/lawweb/avalon/decade/decado51.htm.*

———. 1985. "Maternal Mortality: Helping Women Off the Road to Death." *WHO Chronicle* 40: 175–83.

———. 1995. *Bridging the Gaps.* Geneva: World Health Organization.

———. 1998. *TB: A Crossroads—WHO Report on the Tuberculosis Epidemic.* Geneva: World Health Organization.

———. 1999a. *Coordination of DOTS-Plus Pilot Projects for the Management of MDR-TB.* Geneva: World Health Organization.

———. 1999b. *Report: Basis for the Development of an Evidence-Based Case-Management Strategy for MDR-TB Within the WHO's DOTS Strategy.* Geneva: World Health Organization.

———. 1999c. *Report on Infectious Diseases: Removing Obstacles to Healthy Development.* Geneva: World Health Organization.

———. 1999d. *World Health Report 1999—Making a Difference.* Geneva: World Health Organization.

———. 2000a. *Global Tuberculosis Control: WHO Report 2000.* Geneva: World Health Organization.

———. 2000b. *Tuberculosis and Sustainable Development: The Stop TB Initiative 2000 Report.* Geneva: World Health Organization.

———. 2000c. *World Health Report 2000. Health Systems: Improving Performance.* Geneva: World Health Organization.

———. 2001. *World Health Report 2001: Mental Health—New Understanding, New Hope.* Geneva: World Health Organization.

World Health Organization, Partners In Health, Open Society Institute, et al. 2002. *The Global Plan to Stop Tuberculosis.* Geneva: World Health Organization.

World Health Organization, United Nations Children's Fund, United Nations Population Fund. 2001. *Maternal Mortality in 1995: Estimates Developed by WHO, UNICEF, UNFPA.* Geneva: World Health Organization.

World Medical Association. 1983. World Medical Association International Code of Medical Ethics. Amended by the Twenty-Second World Medical Assembly, Sydney, Australia, August 1968; and the Thirty-Fifth World Medical Assembly, Venice, Italy, October 1983. Available at *http://www.wma.net/e/policy/17-a_e.html.*

Wright, S. 2002. "Les États-Unis et la menace biologique." *Le Monde diplomatique,* 29 January. Available at *http://www.monde-diplomatique.fr/dossiers/armesbiologiques/.*

Wronka, J. 1997. "Toward Building Peace/Human Rights Cultures: Why Is the United States So Resistant?" *American Society of International Law* 13. Available at *http://www.lawschool.cornell.edu/lawlibrary/asil/issue13.htm.*

Wurtz, R., and W. White. 1999. "The Cost of Tuberculosis: Utilization and Estimated Charges for the Diagnosis and Treatment of Tuberculosis in a Public Health System." *International Journal of Tuberculosis and Lung Disease* 3 (5): 382–87.

Yach, D., and D. Bettcher. 1998a. "The Globalization of Public Health, I: Threats and Opportunities." *American Journal of Public Health* 88 (5): 735–38.

———. 1998b. "The Globalization of Public Health, II: The Convergence of Self-Interest and Altruism." *American Journal of Public Health* 88 (5): 738–41.

Zechenter, E. M. 1997. "In the Name of Culture: Cultural Relativism and the Abuse of the Individual." *Journal of Anthropological Research* 53: 319–47.

Zonana, V. F. 1988. "Cuba's AIDS Quarantine Center Called 'Frightening.'" *Los Angeles Times,* 4 November, p. 1.

Zuger, A. 2000. "Russia Has Few Weapons as Infectious Diseases Surge." *New York Times,* 5 December, p. F1.

CREDITS

Against Ethics: Contributions to a Poetics of Obligation with Constant Reference to Deconstructions by John D. Caputo, Indiana University Press, 1993.

El Mozote Massacre: Anthropology and Human Rights by Leigh Binford. © 1996 The Arizona Board of Regents. Reprinted by permission of the University of Arizona Press.

The Earth Is a Satellite of the Moon by Leonel Rugama. Curbstone Press, 1984. Distributed by Consortium.

"Will There Be Any Hope for the Poor?" by Amartya Sen. © 1983 Time Inc., reprinted by permission.

"Voices from Lemnos" in *The Cure at Troy: A Version of Sophocles' Philoctetes* by Seamus Heaney. Copyright © 1990 by Seamus Heaney. Reprinted by permission of Farrar, Straus and Giroux, LLC.

"Weathervane": *Veleta, Julio de 1920 (Fuente Vaqueros, Granada)* by Federico García Lorca, © Herederos de Federico García Lorca, from Obras Completas (Galaxia Gutenberg, 1996 edition). Translation © Herederos de Federico García Lorca and Catherine Brown. All rights reserved. For information regarding rights and permissions, please contact lorca@argslaw.co.uk or William Peter Kosmas, Esq., 8 Franklin Square, London W14 9UU.

INDEX

Text: 10/13 Sabon
Display: Interstate Light
Compositor: Impressions Book and Journal Services, Inc.
Printer and binder: Edwards Brothers, Inc.

More Paul Farmer paperbacks from California

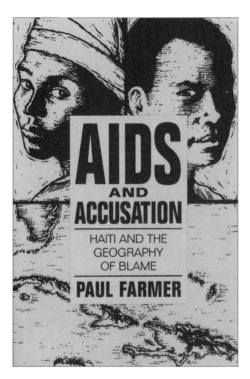

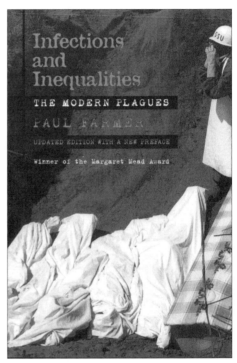

AIDS and Accusation
Haiti and the
Geography of Blame
(1992)

Infections and Inequalities
The Modern Plagues
(2001)

California

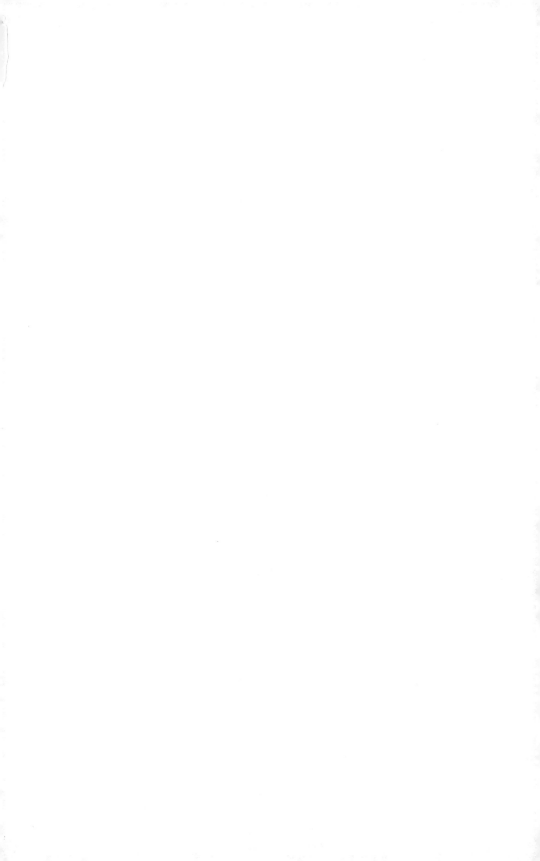